EXPERIMENTAL STUDIES IN REGENERATION OF SPINAL NEURONS

EXPERIMENTAL STUDIES IN REGENERATION OF SPINAL NEURONS

TAT'YANA N. NESMEYANOVA

with an
introduction and editorial contributions
by

Donald Scott, Jr.

1977
V. H. WINSTON & SONS
Washington, D.C.

A HALSTED PRESS BOOK

JOHN WILEY & SONS
New York Toronto London Sydney

V. H. Winston & Sons, a Division of Scripta Technica, Inc., Publishers
1511 K Street, N.W., Washington, D.C. 20005

Distributed solely by Halsted Press, a Division of John Wiley & Sons, Inc.

Translation of this study was supported through the Special Foreign Currency Program of the National Library of Medicine, National Institutes of Health, Public Health Service, U.S. Department of Health, Education, and Welfare, Bethesda, MD. Translated from the Russian *Stimulyatsiya vosstanovitel'nykh protsessov pri travme spinnogo mozga.*

Library of Congress Cataloging in Publication Data

Nesmei͡anova, Tat'ti͡ana Nikolaevna.
Experimental studies in regeneration of spinal neurons.

1. Nervous system–Regeneration. 2. Spinal cord.
3. Neurons. I. Title. [DNLM: 1. Spinal cord injuries.
2. Spinal nerves–Physiology. 3. Neurons–Physiology.
4. Regeneration. WL400 N462e]
QP374.N42 599'.01'88 77-22460
ISBN 0-470-99152-6

Composition by **Isabelle Sneeringer**, Scripta Technica, Inc.

CONTENTS

INTRODUCTION TO ENGLISH EDITION

One of the greatest challenges in neurophysiology today lies in the search for solutions to the many problems involved with repair of spinal function after partial or total cord lesion. It is now apparent that several major factors are involved, such as scar formation, nerve growth stimulation, trophic function, etc. Is the problem primarily one of the biochemistry of proteosynthesis or is it one involving the cellular interaction between neurons and glia? May it be centered on the microvascular supply to the scar or may it be related to an immunologic response between the regenerating cells and their environment? More than one author has pointed to the highly specialized mammalian neuron as being far more readily subject to the results of tissue incompatibility than the more primitive cells of lower forms where regeneration has long been known to take place. Possibly more important than any of these, is the fundamental question involving the subtle differences between peripheral and spinal neurons, since the former are known to regenerate successfully after injury or section while the latter seldom do. However, recent results from several directions of investigation related to these problems have been very encouraging and, at times, it has even been thought that the answer to the overall problems was close at hand. It is now appropriate to review the present situation with regard to these problems.

Research in this difficult field has, by its very nature, tended to make slow progress in which there has been only a modest number of strongly positive answers. Some of the results may be familiar from the readily available literature but much has appeared in lesser known journals and a very considerable contribution has been made in the USSR, of which very little has been reported in English due to the scarcity of translation facilities. The work of two prominent Russian investigators has recently become available in English (L. V. Polezhaev, "Loss and Restoration of Regenerative Capacity in Tissues and Organs of Animals," Harvard University Press, 1972; and L. A. Martinian and A. S. Andreasian, "Enzyme Therapy in Organic Lesions of the Spinal Cord," Brain Information Service, 1976).

The present volume includes a summary of recent research throughout the world on the many problems associated with spinal cord damage and repair followed by the results of studies from the laboratory of Dr. T. N. Nesmeyanova of Moscow over a period of 20 years. In this work the author was assisted by colleagues in the fields of biochemistry and histology and she has also included the results of her joint clinical experiments with the neurosurgeon, Dr. A. N. Trankvillitati, which are presented in detail in the Appendix.

The subjects which are discussed include extensive neurologic studies in which the possibility of finding alternate motor and sensory pathways to bypass the damaged area of the cord have been explored. The establishment of new reflex mechanisms to provide movements of the extremities has also been considered. Many of the experimental subjects, both canine and human, received some form of "treatment" subsequent to the operative procedure, which involved physical therapy including extended regimes of excitation by implanted electrical stimulators, often leading to quite successful results.

More than twenty years ago attention was drawn to the formation of a glial blockade following cord transection which inhibited regenerative growth of axons. Several agents were found to inhibit this effect by investigators in the United States, while the problem has also been extensively examined in recent work from the USSR with the objective of obtaining a friable matrix in the scar which could be easily penetrated by regenerating neural fibers.

Among the biochemical studies are those using substances which have been shown to stimulate the proteosynthesis necessary for regenerative growth of nerve which includes a wide variety of substances from simple chemical compounds to complex proteins. The use of nerve growth factor which had been previously described and developed by Dr. Levi-Montalcini is discussed in detail and experiments are presented in which this substance and other growth promoting agents are used, either alone or in conjunction with other agents. Of special interest are many studies in which implants of modified tissue from a donor animal have been shown to have a strong stimulating effect on spinal regeneration.

The results of these procedures have been extensively analyzed by a wide variety of techniques. Biochemical methods to determine incorporation of therapeutic agents have been correlated with extensive histologic studies. Neurophysiological procedures were undertaken to support observations of the behavioral use and movement of muscles previously subject to denervation. Careful clinical examination has been reported on those patients in whom experimental procedures were undertaken. The use of dogs as experimental animals has had the advantage of the extensive literature available on spinal plasticity in these animals. Most importantly, the results of a control and experimental series of animals have been compared after various extended post operative intervals: some as long as 2 to 3 years. Each experimental group shows differences in the degree of recovery and in some, a high level of appropriate motor function is reported to have been regained. These results are compared with those obtained in patients.

For readers who are not familiar with the current research in this field, the author presents the many approaches to this problem through (1) summaries of relevant literature, (2) results from her own extensive experimental studies, and (3) an extensive bibliography of work from the United States, and both East and Western Europe. Investigators having a more specific interest will find detailed reference to the following approaches to the problem of restoration of spinal cord function:

1. Formation of "atypical" reflexes in the transected spinal cord to replace lost functions.
2. Study of the influence of increased afferent stimulation to enhance the function of the spinal cord after transection: excitation and formation of new reflexes in the distal portion.
3. Development of mono- and polysynaptic motor reflexes in the distal system after treatment with physical therapy, 2 to 4 years after cord section.
4. The block of neural growth by scar formation and the prevention of scars by use of pyrogens, hormones, trypsin and corticosteroids.
5. Significance of blood supply in the reparative process after spinal section.
6. Formation of synaptic connections by regenerating nerve fibers in the spinal cord.
7. Enhancement of nerve regeneration through use of degenerated neural tissue.
8. Stimulation of the regenerative process through enhanced synthesis of neuroproteins: nerve growth factor.

9. Nerve growth stimulation by use of dinitrylmalonic acid.

10. Combined procedures for use on human subjects after complete or partial section of the spinal cord.

11. Possible involvement of sympathetic neurons to provide alternative neural pathways after spinal cord lesion.

12. Use of implanted electrical stimulatiors to reduce distrophic muscle changes.

From the reports of the author's experiments, it appears that some of the most promising results involve several of the above techniques in a carefully programmed sequence. It is my hope that this book may encourage investigators to extend the work which is reported here and to seek new approaches which may be developed from the present results.

The text of this book has been carefully translated and subsequently suitably revised and edited to make its meaning as clear as possible, in a form which is easily readable. In a few cases, unfamiliar concepts have appeared in the text, in which case, an editorial note has been inserted to provide explanation.

Although the material in this book has been reasonably familiar to me since I have contributed some of the original research, there have been many points on which I have had to seek clarification from my colleagues in the Departments of Anatomy and Physiology at the University of Pennsylvania for which I express my appreciation. I am also very grateful for the sponsorship of this project by the National Library of Medicine and, in particular, to Dr. Galina Zarechnak, whose office kindly provided the retyping of the edited manuscript and much valuable advice.

Donald Scott, Jr., Ph.D.

AUTHOR'S INTRODUCTION

An attempt has been made in this monograph to describe the possible means of restoring motor function which may have been lost as a result of spinal cord transection. It is based on the author's experimental and clinical studies with her colleagues carried out in the last 17 years.

Is there any chance of restoration of motor or sensory function after transection of the spinal cord?

In the process of animal evolution, injury has had a great role to play in the development of new adaptive properties without which a particular physiological member might fail. In lower vertebrates, which are mainly of primitive types, there is the capacity to restore organs which have failed and this is mainly due to adaptive properties which may make regeneration possible. Thus, the tail and extremities can be regenerated in a number of amphibians. Even the implantation of an additional new limb is possible in these animals. However, this unique property has been rapidly lost during the process of evolution. In frogs, regeneration of organs only takes place during the tadpole stage and mammals have completely lost the ability needed for reparative regeneration of their organs. It seems that possibilities for repair have diminished in the fight for the existence of the species. However, it is clear that the highest evolutionary development has taken place in mammals among all other animals. When the problem of regeneration is considered from the standpoint of injury to mammals, what characteristics have helped to place them above other forms of life?

To begin with, all the physiological members essential for preserving life in mammals are found to be covered with bone. The brain and the spinal cord are protected, as though they were in armour. The heart is protected by the thoracic cage. In contrast, the capacity for regeneration is highly developed in all peripheral tissues like skin, muscles and nerves which are subjected to trauma.

When essential functions are lost in mammals during injury, this may be compensated by modification of other tissues. For example, loss of the ability to move as a result of a spinal hemisection may be completely compensated by involving spinal neurons which remained intact in the opposite side of the spinal cord. The cerebral cortex plays an important role in the development of compensatory functions, and if an animal becomes decorticate, this leads to a complete failure of functional compensation (Asratyan, 1963, 1953; Goncharova, 1959; Ivanova, 1953; Nezlina, 1957).

If a spinal hemisection is done in a decerebrate dog, the restoration of motor functions does not take place (Asratyan, 1937). Also there is practically no restoration of the weight-bearing and locomotor functions in mammals following a complete transection of the spinal cord. The severance of nervous connections between the brain and the periphery is an insuperable obstacle, which prevents the influence of the cortex. Both the ability to walk and also weight-bearing were affected by (1) loss in voluntary movement of the lower extremities, (2) their sensation, (3) an absence of a constant and stable tone of the antigravity muscles as well as, (4) the rapid development of dystrophic processes. All of these resulted in complete invalidism of man or animal.

Traumatic transection of the spinal cord is not a rare phenomenon and the ability to restore function following this injury is of great importance in clinical practice, in addition to its theoretical interest.

Is it possible to achieve even a partial restoration of function by a compensatory method following complete transection of the spinal cord and, if so, how? Does the distal segment of the spinal cord take over lost functions? What happens there? What are its functional peculiarities?

The unique properties of the spinal cord have to be considered, mainly its plastic characteristics in different phases of phylo- and ontogenetic development. Such a comparison will be useful for evaluating the physiological functions of a mature mammal both in normal and pathological conditions, according to the observations of L. A. Orbeli (1938, 1942). Investigation of the development of motor activity in animals during ontogenesis has shown that reflex movements are possible even in their prenatal life (Volokhov, 1951).

Consequently, the central nervous system has already begun to play a positive role in organizing movements during fetal life. However, only after birth is the brain gradually turned into the key organ for this process. It became clear from observations made in experiments with newly-born rabbits that in the first weeks of postnatal life the character of their movements is already quite well developed. If spontaneous and evoked irregular movements of the extremities and trunk are characteristic of tactile stimulation for newly-born animals it is found that after the sixth week the evoked movements became localized and the spontaneous movements disappeared. Transection of the spinal cord restores the same character of motor activity as was noticed earlier (Deryabin, 1964, 1966). The summation phenomenon and the loss of paths in a spinal cord, which are observed in the first week of postnatal life, are suppressed in adult animals by supraspinal influences (Malakhovskaya, 1960).

The prominent role of the spinal cord in organizing movements in the early phase of animal life is very clear. Thus, transection of the spinal cord in a kitten or puppy in the first few days of their postnatal life, before they have learned to walk, does not prevent them from learning to walk without any difficulty (Shurrager, 1950, 1955; Shurrager and Dykman, 1951). If the same operation is done, two weeks after birth or later, there is no restoration of motor function and the animals fail to learn walking. In other words, until the brain is sufficiently developed to command the spinal cord activity, the latter is able to cause restoration of the animal's motor function. At a later stage of ontogenetic development, the restoration of function without the participation of the cortex is extremely difficult, if not impossible. The significance of the lower parts of the central nervous system (e.g., the spinal cord) is more marked in the process of compensation for motor functions in animals, situated at a lower level of phylogenetic development, in which the process of corticalization has not yet fully developed (Karamyan, 1947; Baru, 1955; Matinyan, 1960; Stefantsov, 1961).

Thus, the spinal cord of animals in the early phase of ontogenesis and phylogenesis possesses a number of properties which are subsequently lost in the course of devlopment of the nervous system. These characteristics, which indicate a great plasticity and some independence of the spinal cord, in the early phases of phylo- and ontogenetic development of an organism, may be utilized for the compensatory development of motor function if the cord is separated from higher centers of the central nervous system. However, the development of dystrophic processes due to disuse, which inevitably happens during paralysis, is an important obstacle to the utilization of the plastic properties of the spinal cord.

In cases of partial transection of a mammalian spinal cord, there is self-training of the motor apparatus which causes restoration of function, though it is not complete. The dog instinctively learns to stand on its legs and steps forward. As a result, the reflex apparatus of the spinal cord is, usually, protected from the rapid onset of a pronounced dystrophy. In these conditions, restriction of movement is delayed due to the development of compensatory neural processes in the animals (Dmitriev, 1951).

Additional afferent stimulation is essential in order to facilitate the plastic properties of an isolated spinal cord. The significance of afferent signals for carrying out locomotion has been emphasized by a number of investigators (Anokhin, 1947; Koshtoyants, 1957; Uflyand, 1965). This phenomenon has also been shown on several occasions in lower vertebrates. Muscular contraction can be noticed in the whole body of the dog fish after transection of the spinal cord, both above and below the level of transection. However, this result was prevented when a double transection was performed.

From these facts, it may be suggested that one of the essential conditions for the restoration of motor function after complete transection is the prevention of dystrophic process in the neuronal apparatus of the spinal cord.

Can motor activity be restored by other means, apart from the compensatory development of additional neural pathways, especially after a complete transection of the spinal cord? Is it possible to restore the regenerating capability of conducting fibers in the central nervous system which could help in the true recovery of the lost functions?

During the last decade, interest in the regeneration of organs has increased considerably, particularly involving the central conducting neurons in mammals. The discovery of new methods in the nineteen-twenties produced a new spurt of interest in histological investigation under the leadership of Ramon-y-Cajal and Samarin. They were able to show that although the problem of regeneration is very difficult to study, one should not give up hope. However, the work in this direction was not continued. Scientists were encouraged to take up this important problem with the vast clinical material during the war, with the need to help the injured as early as possible. The factors interfering with regeneration became clearer and as soon as they were known, people started to find ways of overcoming them. Many investigators engaged themselves in finding methods for regenerating the central conducting fibers (Guth & Windle, 1970, 1973; Illis, 1973a). We, also, started to work on this problem.

The result of experimental investigation, connected with the problem of functional restoration after complete transection of the spinal cord, has been described in the present monograph in four chapters:

1. Characteristics of motor reflexes in the hind limbs of dogs after transection of the spinal cord.

2. Significance of additional afferent stimuli for reconditioning the neuronal apparatus of a transected spinal cord.
3. Regeneration of the intraspinal axons in mammals.
4. Stimulation of the growth of intraspinal axons.

The experimental results were correlated with clinical findings. Spinal patients were treated by the renowned physician of the Republic, Dr. A. N. Trankvillitati. The results of these clinico-experimental investigations are presented in the fifth chapter of the monograph.

I will be failing in my duties, unless I express sincere gratitude to all my colleagues who participated in the experimental and clinico-experimental investigations in order to collect material for this monograph. I am particularly grateful to F. A. Brazovskaya who conducted the whole morphological investigation and aslo to E. N. Aranautova who devoted most of her time to investigating the synaptic connections of the regenerating fibers and the mechanism of Pyrogenal action.

Tat'yana Nesmeyanova

CHAPTER I

MOTOR REFLEXES IN THE HIND LIMBS OF DOGS AFTER SPINAL CORD TRANSECTION

Possibility of Developing New Reflex Motor Responses in the Transected Spinal Cord and Their Characteristics

As early as 1909 the integrative action of the spinal cord was shown to be capable of functional modification (Vvedenskii, 1912; Ukhtomskii, 1927). Sechenov (1864) reported that spinal centers involved in reflex activity are capable of retaining positive signs of motor excitation for a long time after external stimulation even when these centers have been isolated from cerebral control (1952b, Part III, p. 65). However, it was long believed that the spinal cord was continuously developing a set of reflexes and was incapable of changing them (Bolton, 1939).

Meanwhile, many studies have been published which conclusively prove that acquired functional relations can be reinforced in the spinal cord (Bete, 1934). In frogs, behavioral asymmetry after unilateral destruction of the labyrinth is retained even when the cerebral cortex has been separated from the spinal cord by transection (Zimkin, 1947). Moruzzi (1951) concluded that functional changes in the isolated spinal cord can be retained for a long time, as would be expected if the activity of the spinal neurons had returned to their original state. These conclusions were based on the works of Menni (1948a, 1948b) and Di Giorgio (1948a, 1948b) showing the retention of asymmetry of movements caused by unilateral destruction of the cerebellum, which did not disappear after the transection of the spinal cord. This implies that in such experimental conditions the traces of excitation which were previously developed in the intact spinal cord are retained in the isolated spinal cord.

This ability to retain the pattern of activity was demonstrated more concretely by Shamarina. The flexor muscle, when transplanted in place of the extensor, performed the latter's function and this readjustment was retained even after the removal of the cerebral cortex. Moreover, it appeared possible to achieve a similar type of readjustment of the muscular function in decerebrated rabbits, though a little more time was necessary (Shamarina, 1960a, 1960b).

These studies pose two questions: (1) whether the intect spinal cord can carry out motor functions independent of the control of the higher segments of the central nervous system; and (2) whether the characteristics of an isolated segment of the spinal cord can be utilized for developing motor functions.

In reply to the first question, many facts have accumulated up to the present time demonstrating the importance of the spinal segmental apparatus during the development of voluntary movements in an intact organism (Gurfinkel', Kots, & Shik, 1965; Gurfinkel' & Pal'tsev, 1965; Naidel & Pal'tsev, 1965). There appears to be activity in the muscles of the extremities before the development of voluntary movements which is preparatory for their coordination since it provides the body equilibrium necessary for the new activity (Belen'kii, Gurfinkel', & Pal'tsev, 1967). It has been suggested that initiation of the walking process in an intact organism is carried out by higher segments of the central nervous system, but the actual process is initiated by the segmental apparatus of the spinal cord (Austin, 1972; Pal'tsev, 1967).

To answer the second question it is necessary to demonstrate the possibility of developing new reflex motor reactions and their effective function in the distal part of the transected spinal cord. A great deal of work has been carried out in this direction (Taylor, 1974).

The first experiments were conducted on dogs by a group of American psychologists. Initially, this included the works of Culler and Mettler (1934) who thought that they were successful in developing the conditioned motor reflex with sound in decerebrate dogs. This reflex was a diffused one and appeared irregularly, with difficulty. Based on the assumption of the authors that the cerebral cortex was not essential for the development of conditioned reflexes, an attempt was made to develop these in the spinal cord when separated from the brain.

Shurrager and his associates (Shurrager, 1939a, 1939b; Shurrager & Culler,

1938, 1940; Shurrager & Shurrager, 1941) transected the spinal cord of dogs of various ages (2 months to 2 years) at the level of L_3 and developed motor reflexes in the semitendinosus muscles during acute experiments. The procedure consisted of applying a conditioned stimulus (CS) to the tail with weak alternating current or rubbing with a brush. The unconditioned stimulus (UCS) was applied to the skin of the paw by a strong shock of direct current which produced complete contraction of the semitendinosus muscle. The stimuli were applied in the following sequences–three CS at an interval of 1 sec plus the UCS which coincided with the third CS. The application of this group of combined stimuli was repeated at intervals of 15, 30, and 60 sec. Before starting the training, it was confirmed that the new reflex (CR) did not appear by the application of the CS alone. After 10 min rest, following a series of training procedures a number of inhibitory stimuli were applied to the tail. Initially, twitching appeared in both the semitendinosus muscles in response to the paired stimuli. However, if the stimulation was continued, the response disappeared in the contralateral extremity, while it progressed and was strengthened on the ipsilateral side. Repeated conditioning and repeated inhibitions required a decreasing number of paired stimuli and it was possible to obtain the reflex response of the muscles following inhibition even with the application of only a single stimulus (Fig. 1). The reflex reactions developed

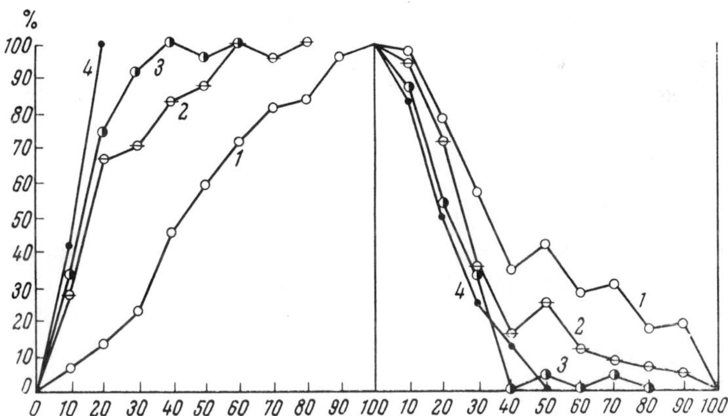

FIG. 1. The development of the spinal conditioned reflex and its inhibition in spinal dogs (adopted from *Shurrager & Culler*, 1940).

Abscissa–number of paired stimuli during conditioning (left) and single stimulation during inhibition (right); ordinate–degree of successful responses (in %). The curves based on the results of three consecutive series of experiments performed on six dogs: 1 = usual form of development and inhibition of the conditioned reflex; 2 = first series of development and subsequent inhibition; 3 = second series of development and subsequent inhibition; 4 = third series of development and subsequent inhibition.

in this way were considered analogous to the cortical conditioned reflex by the authors. In their opinion, the only difference was that the cortical conditioned reflex was generalized in the beginning and gradually became localized with training. However, in these experiments it was the reverse, i.e., the response was more localized in the beginning (individual muscle fibers) and then became generalized (the whole muscle reacted).

Based on these experiments, the authors came to the conclusion that all segments of the central nervous system were capable of developing conditioned reflexes.

To elaborate this concept, Shurrager and Shurrager (1946) conducted a series of experiments by the same method but applied weaker stimuli and noted only twitching of the individual fibers of the semitendinosus muscle. These results were similar to those obtained in the whole muscle, i.e., a new response appeared earlier with each new series of conditioning. Based on the fact that a single muscle fiber reacted to the CS, the authors concluded that a single motoneuron participated during the conditioning and was solely responsible for the response. If the interneurons had participated, more than one motoneuron and several muscle fibers should have been involved in the response. In their opinion, from these observations it was concluded that motoneurons of the spinal cord were capable of developing a conditioned reflex to the same degree as neurons of the cerebral cortex.

Another group of American investigators, headed by Kellogg, carried out similar experiments in subacute preparations lasting for 2-3 weeks. Beyond this time it was not possible to prolong the life of the spinal dogs. During this period a special stand was constructed where the animal was suspended for the rest of its life, with its hind legs supported by a stool when necessary (Kellogg, 1946).

They first conditioned the intact dogs and then transected their spinal cords. The conditioning was given in the following manner: The CS was applied to the front paw with a weak electric shock lasting for a short period and followed by stimulation of the hind paw after an interval of 1 sec with a prolonged double shock of electric current which served as the UCS. The intensity of the shock that was applied was judged by noting the degree of withdrawal of the paw. In intact dogs, the conditioned reflex was evident first by the twitching of the muscles and subsequently by flexion of the whole front leg. The latent period of the first phase of the response (twitching) was 200 msec and that of the subsequent flexor response varied from 400-1200 msec. The degree of twitching was constant but the amplitude of flexion increased with training (Pronko & Kellogg, 1942a).

The conditioned responses disappeared after transection of the spinal cord. The training was continued in these dogs but this time the investigators applied the conditioned stimuli (CS) to the other hind paw instead of the front paw and obtained the usual response. They confirmed that the conclusions made by Shurrager and Culler were correct and that the conditioned motor reflex which results in twitching of the muscle can be developed in the same manner in a spinal dog as in a normal animal (Pronko & Kellogg, 1942b). Later, these investigators analyzed the nature of the response in detail and came to the conclusion that spinal dogs were capable of performing extensive complicated movements, for which coordination of the higher segments of the central nervous system was not essential (Kellogg, Deese, & Pronko, 1946).

After continuing their work with spinal preparations, the same authors doubted whether it was correct to define the results they obtained as a conditioned reflex (Kellogg, Deese, Pronko, & Feinberg, 1947). In their experiments, the CR varied in degree and was inconstant. Occasionally twitching appeared in other muscles which had never been stimulated. The authors suggested that these phenomenon might be explained by the increased sensitivity of the spinal cord which might be obtained without the application of paired stimuli. In a discussion with Shurrager, Kellogg (1947) agreed that the development of spinal sensitivity was a great discovery; nevertheless, he did not consider it as a conditioned reflex. In fact, it was later possible to demonstrate that the twitching of muscles, which was previously considered as a conditioned response, was nothing but a direct response to the CS. It only showed that this was diffuse and not restricted to any particular organ which had been previously stimulated. The main factor determining the appearance of a conditioned response was the intensity of the CS. By changing the intensity of the stimulus it was possible to obtain the "conditioning" or the "inhibition" curves. The authors came to the conclusion that not only conditioned reflexes but also other motor reactions generally cannot be developed in the spinal cord (Deese & Kellogg, 1949). Thus these investigators arrived at a new stand, contradicting the possibility of the formation of new reflex responses.

Shurrager did not agree with the conclusions made by Kellogg and doubted the correctness of his experimental techniques. He thought that Kellogg recorded the generalized reflex instead of the conditioned response which should be increased by increasing the intensity of the electric shock applied to the tail. Shurrager himself did not consider this as a conditioned reflex since this was evoked by the application of a strong CS. Moreover, he suggested that the variations in Kellogg's results might be explained by the fact that his experiments were performed in chronic conditions.

However, the work of the other investigators who repeated Shurrager's experiments led to a similar conclusion, namely, that it was simply increased excitability of the neural tissues which was responsible for the reactions of the muscles of an extremity in response to stimulation of the tail (Pinto & Bromiley, 1950). Shurrager and his associates did not agree with these conclusions and considered that these investigators were unable, like Kellogg, to develop as true a conditioned reflex as they had observed (Shurrager, 1947; Shurrager & Shurrager, 1950). This conclusion was derived from the results of the experiments where the latent period of the conditioned reflex (CR) was more than that of the unconditioned (UCR). This was observed during the development of the cortical conditioned reflex (Shurrager & Culler, 1941).

Dykman and Shurrager (1956) verified their own hypothesis in a later work involving kittens and puppies, not only with acute preparations but also using chronic experimental conditions. In this work they confirmed the results obtained in acute experiments. After developing motor reaction in the right extremity, the latent periods of the reflexes were determined and they showed a great variation. In the CR this was equal to 96 msec and after inhibition this was increased to 115 msec. The latency of the UCR was constant and was equal to 28 msec. As a result, the authors were able to confirm their own conclusion that the resulting reflex was analogous to the cortical conditioned reflex.

The work of Shurrager and his colleagues aroused a great deal of interest among physiologists.

In the early 1950's Franzisket (1951, 1953) reported the development of conditioned reflexes in spinal frogs using chronic experimental conditions. Both Franzisket and Shurrager considered that the response they obtained was similar to the conditioned reflex because it did not correspond with the stimulation of a respective receptive field. Rensch and Franzisket (1954) found that these reflexes could be preserved for a long time.

Danilov (1952, 1953) repeated some of the experiments under similar situations. As a result of pairing during the stimulation of the paw and sacrum in a spinal frog, he noticed a response in the paw, in response to the stimulation of the tail. He explained that this effect was due to the summation of traces of the excitation process in the corresponding centers and found that the reflex response which was obtained was the same as that reported by Shurrager. However, this was solely related to the reflex activity of the spinal cord and it was unnecessary to bring in the idea of a conditioned reflex in order to understand its mechanism.

Experiments in our laboratory attempted investigating the plastic properties of the spinal cord, to confirm the possibility of developing reflex reactions and their inhibition. The essential factor in consideration of the utilization of the ability to reorganize the function of the cord might be the nature of formation and distribution of the resulting reactions, and also the analysis of the mechanism of their appearance and inhibition.

In acute experiments that we conducted on dogs (Nesmeyanova & Shamarina, 1953a, 1953b; Shamarina & Nesmeyanova, 1953), according to Shurrager's method, we never obtained the uniform response which this author reported, i.e., contraction of the semitendinosus muscle or twitching of its individual fibers.

The following types of responses were obtained: (1) contraction of the semitendinosus muscle in response to stimulation of the tail (Fig. 2, A, B); (2) movement of the tail in response to stimulation of the paw (Fig. 2, C, D); (3) inhibition of the tail movement at the moment of stimulation of the paw (Fig. 2E); (4) additional partial contraction of the tail muscles known as "recoiling," following simultaneous stimulation of the tail and paw. Here the nature of responses varied not only in different experiments but also during the course of a single experiment. The appearance and stability of the response depended on the intensity of the stimuli which were applied; the response to weak stimulation usually disappeared initially during development but, after reinforcement by repeated stimulation, less intense stimuli were required. The appearance of either response was found to be related to a significant lowering of the threshold of stimulation for a particular reflex while, on the other hand, the inhibition of the response was related to an increase in the threshold. Likewise, an increase in the intensity of the stimulus, to a certain extent, led to the appearance of a response in the semitendinosus muscle of the contralateral extremity, which had not been subjected to stimulation (Fig. 2B).

The results which were obtained posed the question of whether the expected atypical reaction we obtained could be produced by an isolated stimulus without the application of a paired one. In fact, after the application of 1200 stimuli on the skin of a particular paw, movement of the tail muscle was noticed. This was associated with a lowering in the threshold of stimulation. This reaction did not disappear after a 12-hr rest but after stimulating the right paw for 20 min, movement of the tail started even during stimulation of the left paw (Fig. 2F).

Experiments, which were considered atypical, were repeated on chronic spinal dogs in order to exclude the deficiency of an acute preparation and to follow the course of the newly developed reactions (Nesmeyanova & Shamarina, 1954a, 1954b).

These experiments were conducted in the following manner. The dog was placed on a stand and the hind legs were suspended by straps. In some dogs, paired stimuli were applied in two receptive fields, and in others, an unpaired stimulus in one receptive field. In the first case, three tetani, each lasting for 0.4-0.5 sec with an interval of 0.5 sec between each stimulus, were applied from an induction coil to the skin of the tail. Another electric shock was applied to the skin of the toe simultaneously with the last stimulus to the tail. The stimuli on the tail skin were applied with an intensity 1.5 times threshold, whereas, those on the paw were with 2-3 times threshold. These stimulations were usually given in a group of 25

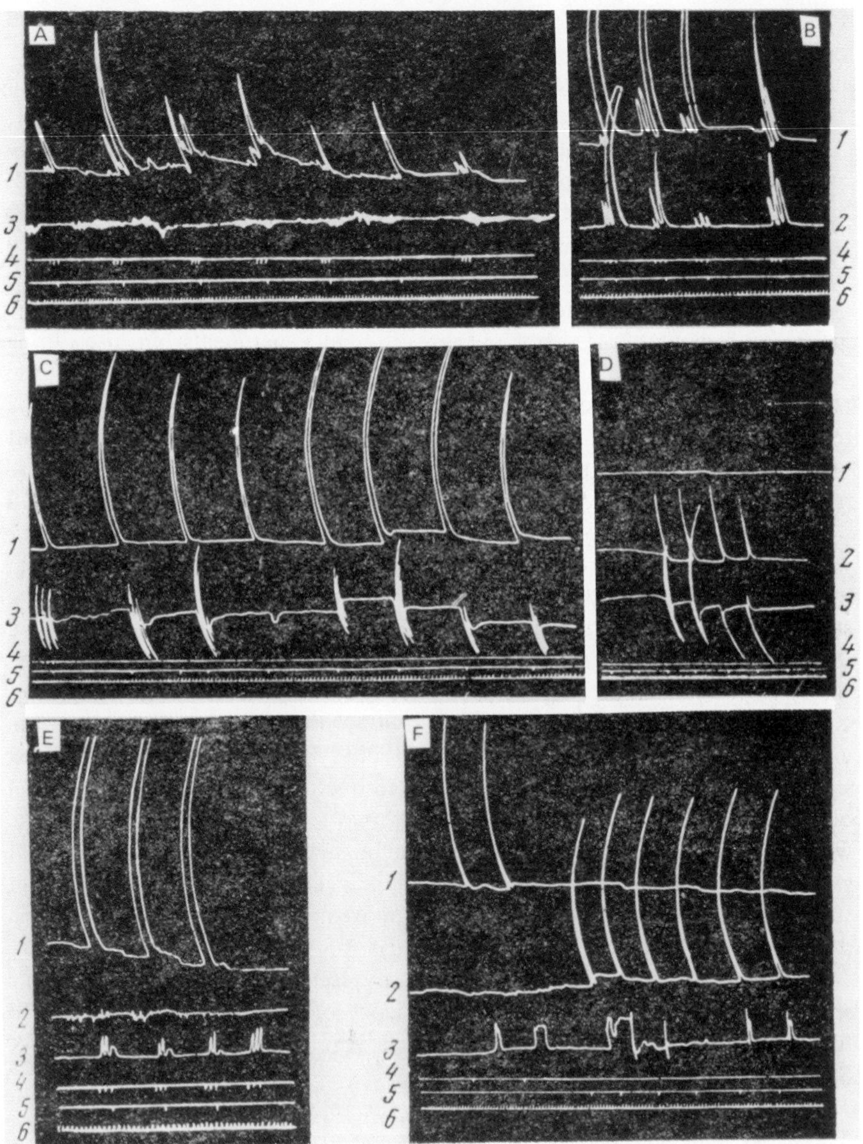

FIG. 2. Character of the developed motor reactions in spinal dogs.

A = contraction of right semitendinosus muscle in response to first two stimulations on the tail after a prolonged application of the paired stimuli; B = contraction of semitendinosus muscles right and left in response to tail stimulation; C = reaction in the tail muscles in response to stimulation of the right paw; D = reaction in the tail muscles in response to stimulation of the left paw (nonsystematic); E = inhibition in the contraction of the tail muscles in response to stimulation of the right paw; F = reaction in the tail muscles in response to stimulation of the reight and then left paw, after a prolonged stimulation of only the right paw.

1 = right semitendinosus muscle; 2 = left semitendinosus muscle; 3 = movement of the tail; 4 = mark of stimulation of the tail; 5 = mark of stimulation of the paw; 6 = time (in sec).

successive stimuli per experiment, with an interval of 1.5 min. In these experiments where one receptive field was stimulated, a single stimulus was given instead of three, with an interval of about 1.5 min with an intensity of 2–3 times the threshold. This work was done on six spinal dogs.

It was found that in the case of repeated experiments, the atypical reaction appeared in response to paired stimuli in two receptive fields in chronic spinal dogs. A novel characteristic of the above experiments was that when the stimulation was continued, the new reaction was reinforced and became permanent. The appearance of the atypical reaction was observed in both experiments, with electrical stimulation of the skin of the toe and tail (Fig. 3A) and also by scratching the side skin instead of by electrical stimulation (Fig. 3B).

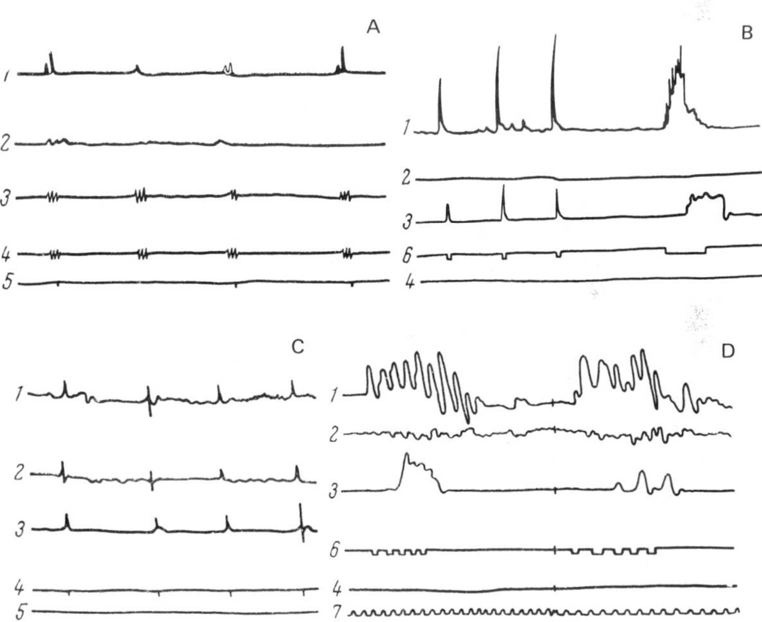

FIG. 3. Reaction developed as a result of stimulating two receptive fields (A, B) and a single receptive field (C, D).

A = reaction of the right paw and tail in response to stimulation of the tail skin; B = reaction of the right paw and tail in response to scratching of the side skin; C = reaction of the right and left paws and of the tail, in response to stimulation of the tail skin; D = reaction of the paws and the tail in response to scratching of the side skin.

1 = movement of the right paw; 2 = movement of the left paw; 3 = movement of the tail; 4 = mark of stimulating the tail; 5 = mark of stimulating the paw; 6 = mark of scratching; 7 = time (in sec).

The experiments where one receptive field was stimulated also gave positive results, i.e., new reactions appeared; but in this case, it was noticed that the atypical reaction appeared in response to a smaller number of stimuli than in the other case, where paired stimuli were given. Thus, after the application of 400 stimuli the response appeared on the right and then on the left paw in response to the stimulation of the tail skin (Fig. 3C). Scratching the side skin led to the appearance of a reaction in the tail instead of the paw. This reaction became permanent very quickly (Fig. 3D). During the application of stimuli in two receptive field, it was necessary to give approximately the same number of 400 stimuli but in pairs, which means double stimuli in order to evoke the appearance of an atypical reaction. It was noted that the application of strong or multiple stimuli hampered the development of the atypical reactions.

It was interesting to consider to what extent the atypical reactions were stable. To explore this, the spinal dogs which developed atypical reactions were examined during the periods of stimulation, as well as during the intervals between them, in the course of 1-2 years observation. The results showed that, as a rule, short intervals of up to one month without stimulation did not abolish the reinforced atypical reaction; it was only somewhat weakened. It increased again after the application of several new stimuli. However, unstable reactions which appeared very recently were completely abolished after an interval of one month. More prolonged intervals of, say, three to four months, of course, caused the abolition of the nonreinforced reaction, but after a small number of stimuli this reaction appeared again after a relatively short interval. When the reaction was reinforced, not even a prolonged interval could abolish it. The reaction appeared occasionally, although in a less intense form, even with the application of the initial stimulus. Our observations revealed that the factor deciding the preservation was the number of stimuli applied after the appearance of such an atypical reaction which had the effect of reinforcing it (Nesmeyanova & Shamarina, 1954b, 1956).

All the above facts indicate that the isolated spinal cord is capable of reorganizing motor functions and can evoke new reflex reactions which are preserved for a long time.

The possibility of establishing these reactions after the prolonged stimulation of one organ led us to think that the main basis of this phenomenon was the activation of the excitation processes. In fact, when the threshold for evoking the reflex was considerably lowered, the receptive field in the zone of the afferent input was widened and spread to new elements of the spinal cord. Consequently, additional atypical reactions were produced. In all probability, the prolonged and intense stimulation of a single receptive field produced a condition favorable for the spread of excitation. As a result of this, the dog gave a similar type of reaction to that reported by Vvedenskii (1938) in animals with strychnine poisoning. The character of the evoked response might change depending on the functional status of the components of the reflex arc participating in this reaction, which might fail to make normal connections, as reported by Exner (1882). The resultant diversity of reactions also included excitation of the type of Ukhtomskii's dominants, when the response reaction of one extremity (leg or tail) developed as a result of stimulation of various receptor fields.

The observations of Afelt (1963, 1964, 1965, 1966) regarding the transformation of twitching into a locomotor reflex caused by the systematic stimulation of cutaneous receptors mediating the earlier reflex in a spinal frog led her to conclude that excitability of the reflex centers was continuously increased. The earlier appearance of an atypical reaction in response to stimulation of a single receptive field, in our experiments, was apparently explained by the fact that stimulation of two different parts of the skin resulted in the formation of two different centers of excitation in the spinal cord. The presence of a second strong center of excitation prevented its activation from the first one. However, in certain selective cases, this second center of excitation helped in the development of a response. Therefore, in a number of our experiments, during the stimulation of one receptive field, the stimulation threshold of the other was systematically determined. For example, during systematic stimulation of the tail, the threshold was measured from the sk n of the right toe; the results showed that weak repetitive stimuli given several times during an experiment produced the quick appearance of atypical reactions, especially in the right paw. The atypical reaction developed rather slowly in those experiments where one receptive field was stimulated and the stimulation threshold of the other was not measured. Probably weak and less frequent stimuli helped in the formation of a particular spinal center. As a result, its excitability was somewhat increased and the excitation spreading from the second center initially had a great effect on the primary center. Thus, a response appeared in the motor area corresponding to the second receptive field, in response to stimulation of the first receptive field.

It is necessary to note that in the experiments of several investigators, combined stimulation produced a considerable increase in maximal muscle tension (expressed in gm). Similarly, no pronounced increase in the response was observed if no combinations were allowed during the cutaneous stimulation of the thigh and toe. The same type of correlation was also noted during inhibition (Fitzgerald & Thompson, 1967). It was characteristic of the results of these acute experiments that the maximum increase in the response was observed in the sixth series of stimulations. This was followed by abolition when the experiment was continued (Fig. 4). It is probable that combinations during the time of stimulation increased both the excitability

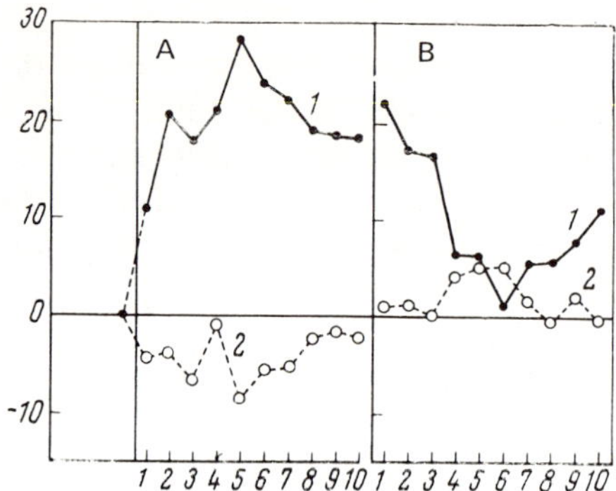

FIG. 4. Difference in the development (A) in the inhibition (B) by use of combination (1) and noncombination (2) during the time of stimulation (adopted from *Fitzgerald & Thompson*, 1967).

On the abscissa–successive stimulation; on the ordinate–amplitude of the response expressed as percent of control; 1 = conditioned reflex group; 2 = control group.

which was often observed in the first phase of the development as well as the inhibition.

The important factor for the establishment of an atypical reaction probably was the activation of synapses in neurons of the spinal cord as a result of the phenomenon which resulted when repeated stimulation facilitated the spreading of impulses along the same path, owing to a more effective synaptic influence over all those neurons which were influenced earlier (Eccles, 1953; Konorski, 1950; McIntyre, 1953, Young, 1951).

The stability of the evoked responses that we observed indicates that a new functional state in the different segments of a particular reflex arc was maintained for an indefinite period. Probably this was basically due to the absence of supraspinal influences. This effect resulted in the withdrawal of the excitatory influences of pyramidal impulses from the flexor motoneurons and the inhibitory influences from extensor motoneurons (Lundberg & Voorhoeve, 1962; Maksimova & Sverdlov, 1966; Vasilenko & Kostyuk, 1966). After the withdrawal of the excitatory and inhibitory impulses, a different correlation was established for carrying out segmental reactions. Thus, it was possible to establish new long lasting reflex reactions.

The plastic changes in the function of the transected spinal cord were very pronounced. They might be compared with some of the elements of a cortical conditioned reflex (Kozak & Westerman, 1966). However, these changes were not analogous to a conditioned reflex, as suggested by Shurrager and Culler (1941), as this analogy was neither possible nor necessary. The above hypothesis was confirmed by the fact that the development of the atypical motor reaction in the transected spinal cord was carried out by stimulating one receptive field, without combining it with other stimuli. Apart from this, such phenomena as the appearance of unstable responses in the course of an experiment, and then the spread of the reaction into a new area which had not been stimulated earlier, also suggested that Shurrager's conclusions were incorrect. Moreover, Shurrager noticed the spread of excitation but considered this as the only feature by which an atypical reaction could be distinguished from a conditioned reflex.

The basis for considering the response which was obtained as being a conditioned reflex was based by Shurrager & Shurrager (1950) on the following grounds: (1) absence of a reaction during stimulation of the receptors in a single reflex arc, (2) appearance of a reaction as a result of combination during prolonged stimulation of the receptors of two different reflex arcs, (3) extinction of the reaction if not reinforced, and (4) absence of a summation effect, the presence of which might give an analogous reaction. As can be seen from the above material, these grounds did not justify making such a conclusion. The differences in the results of our experiments (which we observed during the development of an atypical reaction by stimulating the receptors of a single reflex arc) from those of Shurrager could probably be explained by the fact that he gave a total of 30-60 stimuli to a particular area and, without obtaining any result, considered this sufficient to allow interpreting the nature of the response which was evoked by paired stimuli as being a conditioned reflex. Meanwhile, our experiments showed that in order to obtain a response by stimulating a single receptive zone, it was necessary to give not 30-60, but 400-1000 stimuli.

Kellogg, as well as Pinto and Bromiley, studied the reflex activity of the transected spinal cord and initially interpreted the nature of the evoked reaction correctly; but finally they contradicted their earlier observations and remarked that the transected spinal cord was incapable of undergoing any plastic changes and what was seen in the vast majority of literature was incorrect.

Our investigations proved beyond doubt that plastic changes could occur in the distal part of the transected spinal cord. It was important to know how to produce them and it was also necessary to explain the phenomenon in terms of modern physiology. In order to utilize the plastic properties of the spinal cord in the compensatory development of motor functions, it was necessary to describe the elements of the spinal reflex arc which were responsible for the establishment of the new reflexes.

Formation and Localization of Atypical Responses in the Spinal Reflex Arc

The role of interneurons in the majority of reflex reactions has been well known and we have, therefore, suggested that they played an important role in the formation of atypical responses. However, based on experiments using the response of a single muscle fiber, Shurrager and Culler (1940, 1941) have suggested that the motoneurons were responsible for the resulting reaction.

Matyushkin (1953) held the same opinion when he observed repetitive firing in the motoneurons evoked by stimulating the receptive field of monosynaptic reflex. We compared the effects produced by systematically stimulating the receptive fields of the polysynaptic flexor and the monosynaptic knee and ankle reflexes to determine which structures in the spinal cord might be responsible for the development of an atypical reaction.

Let us see what we know about the nature of the knee reflex. Can this reflex be considered similar to an ankle jerk, with a single receptive field? Tsehirjew (1887) showed that the response in the quadriceps muscle of the thigh was slightly delayed following stretch of its tendon. Weiler (1910) found that the latent period of the knee jerk was equal to 0.05–0.07 sec, i.e., it was related with those reflexes which typically have a single receptive field. Therefore, the knee jerk could be considered as a stretch reflex, like the ankle jerk reported by Sherrington. These reflexes appeared as a result of the activation of the muscle spindle during rapid stretching of a muscle produced by a tap on its tendon. After partial or complete interruption of impulse transmission in the spinal cord, it was less affected than the other reflexes. Thus, when the pyramidal tract was damaged, the reflex became more pronounced and its receptive field widened (Rusetskii, 1935). Complete transection of the spinal cord in cats and dogs caused a rapid increase in the amplitude of this reflex instead of its abolition (Krid, Denny-Brown, Eccles, Lidell, & Sherrington, 1935). Thus, rapid stretching of the muscle did not change the responses of the monosynaptic reflexes, even during the first few hours after the transection of the cord. Some inhibition of the reflex response could only be produced by slow and uniform stretching of a muscle and this could be related to the appearance of spinal shock (Bragin, 1966). In man, the first motor reflex reappears 2–3 weeks after spinal injury (Riddoch, 1917).

The flexor reflex produced by stimulating the skin on the plantar surface of the foot is a typical example of a polysynaptic reflex. According to Sherrington (1910), this involves the following muscles in a spinal dog: tibialis anterior, biceps femoris, semitendinosus, and part of the rectus femoris. The receptive field of this flexor reflex is covered by the skin of the foot and by that over the anterior of the tibia.

Experimental Procedure

We examined this problem on seven adult dogs with their spinal cords transected at the level of T_{10}. Two intact dogs served as control (Nesmeyanova, 1966, 1968b).

The work also included a new group of muscles by repeatedly stimulating the receptive fields of the polysynaptic flexor and the monosynaptic (knee and ankle) reflexes. A recording of muscle potentials was made by inserting electrodes at a depth of 2-3 mm. The muscle potentials were led to a preamplifier UBP 1-01 and then recorded with the help of an oscillograph N_{102}.

Flexor reflex. The experiments were performed three to four months after transection of the spinal cord, at which time the skin of the right paw was systematically stimulated with rectangular impulses at a frequency of 1 and 3 impulses/sec using a current which was above threshold. During each one of the series of experimental procedures (on alternate days), about 1000 stimuli were given, followed by 1500 stimuli.

The positive results were obtained by stimulating the receptive field of the flexor reflex. During the second procedure, gastrocnemius and vastus lateralis of the ipsilateral side were included in the response. This was initially unstable and disappeared in the middle of the period of stimulation but reappeared in the beginning of the next procedure and stabilized in the fifth procedure.

The biceps femoris and tibalis anterior muscles of the contralateral extremity which do not participate in the crossed reflex were included in this reaction during the third procedure and in one dog during the fourth procedure (Fig. 5). Beginning with the sixth and seventh procedures, all these muscles participated regularly in this reflex. The latent period of the response

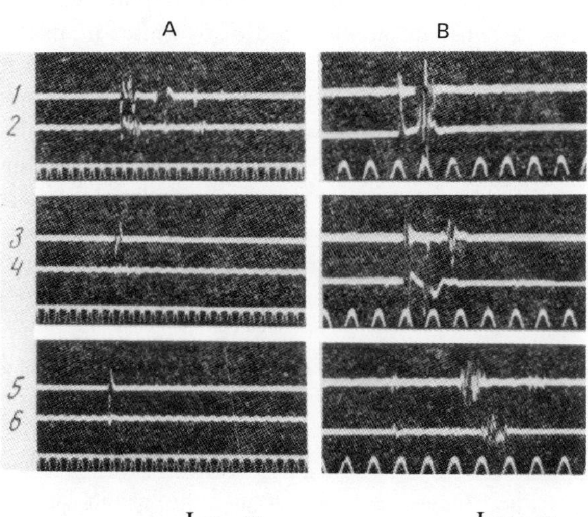

FIG. 5. Inclusion of new muscles in the flexor reflex of the left extremity.

A = first experiment; B = sixth experiment (6500 stimuli). 1 = biceps femoris (left); 2 = tibialis anterior (left); 3 = vastus lateralis (left); 4 = gastrocnemius (left); 5 = biceps femoris (right); 6 = tibialia anterior (right). Time = 20 msec.

in the gastrocnemius of the ipsilateral extremity was 18-22 msec and in the vastus lateralis it was 26-30 msec. This latent period varied from 35-50 msec for the muscles of the contralateral extremity (Table 1).

The latent periods shown in Table 1 had the characteristics of a polysynaptic reflex with inclusion of associated synaptic delays. The patella reflex was evoked by striking with a mechanical hammer at a frequency of 3 per sec. These experiments were performed on two dogs during a period when only the quadriceps responded to the application to the above stimuli. They were conducted at intervals of 1-2 days and during each procedure about 2000 stimuli were applied. Altogether seven experiments were performed on each dog. The reaction of the following muscles was investigated: biceps femoris, tibialis anterior, gastrocnemius and rectus femoris of both the ipsilateral and contralateral extremities. These procedures eventually resulted in contraction.

In both dogs, the response to stimulation was only observed in the heads of quadriceps initially. In the second procedure, after 1600-1800 stimuli, the tibialis anterior and the gastrocnemius were found to be included in this response. The ipsilateral biceps femoris and the contralateral rectus femoris responded a little later, after approximately 2200-2400 stimuli (Fig. 6). The reaction of these muscles was initially unstable and disappeared during the course of each procedure. It reappeared at the beginning of the next and then became stable in the fourth procedure (about 5000 stimuli). However, the latent periods of the individual muscles were different. Vastus lateralis and rectus femoris had a constant latent period of 5-7 msec in all the cases, while in biceps femoris, gastrocnemius and tibialis anterior of the ipsilateral extremity, the latent period was 16-17 msec. In the contralateral rectus this was 35-50 msec (Fig. 7). In other words, whether stimulating a receptive field in a monosynaptic or a polysynaptic reflex, the excitation process in the muscles participating in the reflex was transmitted along a polysynaptic arc.

The method of post-tetanic potentiation is one of the methods of choice in modern electrophysiology, and characterizes the changes in synaptic conduction of a particular reflex arc. Post-tetanic potentiation is usually

TABLE 1. Latent Period (in msec) of the Muscles Participating in Different Spinal Reflexes

Reflexes	Muscles of the extremity					Muscles of the contralateral extremity			
	rectus femoris	vastus lateralis	biceps femoris	gastrocnemius	tibialis anterior	rectus femoris	biceps femoris	gastrocnemius	tibialis anterior
Flexor	16–17	26–30	15–17	18–22	16–17	45–50	35–50	–	45–50
Knee	5–7	5–7	16–17	16–17	16–17	35–50	–	–	–
Ankle	16–17	–	16–17	5–7	16–17	–	–	35–50	–

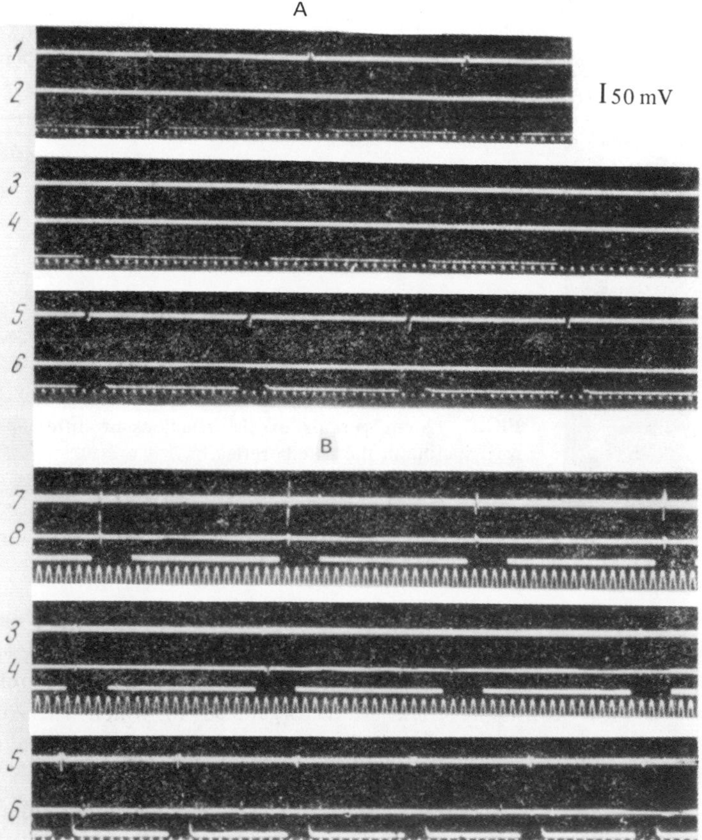

FIG. 6. Involvement of new muscles for carrying out the knee reflex in the left extremity.

A = first experiment; B = fourth experiment (6000 stimuli). 1 = left rectus femoris; 2 = left biceps femoris; 3 = left gastrocnemius; 4 = left tibialis anterior; 5 = left rectus femoris; 6 = right rectus femoris; 7 = left biceps femoris; 8 = left rectus femoris. Third line = stimulation mark; fourth line = time, 20 msec.

observed as homosynaptic, i.e., recorded from the synaptic terminals of those afferents which are subjected to earlier tetanization. However, several investigators have reported that post-tetanic potentiation may also be heterosynaptic (Afelt & Weber, 1970; Kandel & Tauc, 1965a, 1965b). A more prolonged potentiation might indicate the increased state of excitability of the neurons in particular reflex arcs, i.e., their ability to be involved in the reflex motor response. This property may be considered essential for the development of a new reflex response. It follows that heterosynaptic potentiation is not normally observed (Kostyuk, 1959).

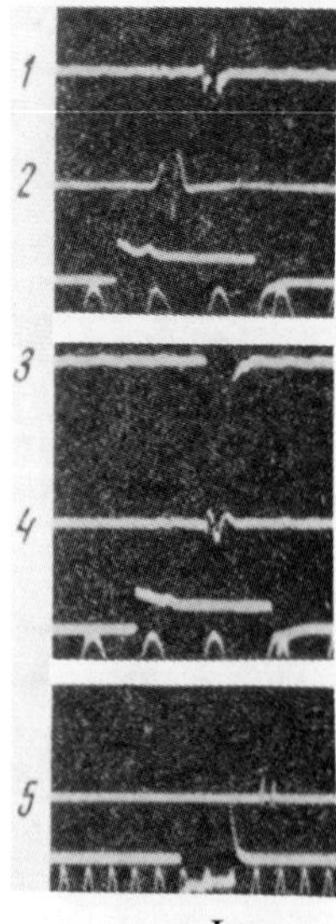

FIG. 7. Latent periods of the reactions of different muscles participating in the patella reflex.

Ipsilateral extremity: 1 = biceps femoris; 2 = rectus femoris; 3 = gastrocnemius; 4 = tibialis anterior: contralateral extremity; 5 = rectus femoris. Third line = stimulation mark; fourth line = time, 20 msec.

The response involving new muscles in a motor reflex might be considered analogous to an atypical reaction. Stimulation of a receptive field activates new nerve elements which had previously not been included in the reflex. As a result, a more complex reflex arc is organized in which two or more intervening neurons may be included. This reflex then turns into a polysynaptic one.

Involvement of new muscles in the reflex was not dependent on whether the receptive field of a mono- or a polysynaptic reflex was stimulated. In both cases, the involvement of new muscles in this response was caused by stimulation with a low frequency electric current which was above threshold. As can be seen from Table 1, the latent periods of the responses produced during the stimulation of the receptive field of a polysynaptic reflex, were longer for the muscles newly involved in the reaction than for the muscles regularly participating in the reflex. Therefore, the new arc always contains more synapses than the one which was functioning previously. The results of Dykman and Shurrager (1956) could be explained by an increase in the latent period of the "conditioned reflex" as compared with that which was "unconditioned." The new reflex always possesses a more complicated reflex arc.

What important components of the nervous system may be primarily responsible for producing this new type of response? On the basis of the data obtained about the polysynaptic nature of the atypical motor reactions, it might be suggested that the essential factor for its arousal was stimulation of the skin which exclusively activates the spinal interneurons. It is a known fact that stimulation of the skin produces contraction of the muscle lying just below the area of stimulation and this inhibits the response of the antagonist muscles. For this phenomenon, both the α- as well as γ-motoneurons are responsible. Threshold excitation of the γ-motoneurons is comparatively less effective and is activated by stimulating the cutaneous nerves (Eldred & Hagbarth, 1955; Hagbarth, 1952).

The experiments we conducted (Nesmeyanova, 1967, 1968b) showed that it was necessary to stimulate the skin even when the monosynaptic reflex had been repeatedly developed in order to develop an atypical response. The development of these responses was investigated in two dogs by systematically stimulating the skin over the Achilles tendon with a mechanical hammer at a frequency of 3 per sec. Before starting the experiment, the area of skin which was to be stimulated was anesthetized. For this purpose, 0.7 ml of 1% novocain was given subcutaneously over the Achilles tendon. After the absorption of the wheal, which required about 5-7 min, the experiment began and continued for 15 min. According to data from the Institute of Pharmacology, the action of novocain usually lasts for 30 min after subcutaneous injection. These experiments with novocain were performed on alternate days for three weeks. The response was observed in the gastrocnemius, tibialis anterior, rectus femoris, and biceps femoris on the left or ipsilateral extremity and in the rectus femoris and gastrocnemius of the contralateral or right extremity.

The results of experiments to determine the involvement of additional muscles in the ankle reflex were negative during the period when the skin was anesthetized. Initially the response to stimulation appeared in the gastrocnemius and tibialis anterior muscles of the ipsilateral extremity. No change was noticed after seven experiments (1400 stimuli), when the response to stimulation appeared in the same group of muscles (Fig. 8). In contrast, the results of experiments concerned with the involvement of new muscles in the reflex where the skin was not anesthetized were positive. In these spinal dogs, the ipsilateral rectus femoris, biceps femoris, and the contralateral gastrocnemius participated in this reflex during the second series of stimuli (after 1200 stimuli), as well as the ipsilateral gastrocnemius and tibialis anterior.

These experiments established the importance of stimulating the skin in order to involve new muscles in the motor reflexes. However, no one has reported the formation of an atypical motor reaction in response to stimulation of the muscular afferents. It is difficult to believe that the spike potentials evoked in the muscle afferents, in spinal as well as in normal animals, only come from motoneurons. The excitation from muscle afferents is, in all probability, transmitted to the interneurons from some other pathway. In fact, there are reports that in spinal animals monosynaptic

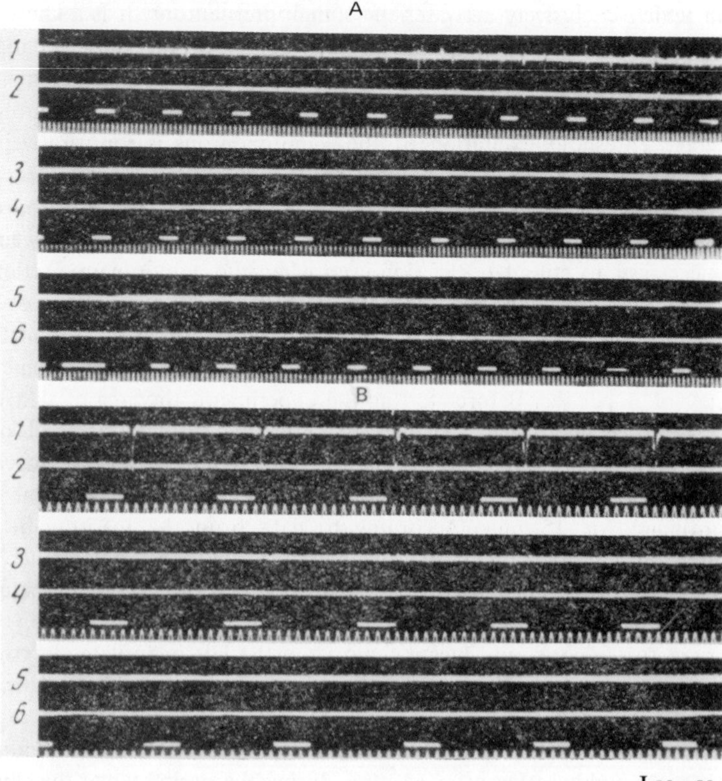

FIG. 8. Absence of the involvement of new muscles in the ankle reflex following stimulation of the anesthetized skin.

A = first experiment; B = sixth experiment (10,000 stimuli). 1 = left gastrocnemius; 2 = left tibialis anterior; 3 = left rectus femoris; 4 = left biceps femoris; 5 = right rectus femoris; 6 = right gastrocnemius. Third line = stimulation mark; fourth line = time, 20 msec.

conduction is transformed into a polysynaptic form in response to weak stimulation of a motor nerve (Sumi, 1959). Interaction between the different motor nerves was observed by Afelt and Weber (1970). Conditioned (tetanic) and test (single) stimuli were applied to different nerves in the caudal part of the spinal cord of a cat, five months after a double transection. In one case, a cutaneous and a motor nerve, and in another case, two different motor nerves of group I, were subjected to stimulation. In both cases, heterosynaptic post-tetanic potentiation was noted, though in the second case, this potentiation was less pronounced than in the first. A phenomenon very close to this was observed by Kandel and Tauc (1965a, 1965b) who studied the after-effects by simultaneously stimulating two afferents to a giant neuron isolated from the abdominal ganglion of a mollusca *Aplysia depilans.* They observed heterosynaptic facilitation in this particular experimental situation.

These results, besides explaining the new fact that different nerves may interact among themselves, also help in understanding the cellular mechanism responsible for the development of new reflexes. Kandel and Tauc believed that the phenomenon they observed was facilitated by a presynaptic process. Fitzgerald and Thompson (1967) simultaneously stimulated two different cutaneous receptive fields in acute spinal cats, and considered that the basis for the development of the above process and the new reflexes was analogous to the hyperpolarization of the presynaptic afferent terminals.

Though the cellular mechanism for the development of the new reflex is not sufficiently clear, the end result indicates a great variation in the coordination between excitatory and inhibitory processes in the spinal cord. The strict reciprocal relations between antagonist muscles can be disturbed. Thus, judging from our results, excitation might appear simultaneously in a series of antagonist muscles either in one or both extremities.

The disturbance in such reciprocal relations has also been reported by a number of physiologists in other cases—such as after prolonged stimulation of afferent nerves in a decerebrate preparation (Skuratova, 1956) and in experiments with patients having a slight hemiparesis (Person, 1960, 1965). Saf'yants (1964a, 1964b) described the presence of synergism simultaneously with antagonism between the flexor centers of the two extremities. It may be suggested that after transection of the spinal cord, synergistic relations are to some extent improved and prevail over the antagonistic ones. Along with disturbances of reciprocity in the isolated spinal cord (separated from the higher segments of the central nervous system), some other unknown phenomena may take place which are characterized by increased sensitivity to stimulation and mediator substance. Cannon and his associates have reported that this phenomenon is typical for denervated structures (Cannon & Haimovici, 1939; Cannon & Rosenblueth, 1951).

The increased reactivity of the spinal cord components to various forms of stimulation is a mechanism which could play an important role during the reorganization of recovery processes in a transected spinal cord. The length of the post-operative interval is an important factor in the appearance of increased excitability. In animals which have had a spinal transection for 2–3 weeks or more, the signs of spinal reflex excitability were usually different from those in animals where spinal sections were made immediately before experimental evaluation. Thus, stimulation of a muscle nerve in a spinal cat under chronic experimental condition produced a repetitive firing which could be recorded from isolated fibers of a ventral root (Sumi, 1959). The author considers this similar to the action of strychnine on the nervous system. Experiments using intracellular recording confirmed this and helped in understanding the reported phenomenon. Austin and Sato (1962) reported that motoneurons in the distal part of the spinal cord in cats were more excitable 2–3 weeks after operation than immediately after decerebration or acute spinal transection. Using microelectrodes, they found that this increased excitability of the motoneurons resulted in the appearance of spontaneous activity which was not observed in acute experimental conditions performed immediately after spinal transection. The second sign of excitability, consisting of repetitive firing of motoneurons in response to orthodromic volleys of impulses, was observed from 2–10 sec after stimulation.

These observations indicate that excitability is gradually changed after spinal transection. There are many studies where changes in the pattern of interneuronal activity have been reported under these conditions. This fact might have an important bearing on the reorganization of spinal activity. The increased excitability of the spinal reflexes on the hemisected side of the spinal cord was characterized by a prolonged excitatory after discharge in the polysynaptic arc and its absence in the monosynaptic pathway (Cannon, Rosenblueth, & Carsia, 1945). It was reported that strong stimulation of a cutaneous nerve, particularly the sural nerve, produced such a response for a considerably longer time in experiments with chronic spinal cats than in acute experiments. Kozak and Westerman (1966) found that the response was particularly prolonged in the flexor nerve of the ipsilateral extremity (Fig. 9). Thus, interneuronal excitability is not depressed after spinal transection and, in all probability, the excitability of motoneurons is increased. This was also confirmed by our observations.

It is quite possible that the appearance of increased interneuron excitability which was observed as early as two weeks after the transection of a spinal cord (the time accepted by the majority of the investigators for passing into a chronic stage) was related to the initial dystrophy. The dystrophic processes in the interneurons probably produced increased motoneuron excitability after a temporary asphyxia of the spinal cord in animals (Gelfan & Tarlov, 1959; Van Harreveld & Schade, 1962).

How may the above-mentioned functional characteristics in the distal part of the transected spinal cord be utilized in the process of compensatory restoration of the motor function? Let us examine this in relation to the act of weight-bearing. In man, this is carried out mainly by the muscles of the leg (Gurfinkel', 1961). According to our findings, there was a constant fluctuation of the activity in the calf muscles of both extremities in *intact* dogs. The activity in the vastus lateralis and in the longissimus dorsi was only represented by isolated firing (Fig. 10A). However, in *spinal* dogs all the muscles of the extremity participated in the weight-bearing reflex, excepting the flexors of the knee and the long muscles of the spine (Fig. 10B). Tension in the last group of muscles helped to hold the pelvis of the animal in a horizontal

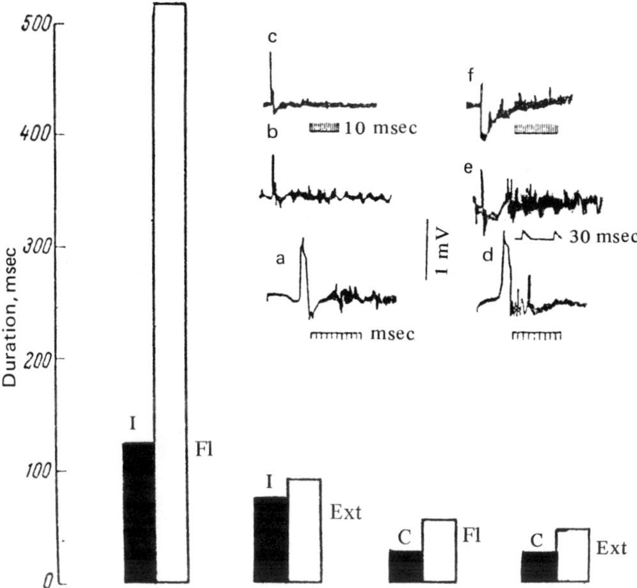

FIG. 9. Reflexes evoked in response to stimulation of cutaneous nerves in chronic and in acute spinal cats with spinal transection at the lumbar region (adopted from *Kozak & Westerman,* 1966).

a–f: type of the reflex discharges recorded from the flexor nerves in acute (a–c– and in chronic (d–f) spinal cats in response to a single stimulus with an intensity of 20 times threshold applied to an ipsilateral sural nerve. Three times scales were utilized.

Columns: duration of reflex response in acute (black) and in chronic (white) spinal cats; I = ipsilateral stimulation; C = contralateral stimulation; Fl = flexor; Ext = extensors.

position, but, at the same time, the activity of the extensors and some of the flexors was responsible for the unstable weight-bearing which we observed. Other examples utilizing the characteristics of the transected spinal cord for functional reorganization will be reported below, in relation to other problems.

Inhibition of Muscular Activity in the Hind Limbs in Spinal Dogs

The characteristics of the reflex activity of a transected spinal cord affect both the excitatory and inhibitory processes. Coordination is maintained in an intact spinal cord by way of continuous interaction between these processes. Reciprocal inhibition is manifested by hyperpolarization of the neuronal membrane due to the action of inhibitory impulses. Such inhibition is essentially postsynaptic (Eccles, 1966; Kostyuk, 1958a, 1958b).

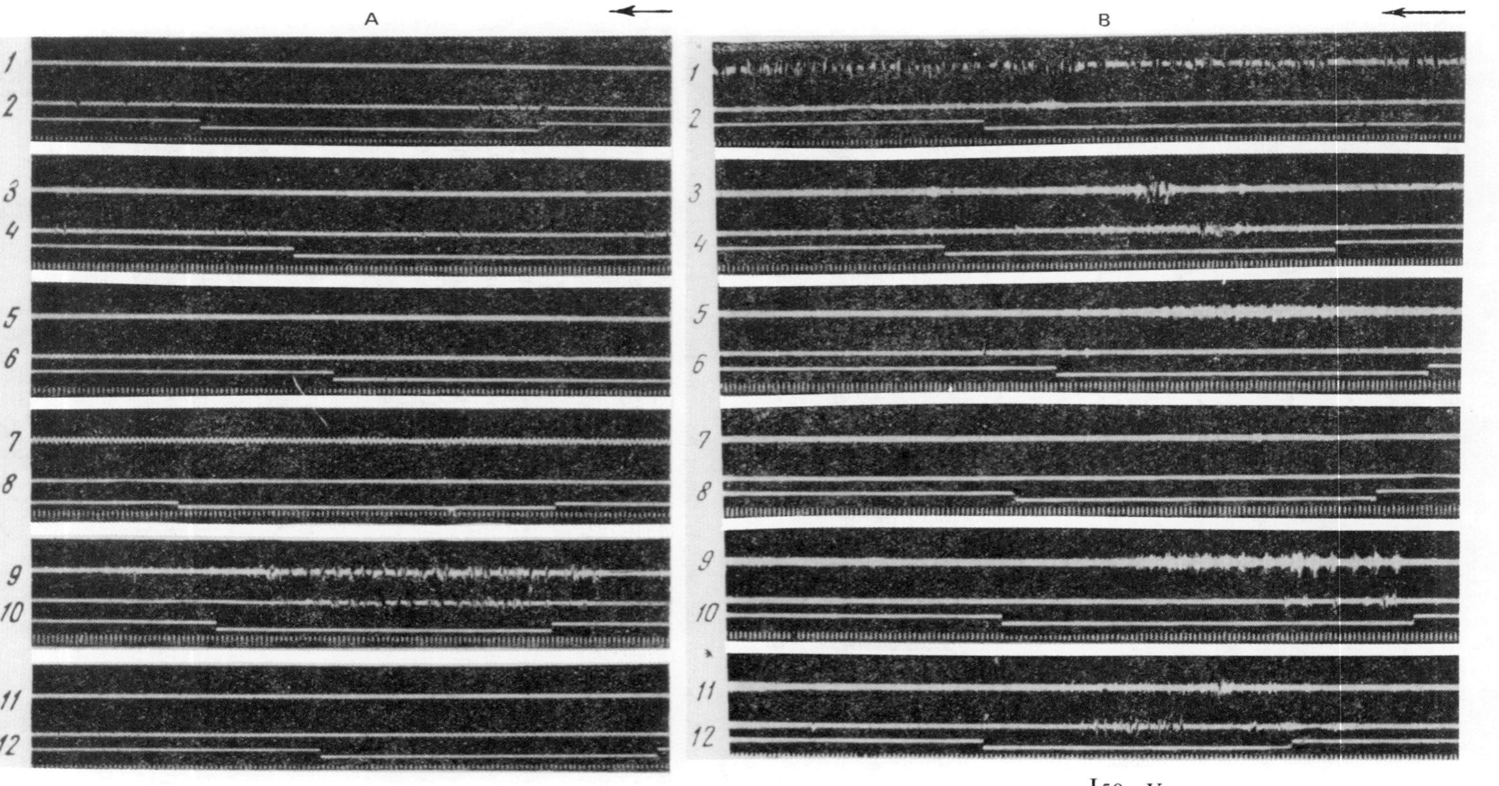

FIG. 10. Activity in the muscles of the trunk and of the extremities during weight-bearing in intact (A) and in spinal (B) dogs.

1 = right longissimus dorsi; 2 = left longissimus dorsi; 3 = right rectus femoris; 4 = left rectus femoris; 5 = right vastus lateralis; 6 = left vastus lateralis; 7 = right biceps femoris; 8 = left biceps femoris; 9 = right gastrocnemius; 10 = left gastrocnemius; 11 = right tibialis anterior; 12 = left tibialis anterior. Third line = mark indicating the commencement of weight-bearing; fourth line = time, 20 msec.

In addition, other types of inhibition lasting for prolonged periods and affecting a number of reflex arcs have been reported in preparations involving a transected spinal cord, such as the overflowing of inhibition in the cerebral cortex (Pavlov, 1951a, 1951b, 1951c).

Sechenov (1868) first reported the phenomenon of extinction in a decerebrate frog (below the level of the fourth ventricle) in response to stimulation of a sensory nerve using a strong tetanic current which, when stopped, evoked a revival of motor activity. From this observation it may be concluded that such extinction was due to inhibition of the motor reflexes and was not due to fatigue. Sherrington (1906), working with spinal cats, noted that partial stimulation of a particular cutaneous area produced a decrease in the response amplitude to the point where it disappeared.

Prosser and Hunter (1936) in spinal rats and Franzisket (1953) in frogs observed extinction of spinal reflexes when they were evoked at a particular frequency. Motor reactions evoked in spinal cats and dogs have been similarly inhibited (Culler, 1938; Shurrager, 1939a, 1939b). This was achieved by the application of a single unpaired stimulus (CS) instead of the paired stimuli necessary for the development of such reactions as those described above. As a result, there was extinction of the evoked response in the semitendinosus muscle after application of a series of such single stimuli. The curves of development and extinction were symmetrical (Shurranger & Culler, 1940) and this fact led the authors to conclude that development and extinction take place in the same structures and probably at the synapses of the motoneurons (Shurrager & Culler, 1941).

The object of this part of our work was to test whether or not the reported inhibition of motor reactions was specific for the transected spinal cord (Nesmeyanova, 1955a, 1955b; 1957). Based on the idea that in this particular case one has to deal with the central processes, we simply applied the term "adaptation" to indicate the phenomenon we reported as inhibition or extinction.

The experiments were performed in two series using four dogs in each group, with spinal transections at the level of T_3-T_6.

The possibility of inhibiting the atypical motor reactions and the spinal reflex was essentially verified in the first series of experiments. Inhibition was produced by a light scratch on the side skin at a frequency of one in two sec, which usually produced a moderate motor response. The spinal reflexes and atypical motor reactions were well developed in these dogs before starting the experiments. In the first series of experiments, the stimuli were applied in series of 6-10 groups per experiment and 10-50 scratches were given in each group. An interval of 2-5 min was given in between each group of stimuli. The experiments were performed 4-6 times per week. The control stimuli, in the form of strong scratching on the skin or pinching of the foot pad, were applied in approximately every fifth experiment. The condition of other motor reflexes evoked by stimulating different areas of the skin was systematically examined.

In the experiments of the second series, an attempt was made to inhibit the extensor jerk—the reflex connected with weight-bearing of the animal. According to our findings, the latent period of this reflex was 16–18 msec, indicating that it was polysynaptic. To produce inhibition, the same light strokes were applied on the foot pads of the hind legs with a frequency of 1–2 per sec and about 25–500 strokes were applied during an experiment. The rest of the work was carried out in the same manner as in the experiments of the first series.

The results in both series of experiments showed that, initially, weak stimuli increased the excitability of a particular reflex arc, and the subthreshold stimulus became a threshold one. This condition continued during the course of several experiments—after which the excitability started decreasing until there was a complete disappearance of the response to test stimulation. During the systematic stimulation of any receptive field, the atypical motor reactions (physiologically less significant polysynaptic reflexes which appeared at a late stage) were initially inhibited, followed by the scratch reflex. There was incomplete inhibition of the flexor reflex and the extensor jerk. They appeared occasionally, even after the application of 10,000 stimuli, i.e., their inhibition was incomplete. The monosynaptic reflexes, such as the knee and the ankle jerks, were not inhibited; they remained constant and rather pronounced.

This type of inhibition was characterized by spreading later to other reflex arcs which could be stimulated by their own receptive fields.

The inhibition was initially not very stable and the reflexes were reestablished very easily. However, after the application of about 500 stimuli, the scratch reflex and the atypical reactions were not reestablished even after a 10-day rest. All the reflexes were reestablished only after a lapse of one and a half months. The order of their reappearance was opposite to the order of their inhibition. First, the inborn reflexes associated with the weight-bearing reappeared, i.e., the flexor, the extensor jerks, then the scratch reflex and, last of all, the atypical motor reactions. Initially, when the reflexes were reestablished, they were unusually prominent and stable. However, this condition was changed after a month's rest and a second wave of inhibition was observed which lasted for about three weeks. These results confirmed that the ability to reorganize the functions in a transected spinal cord is also distributed among the inhibitory processes.

The success of inhibition in our experiments was mainly determined by the type of reflex. All the polysynaptic reflexes were inhibited, though the rate of inhibition varied. In one case, the inhibition was deep but in other cases, it was very superficial. This difference was dependent on the physiological significance of the reflex. Reflexes connected with weight-bearing and locomotion were inhibited with great difficulty in comparison to a pure scratch reflex. According to Kozak and Westerman (1966), the scratch reflex was inhibited even by repeated application of stimuli above threshold level.

This type of reflex inhibition might be related to a central process and not due to the adaptation of receptors as a result of prolonged stimulation. This was proven by the fact that in the initial application of weak stimuli, an increase in the excitability of that particular reflex was observed where the threshold was lowered and the response increased. Later, when there was extinction of the reflex, application of a strong stimulus could evoke the reflex again. The possibility of spreading the inhibitory process in other reflex arcs, and similarly the appearance of second and third waves of inhibition without the application of additional stimuli, indicates that the above process may be a central one. The majority of investigators working with a similar type of inhibition noted the importance of applying weak stimuli at a low frequency for successful inhibition. The role of these parameters was thoroughly studied by Afelt (1965, 1966). In her experiments with frogs, she reported that the percentage of extinction was greater when giving tactile stimulation to a localized area with the help of Frey's hairs than when stimulating a wider area of skin with the help of a brush. Similarly, another essential condition for producing inhibition in her experiments was selection of the interval between stimuli. With an interval of 20 sec, there was extinction of the reflex whereas with 10 sec the response was intensified.

The importance of low frequency stimulation was similarly observed in experiments by other investigators (Kozak, Macfarlane, & Westerman, 1962). Nevertheless, in those cases, the frequency was always more than 1 per 10 sec. The necessity of such precise localization of stimulus to a small receptive zone, as in the experiments of Afelt, was not reported by others, and we did not notice the importance of such localization. It is difficult to explain the above discrepancy, but it is possible that the type of animal had an important role. Afelt worked with frogs but most other investigators used cats and dogs. Cutaneous receptors of cats and dogs differ significantly from those of frogs; tactile stimulation by the movement of hairs covering the skin appears to be one of the important type of cutaneous stimulation in mammals, but this is not so in the case of frogs.

The most sensitive cutaneous neurons are the large afferents and their receptors adapt rapidly to repeated stimulation. A group of such fibers already form a bundle in the periphery, and converge on a single interneuron (Woll, 1964). Therefore, cutaneous stimulation is not strictly localized and in mammals it may be directed either to a single cell or to a small number of interneuronal cells; this probably helps in the development of the process of extinction.

This fact was, to some extent, confirmed by the results of our experiments in untrained spinal dogs, where a thin layer of dichloramine was applied to the skin covering the gastrocnemius muscle to serve as inhibitory stimulus. As a rule, there was a violent motor reaction in the hind limbs after the first application. The second application, made after two to three days, produced a considerably diminished reaction and the third or fourth application usually failed to produce a response.

The less frequent stimuli may be more effective for extinction of the reaction because the residual phenomena in the afferent part of the reflex arc continue for about 100 msec after receiving a volley of afferent impulses, particularly during the state of increased excitability (Eccles, 1966). Residual phenomena in the efferent part of the reflex arc were observed during a period of 15-45 sec in the form of a reduced frequency of discharge from the phasic motoneurons, and a decrease in their amplitude when evoked by tetanic stimulation of the skin (Buchwald, Halas, & Schramn, 1965). It is quite possible that the effective factors for extinction of previously developed responses are the repeated stimuli which may be applied during the absence of increased efferent excitability, and the persistence of decreased excitability in the efferent segment of the reflex which is continued for a fairly long time.

What are the various parts of the spinal reflex arc which were responsible for inhibition resulting from weak and low frequency cutaneous stimulation? Cutaneous stimulation was essential for the appearance of inhibition where the excitation was transmitted to the interneurons. In our experiments, the monosynaptic reflexes were not inhibited. There are reports of the appearance of inhibition in response to stimulation of the cutaneous afferents. In the work of the Italian scientists (Giaguinto & Pompeiano, 1963; Pompeiano & Swett, 1962a, 1962b), it was reported that stimulation of the cutaneous afferents of group II with an electric current at low frequency (1-10 per sec) in unanesthetized cats produces a partial inhibition of the spontaneous as well as the reflex muscular activity. Here the inhibition was observed in both the mono- and polysynaptic spinal reflexes. This inhibition did not appear in response to stimulation of group I afferent muscular fibers, in even a single case. When muscular contraction alone produced a displacement of the skin, it did not prevent this type of response.

It is very likely that inhibition noticed in spinal animals develops in the afferent segment of the spinal reflex arc or, in other words, it is presynaptic. This type of inhibition was discovered fairly recently (Frank & Fourtes, 1957). When investigating the mechanism, it was shown that it is mediated by depolarization of the presynaptic afferent terminals (Eccles, Kostyuk, & Schmidt, 1962a). Presynaptic inhibition probably has a great role in carrying out spinal reflexes (Eccles, 1966), as indicated by its appearance in the response to strychnine (Eccles, Schmidt, & Willis, 1963). Results of various investigators confirm the belief that inhibition from a weak stimulus involves the afferent segment of the reflex arc and probably is presynaptic.

Kozak and Westerman (1964, 1966) reported that the scratch reflex was inhibited after administration of meprobamate. It is well known that meprobamate decreases the excitability of interneurons in the spinal cord. Consequently, according to the opinion of these authors, extinction of the reflex in this particular case was associated with decreased excitability of the interneurons where its effect was localized. Other investigators working with the problem of "adaptation" in the transected spinal cord have concluded that in this case the activity of interneurons in the polysynaptic reflexes is suppressed or, in other words, the inhibition is localized in the afferent segment of the reflex arc (Hernandez Peon & Brust-Carmena, 1961; Spenser, Thompson, & Neilson, 1964, 1966a, 1966b; Thompson & Spenser, 1966).

The monosynaptic reflex response in flexor motoneurons evoked by repeated stimulation of muscular nerves was unchanged. The participation of presynaptic inhibition during the "adaptation" process in the neurons of Prudovik *Limnaea stagnalis* was shown by the repeated application of low frequency orthodromic impulses with a small amplitude electric current (Sokolov, Arakelov, & Levinson, 1967).

Experimental Procedure

In order to clarify the cellular mechanism of inhibition evoked by weak cutaneous stimuli in a transected spinal cord, we performed experiments where inhibition was produced in the presence of strychnine (Nesmayanova, 1968). It is well known that strychnine blocks postsynaptic inhibition by reducing the excitability of the subsynaptic membranes (Curtis, 1959; Eccles, 1959). Accordingly, the ability to inhibit the reflexes during the application of weak stimuli in the presence of strychnine confirmed that this specific inhibition is not postsynaptic. In a spinal dog, a one percent solution of strychnine in a dose of 0.01 ml/kg was administered intramuscularly. The experiment was performed after the appearance of the strychnine effect when swaying movements in the hind legs and a tremor were noticed. The total muscle activity of the gastrocnemius of the left paw was recorded by indwelling electrodes: The biopotentials were led through a preamplifier (UBP 1–01) and were fed to an integrator which recorded the product of the potentials (amplitude and frequency of impulses) on a digital counter.

The mean arithmetic values from several measurments, each of which was recorded for 10 sec, were utilized for preparing the graphs. Inhibition of the swaying movements and the tremor caused by strychnine were produced by lightly scratching the skin of the ipsilateral thigh at a frequency of 1-3 per sec. Kozak and Westerman (1966), as well as our observations, showed that strong pressure over the sacrum produced a quick and complete stoppage of

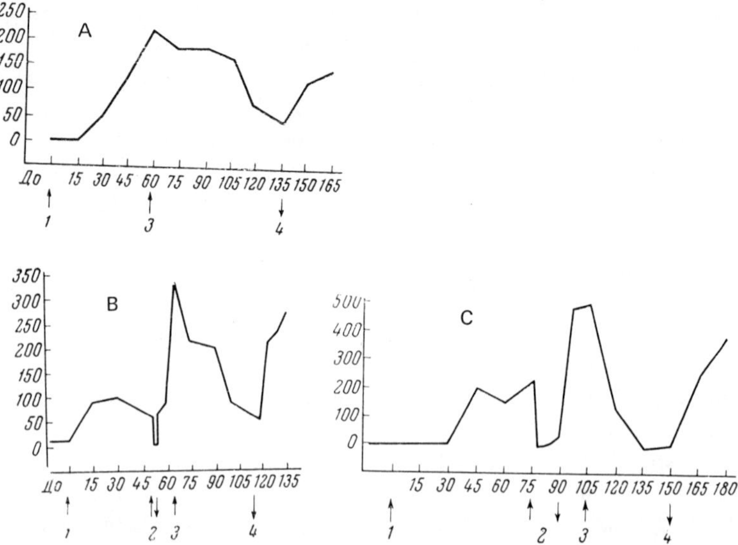

FIG. 11. Inhibition of activity in the calf muscle in spinal dogs.

A = in response to weak stimulation in the skin of the thigh; B, C = in response to strong pressure over the thigh followed by weak cutaneous stimulation.

Arrows: 1 = administration of strychnine; 2 = application of pressure over the thigh; 3 = scratching of the skin of the thigh; 4 = termination of the scratching.

On the abscissa–time (in min); on the ordinate–Electromyogram (average number of impulses in 10 sec); calibration: 20 mv–30 impulses in 10 sec.

spontaneous activity. This series of experiments was conducted with five dogs. The results of these experiments are presented in Fig. 11A.

It can be seen from Fig. 11 that the activity of the gastrocnemius muscle gradually increased with strychnine. The application of weak cutaneous stimulus in the form of scratching led to a decrease in the acitvity, which was reduced to nearly zero when it was continued for 75 min. When the stimulation was stopped, the activity again reached the original value.

In the first half of Figs. 11B and 11C, the results of the application of weak scratching were presented. This resulted in a gradual decrease of the response, but it actually never reached zero. When stimulation was stopped, the activity gradually returned to its original level. From these experiments, it may be concluded that inhibition from weak stimulation cannot be related to a postsynaptic site as it appears in the presence of strychnine.

It is not possible to make any final conclusion regarding the mechanism of this phenomena on the basis of the available data. It is suggested that homosynaptic depression has a definite role here, i.e., the depression in the activity of the interneuronal paths of a reflex arc (Spenser et al., 1966b). One of the mechanisms for depression is presynaptic inhibition. There may also be exhaustion of the mediator at a critical time during the development of "adaptation" (Sharpless, 1964).

The results of experiments in which inhibition was produced by strong pressure over the thigh are presented in the left half of Figs. 11B and 11C. It can be seen that there was a complete and immediate block of activity in the muscle with the application of pressure, and after withdrawal of pressure, the activity was restored very quickly and the height of the activity became much greater than it was originally. If pressure was applied for a longer time, say 10-15 min (Fig. 11C), inhibition was continued during this period but very weak activity might appear in the last minutes. Withdrawal of the pressure led to a quick restoration of the activity.

Appearance of a similar type of inhibition in spinal animals has often been reported. Sechenov (1864) noted the inhibition of motor activity in frogs by a strong tetanic current: The spinal frog was motionless during the stimulation but in the interval between periods of stimulation an increase in activity was observed. In the experiments of Kozak and Westerman (1966), epileptic seizures in spinal cats were stopped by the application of strong pressure over the sacrum. The inhibition was continued during the period of pressure and after withdrawal of pressure the seizure reappeared. This type of inhibition was also reported in intact animals, although in spinal animals it was more pronounced. Repeated stimulation of a peripheral nerve or a dorsal root, stretching of a muscle or striking a tendon at a frequency of one per second in animals under hexonal anesthesia, produced a sharp decrease in the amplitude of reflex response as recorded from a ventral root. The response was restored by changing to a less frequent stimulus. The authors concluded that a strong stimulation was less effective for inhibition than a weaker one (Bazanova, 1963, 1964; Bazanova, Ershova, Merkulova, & Chernigovskii, 1962).

It is possible that the above type of inhibition, noted by us and by other investigators, was related to the phenomenon of "dominance," first reported by Ukhtomskii, who reported that a strong center of excitation produced by the action of strychnine or by a prolonged stimulation inhibits the fixation of any new strong stimulus in the form of pressure over an extremity. "The inhibition appears in an area of prolonged stimulation, particularly due to its high sensitivity to rhythmic impulses with long waves" (Ukhtomskii, 1950, p. 273). The nature of this type of inhibition is unclear.

The inhibition which appeared in the presence of strychnine is considered the same type as that which appeared after the application of a weak stimulus and not postsynaptic. It may be that this inhibition is mainly due to cathodic depression, as reported by Kawai and Sasaki (1964), and resulted in accommodating the motoneurons to prolonged depolarization caused by a strong stimulus.

The adaptation in the above type of inhibition may probably be responsible for protection from overstimulation and appears to be important for self defense (Asratyan, 1955; Pavlov, 1951). This is confirmed by the results of our experiments, where atypical motor reactions were inhibited, as well as by the results of Kozak and Westerman (1966), who showed that weak stimulation of a single cutaneous receptive field in spinal cats initially produced an epileptic seizure which subsequently ceased.

CHAPTER II

THE IMPORTANCE OF ADDITIONAL AFFERENT STIMULATION FOR RECONDITIONING THE NEURAL CONNECTIONS OF THE TRANSECTED SPINAL CORD

The Signficiance of Decreased and Increased Activity for Synaptic Conduction

To insure normal activity and the reconstruction of reflex reactions, it is absolutely necessary to prevent the development of muscular atrophy from disuse. The importance of the latter for reconditioning reflex connections of the spinal cord was unclear for a long time, since an increase of spinal excitability can seriously change the true state of neural connections. Formerly, proper attention was not paid to the significance of decreased or increased activity of the nervous system. It was only during the last decade, after the introduction of new techniques in cyto- and histochemistry, that interest in this problem increased and a large number of papers were published in which the problem was tackled in many ways. The particularly convincing work was that where the picture of changes in the structure and function of nerve cells was studied in cases where inactivity was established on one side and increased functioning on the other. We will examine the data relating to the different parts of the nervous system in view of the fact that there is little literature which illustrates how significant these factors may be for a transected spinal cord.

In order to give a better presentation of the problems and methods to be reported, the literature on various physiological, morphological, cyto- and histochemical changes has been summarized separately. However, in the last few years, more effective results have been obtained when the problem was tackled using a multiple approach.

Physiological Investigations

In order to determine the significance of decreased activity on the condition of neural connections in the spinal cord, physiologists mainly studied the changes of synaptic function during local damage of a motor reflex arc.

Thus, Eccles and McIntyre (1953) studied the effect of disuse resulting from transection of individual dorsal roots just distal to the ganglion on the monosynaptic reflex, 30–40 days after operation. It was found that the reflexes evoked by dorsal root stimulation and recorded from the different motor nerves were either absent or significantly reduced. On the other hand, the polysynaptic reflexes had a tendency to increase in amplitude. It was also found that post-tetanic potentiation of the monosynaptic reflex increased considerably more than normal and continued for a prolonged period. Goldberger (1973) has reported collateral sprouting and functional recovery in cat spinal cord following deafferentation (also Murrey & Goldenberger, 1974).

In another experiment, Eccles, Krnjevic and Meldi (1959) transected the nerves of several synergistic muscles of an extremity. The changes in synaptic function were recorded from the motoneurons by intracellular electrodes at 6–25 days after the operation. The conditioning and the test stimuli were applied to the central end of the transected nerve. The results were more or less similar to the previous studies: The synaptic function of the motoneurons of the damaged reflex arc decreased by about 50 percent. However, the post-tetanic potentiation was increased and continued for 15 min, even after withdrawing stimulation. These characteristics were observed when investigating both the intact motoneurons as well as those showing chromatolysis. The authors suggested that although various factors present as a result of the operation could reflect on the character of synaptic function, the latter mainly depended on the activity of a particular reflex arc and the specific depression of the monosynaptic response which was observed. It was demonstrated in special experiments that the activity of deliberately chromatolyzed neurons did not differ significantly from that of normal ones (Eccles, Libet, & Young, 1958).

In order to get reliable data about the effect of dystrophy on neuronal activity and to produce prolonged inactivation of a monosynaptic spinal reflex arc, Beránek and Hnik (1960) tenotomized the Achilles tendon. After a lapse of 27–36 days, the nerve supplying the gastrocnemius was stimulated in an acute experiment and potentials were recorded from the ventral roots and from the dorsal surface of the spinal cord. As a result of tenotomy, the amplitude of the monosynaptic response increased by 338–370 percent more than the control side and the latent period was considerably shortened. There was no difference in the post-tetanic potentiation when compared with the control side, nor was there any change in the reflexes of the neighboring segments. The authors concluded that tenotomy leads to a plastic change in the central part of the monosynaptic arc of the tenotomized muscle. This may also explain Eccles and McIntyre's findings of chromatolyzed spinal ganglia, as a result of transection distal to the corresponding dorsal root.

Later Beránek and Hnik, along with their colleagues, studied the causes of increased amplitude of the monosynaptic response after tenotomy, and noticed that the latter does not produce significant changes in the peripheral part of the proprioceptive system of the muscle. Although the total number of afferent impulses during passive stretching is reduced, the spontaneous activity of the spindles during rest remains unaltered (Beránek & Hnik, 1959; Beránek, Hnik, Vyklicky, & Zelena, 1961; Hnik, Beránek, Vyklicky, & Zelena, 1963). Or, in other words, the afferent activity from the periphery was sufficient to maintain the neural apparatus in a normal condition. Therefore, the findings of Eccles and McIntyre should not be considered to be solely due to degeneration of the ganglia. Eccles (1961), when discussing this question, once again suggested that a decrease in synaptic function was mainly produced by inactivation and was not due to degenerative changes of the ganglion. The capacity of the dorsal root to regenerate has been described by Ikeda and Campbell (1971).

In order to compare the functional properties of the spinal reflex apparatus and its lack of influence on synaptic conduction in a monosynaptic reflex arc in cats, unilateral tenotomy was applied to the Achilles tendon, m. flexor digitorum and m. flexor hallucis longus. As a result of this, these muscles did not participate in the motor activity of the animal. In some of the cats, the spinal cord was transected at the level of T_{10}, simultaneously with the tenotomy. After 1–5 weeks, the condition of the reflex arcs from the tenotomized and the control muscles were compared. For this purpose, the monosynaptic response, evoked by stimulation of the motor nerves, was recorded from the ventral roots of L_6, L_7, and S_1 and from the spino-cerebellar tracts. The results showed that stimulating the nerve of a teno-tomized muscle increased the monosynaptic reflex 50 percent or more as compared to an intact muscle and, in addition, the latent period of the response was somewhat shortened (Kozak & Westerman, 1966).

The above results were not unexpected as similar results were obtained by

Hnik in his experiments with tenotomized muscles. As already mentioned, the nature of the increase in the monosynaptic reflex after tenotomy is still unclear. If the tendon was transected in a chronic spinal animal, the increase in the monosynaptic responses (evoked in response to stimulation of the motor nerves) did not take place (Kozak & Westerman, 1966). This shows that in the first case, an increase of supraspinal activation of γ-mononeurons associated with increase of discharges in the I*a* fibers could be involved.

When a cat's hind leg was experimentally immobilized, it was found after several weeks of inactivation that the process of muscular atrophy, and amplitude of the contraction recorded either from individual motor units or the total contraction, was decreased due to changes in the central part of the reflex arc (Fudema, Fizzell, & Nelson, 1961). These results confirm Eccles' conclusion that decreased synaptic function is due to muscle inactivation.

Clearer results were obtained by studying synaptic function during an animal's increased motor activity. For this purpose, unilateral denervation was made in all synergistic muscles, i.e., the extensor muscles of an extremity were all denervated excepting one, and the operated animals were subjected to exercise on a treadmill. It was found that the monosynaptic reflex was increased in the muscle with an intact nerve supply (Eccles & Westerman, 1959). In similar types of experiments, spike potentials were recorded from the ventral roots by evoking activity in muscle nerves of group I*a* five weeks after denervation. There was an increase of the monosynaptic response obtained by stimulating the nerve with the intact muscle and even transection of the spinal cord failed to prevent this increase. The authors suggested that the intensity of the monosynaptic reflex in these experiments may depend more on the number of motoneurons which actively participated than on the change of their activity as a result of denervation (Eccles, Kozak, & Westerman, 1962).

As seen from the above studies, the changes due to decreased activity are unclear. Probably, the various surgical interventions produced some abnormalities, whose causes often remained unexplained. At least it is clear that increased motor activity leads to an intensification of synaptic function (Schneider & Johnson, 1972). The attempts to reduce such motor activity by means of tenotomy or deafferentation produced a considerable change in the reflex activity which was not only related to decreased activity. A sequence of new relations appeared in the neuronal connections of the spinal cord, which was responsible for the appearance of new properties. Thus, it was found that the flow of afferent impulses from tenotomized or deafferented muscles might play an important role in producing plastic changes in the central nervous system (Eldred, Granit, & Merton, 1953; Kazakova & Nesmeyanova, 1972).

Morphologic Investigations

Szentágothai and Rajkovits (1955) found that unilateral transection of a dorsal root in puppies led to a reduction of the area of synaptic contacts with the cells in the dorsal horn of the spinal cord, two to four months after the operation. Removal of the long bones of the extremities, while keeping the nerves intact, caused a decrease in the number of nerve fibers and a reduction in their diameter. Plechkova (1961) reported the structural changes of synapses in both the lumbar and thoracic regions of the spinal cord, after putting a tightly fitting ring around the sciatic nerve of a dog.

Even complete isolation of segments of the spinal cord after a double transection and deafferentation may not produce any morphological changes in the neural apparatus (Anderson, 1959; Tower, 1937). However, other observers reported the presence of significant morphological (Barron, 1933) and histological (Young, 1966) changes.

The majority of investigators noted that in lesions of the central nervous system, gross changes are observed in the neural apparatus of the spinal cord in those segments where the interneurons are most affected and the motoneurons are least affected. Thus, in rats, after spinal transection, the greatest changes were noticed in the small and medium sized cells while the big motoneurons were less affected (Yakovleva, 1951). These irreversible changes of the interneurons following transection resulted in lysis or stable atrophy in the neurons (Howe & Bodian, 1941). The change in structure of the neurons appears not only in an area close to the transection of the spinal cord but also in a part distal to it. According to Liu (1953), either a generalized or a centralized chromatolysis was observed in cats soon after transection, once the posterior spinocerebellar tract had been destroyed in the part adjacent to the neurons of Clark's nucleus. Temporary asphyxia of the spinal cord produced by tying the aorta (Gelfan & Tarlov, 1959) or by increasing pressure in the subdural space (Van Harreveld & Shadé, 1962) resulted in gross structural change of the spinal cord. There has been unanimous agreement that motoneurons are more stable than interneurons, particularly during a deficiency in the flow of oxygen.

The effect of the magnitude and duration of activity on the structural changes in a neuron was reported in several investigations. Thus, additional moderate motor activity could lead to a significant increase in the volume of nucleoli—up to 241 percent. When the activity was briefly increased, it may increase the diameter of the cell, but it was not associated with any change in the size of either the nuclei or the nucleolus (Edström 1957). However, if the imposed activity was unusually high, as in a convulsion, the diameter of the nuclei of the motoneurons was decreased as compared with that of neurons supplying resting muscles (Chance, Lucal, & Waterhouse, 1956). Studies in rats have shown that compensatory hyperfunction of one extremity, after amputation of the other, was accompanied by an increase in the size of the nuclei and some of motoneurons, on both sides of a spinal cord, at a later stage (Shchitkov, 1959).

Prolonged stimulation of the vestibular apparatus by rotating the animals was followed by hypertrophy of the interstitial and motor nerve cells in the trigeminal nucleus of the brain stem receiving impulses from the receptors subjected to stimulation (Kosmarskaya, 1962).

Thus, the histological data may indicate the influence of the pattern and magnitude of activity on the metabolic processes in the central nervous system.

Histo- and Cytochemical Studies

It was reported by Hydén (1943) that animals running until exhausted showed a significant lowering in the concentration of RNA and protein in the motoneurons of the spinal cord. Later it was found that supersonic sound stimuli alone decreased the trigroid substance in the Deiters' nucleus cells (Hydén, 1947). Depletion of Nissl substance in the cells of the hypoglossal nucleus after prolonged electrical stimulation of the hypoglossal nerve or after an uninterrupted movement was reported by Barr and Bertram (1951) and by Snesarev (1950). It was shown by Pevzner (1959, 1963) that ischemic hypoxia, lasting for an hour in rats, decreased the cytoplasmic RNA in cells of the optic and motor areas of the cortex to less than half, while the amount of DNA was practically unchanged.

Comparable results were obtained by electrical stimulation with moderate intensity, particularly during prolonged application. According to the findings of Edström (1957), there was an increase in the size of the nucleolus after prolonged activity, which indicates a stimulation of protein synthesis inside the neuron. Moderate stimulation of the vestibular apparatus produced by rotary movement was associated with an increase of 40 percent in the concentration of RNA in cells of the vestibular ganglion. A similar type of stimulation quantitatively increased the nucleotides in the cells of the Deiters' nucleus (Hydén, 1960; Hydén & Hamburger, 1949; Hydén & Pigon, 1960). The authors conclude that the rate of synthesis of cellular RNA and proteins is dependent on the degree of activity. In their opinion, the neuron could be compared to a secretory cell which works continuously and can change the pattern of protein synthesis very quickly. Based on experiments in which it was found that the change in RNA content was dependent on the intensity and duration of light stimuli, Brodskii and Nechaeva (1958) concluded that RNA was essential for the activity of the cells.

Besides cytoplasmic RNA, nuclear RNA was investigated and it was found that nuclear RNA responds to a change of activity more quickly and to a greater extent than cytoplasmic RNA (Brodskii, 1960, 1961). The link between the metabolism and the degree of activity was further developed in the work of Levinson (1961) and later of Jarstedt (1966) and others. The literature on this problem prior to 1965 has been reviewed by Zhobotinskii (1965).

In the last few years, significant achievements were made by a group of scientists using complex methods to study the effects of activity on the characteristics of neural tissue in different parts of the brain. An increase in the diameter of neurons, their nuclei and nucleoli was observed, in the preserved structures of the cerebral cortex (V layer of pyramid of the ipsilateral hemisphere) as a result of a lateral hemisection of the spinal cord in the cervical region, making it possible for them to take over additional functions. At the same time, the morphology of the neurons was altered and their sizes decreased on the side affected by the hemisection (V layer of the pyramid of the contralateral hemisphere) (Kazakova, 1966, 1968).

After transection at the level of T_{11}, the evoked potentials in the sensorimotor area of the cortex were characterized by an increased amplitude of the short latency components of the response to electrocutaneous stimulation of the front paw. This was observed in the initial stages of recovery and was particularly pronounced in the ipsilateral hemisphere (Nezlina & Kazokova, 1968). Similarly, changes in the diameter of the neuronal cell bodies and their nuclei were observed, depending on the activity of the cortical structures responsible for visual discrimination (Brazovskaya, 1967).

Intense metabolism of the neurons which were involved was observed during increased activity, and this was confirmed by a change in the tigroid substance and the RNA. The number of perineuronal glial cells—the cells responsible for carrying out trophic functions in the corresponding neurons—was also significantly increased (Aleksandrovskaya, Geinisman, & Mats, 1965; Kazakova, 1967; Kulenkampff, 1952; Mats, 1969). Based on these facts, it is apparent that inactivity causes a slowing of the metabolic processes in the pathways of the spinal cord, and that increased activity stimulates these processes.

It was essential to investigate the effect of inactivity or of additional afferent stimuli on the condition of neural pathways in the spinal cord, in order to explain the possibility of reorganizing the motor functions of a spinal animal and also in order to study the necessary conditions for regeneration of central neurons.

Functional Changes of the Neural Pathways in a Transected Spinal Cord Resulting from Its Activity

Method of Excitation in the Distal Part of a Transected Spinal Cord

We conducted this investigation on the consequences of dysfunction and systematic activation of the paralyzed part of the body of a spinal animal, from both the physiological and morphologic aspects (Brazovskaya, Nesmeyanova, & Arnautova, 1966; Nesmeyanova, 1956, 1959). The animals' treatment involved the application of electrocutaneous stimuli to the paw of both extremities. This resulted in flexion with subsequent relaxation, which was followed by vigorous massage and passive exercise of the hind legs. The choice of this procedure was based on the following facts: When a short, systematic, electrical stimulation is applied to a muscle after transection of its nerve, this results in the contraction of all the muscle fibers and completely eliminates the loss in weight of the muscle (Ginetsinskii, 1956). This even produces an actual hypertrophy of the muscle in which the dry weight of the denervated muscle is increased. However, a significant difference in its histological structures was observed. In the stimulated muscle, its fibers could be seen crossing each other, while in the control muscles the majority of the fibers remained parallel running only in the longitudinal direction. Furthermore, electrical stimulation of the n. ischiadicus in rats led to a metabolic change in the surrounding Schwann cells, especially where the oxidative processes were not increased (Heller & Hesse, 1961a, 1961b).

Similarly, electrostimulation has a marked effect on conditioning neural pathways in intact animals (Hydén, 1943, 1947). Hoffman (1952) observed stimulation in nerve growth by electrical stimulation of the spinal roots. The author has suggested that under the influence of electrical stimulation there is an increase in the synthesis of protoplasmic granules inside the cell body. Based on these findings, we suggested that a moderately intense stimulus with low frequency impulses which consistently evoked a reflex response would help to keep all the segments of the reflex arc in a relatively normal condition. The main object of passive exercise and massage of the hind legs was to improve the blood supply to all the paralyzed parts of the body and also to maintain the muscles and the joints in a normal condition.

The purpose of this series of experiments was to compare the character of the reflex activity evoked from the distal part of the transected spinal cord in groups of dogs, when such treatment* was either applied or omitted. These observations compared the evoked mono- and polysynaptic reflexes as well as the ability of the cord to organize atypical reflex reactions and determine their stability. The morphologic investigation included dimensional measurement of the different groups of interneurons, and motoneurons and observation of the synapses on them, in dogs of both groups, at different intervals after the operation. The work was conducted on 12 adult spinal dogs where the spinal cords were transected at the level of T_{10}-T_{11}. Half of the dogs were subjected to systematic treatment and the others were not.

*The author uses the word "treatment" to include the exercise of tissues by either electrical stimulation or massage.

The treatment consisted of passive exercise of the hind legs and massage as well as electrocutaneous stimulation of the paw, which evoked a motor reflex. Such treatment was administered 5-6 times a week, initially for 20 min. After a week, the period of treatment was increased to 30 min. At a later stage, 1-2 years after the operation, a rest period of up to 25 days was occasionally given. Initially, the paw of each hind leg was subjected to stimulation with impulses 2-3 msec duration at a frequency of 30-60 min. The massage was started with the proximal joints of the extremity. Movement of the operator's hand was directed from the periphery toward the center and this improved the circulation in the massaged extremity. The passive exercise consisted of flexion and extension of all the joints of the hind legs. It started with the proximal joints and then gradually moved to the distal ones. This was repeated in each of the joints, each time starting with the most distal, and was ended by exercising the hip joints. Besides this, the dog was made to run passively with its hind legs and to make circular movements. Both of the legs were moved sideways and backwards at the same time.

The different parts of the treatment were applied in the following order: First the massage evoked a very mild motor reaction but significantly increased the circulation of the extremities; then the passive exercise; and finally the electrocutaneous stimulations which systematically evoked motor reflexes of the extremities. In the first week of treatment, the massage was applied with mild rubbing. During the passive exercise, each procedure was repeated six times. The electrocutaneous stimulation was applied for 5 min to each paw, i.e., a careful program of procedures was adopted. Later, the massage, along with the initial mild rubbing, included the kneading (petrissage) of muscles with regular relaxation at the end of the massage by the rubbing (effleurage) of each part. Each exercise was repeated 12 times and electrical stimulation of each extremity was continued for up to 10 min. This evoked a moderately good reflex activity.

The dogs were divided into three groups: (1) those not subjected to treatment during the period under observation (physiological experiments on 4 dogs, histological investigations on 16); (2) those subjected to treatment starting with the third postoperative month (physiological experiments on 4 dogs); (3) those subjected to treatment starting with the fourth to seventh day after operation (physiological experiments on 6 dogs, histological investigations on 16 dogs).

The objective observations involved the motor reflexes of spinal animals: (a) polysynaptic reflexes like the flexor, the scratch and the stepping reflex, the extensor thrust, the crossed extensor reflex and the atypical motor reactions, and (b) monosynaptic reflexes like the ankle and patellar reflexes. Besides studying the condition of reflex activity, observations were made on weight-bearing and locomotor functions as well as the condition of the skin, muscles, and joints. The reflex flexion of the extremity was tested by applying a single electrocutaneous stimulus to the paw, with a duration of 1 msec (flexor reflex). The extensor thrust was evoked by pressing the foot-pads. The knee jerk was elicited by striking the quadriceps m. tendon with a rubber tipped mechanical hammer and the ankle jerk by striking the Achilles tendon. The scratch and swaying reflexes were evoked by scratching the respective cutaneous receptive fields.

Initially, the reflex activity was recorded graphically with the help of a pneumatic level. This was also done using the electromyographic method. The muscle potentials were obtained from bipolar electrodes separated by 2 mm. After amplifying the potentials on UBPI-OI, they were recorded on the oscilloscope N_{102}. In several reflexes the activity of two muscles was recorded simultaneously: (a) in the flexor reflex - m. biceps femoris of the ipsilateral and different extensor muscles of the contralateral extremity; (b) in the knee reflex - m. rectus femoris and m. vastus lateralis of the ipsilateral extremity; (c) in the scratch and swaying reflexes - m. biceps femoris and tibialis anterior of the ipsilateral extremity or from the same muscle of both extremities; (d) the crossed-extensor reflex was recorded in m. gastrocnemius of the left and in m. biceps femoris of the right extremity, when producing flexion in the latter and the ankle reflex in m. gastrocnemius. These observations were made over a prolonged period—up to three and a half years after the operation.

The Ability or Failure to Develop New Reflex Reactions During Treatment

Characteristic of reflex activity in the initial period after spinal cord transection was a condition of relative a-reflexia when it was possible to evoke only the knee, ankle, and flexor reflexes. This condition was typical of spinal shock which appeared as a result of separation of the spinal cord from higher segments of the central nervous system (Sherrington, 1906; Ashby, Verrier, & Lightfoot, 1974). In our experiments, the duration of shock depended on the method of transecting the spinal cord, the application of treatment, and the individual character of the animal. The crossed extensor reflex, the extensor thrust, the scratch, and the swaying reflexes reappeared 2 weeks after operation, and full activation of the reflexes 1½-2 months after operation. This was true in all dogs, whether they received treatment or not. The differences in their reflex responses were apparent only 4-6 months after operation. In the dogs in the third group (which were treated 4-7 days after operation), all the innate reflexes were very pronounced and the atypical reactions appeared easily. The condition of the reflex activity was also very similar to that in dogs of the second group, whose treatment started two months after the operation. At the same time, the dogs in the first group, to whom no treatment was given, showed a significant decrease of reflex activity.

Many polysynaptic reflexes like swaying, scratch, and the crossed extensor reflexes were unstable while the atypical reactions were absent. The attempts to develop the latter were unsuccessful, however, despite the application of 8,000 new stimuli, and this was completely discontinued. Some of the inborn reflexes were easily activated during such treatment. Participating in a four month course of massage and passive exercise and electrical stimulation, the dogs of the first group (control) showed a significant improvement in the condition of the muscles and joints of the hind legs but the activation of the atypical as well as the inborn reflexes was minimal.

These findings demonstrated that electrocutaneous stimuli, which evoke motor reflexes are particularly important for conditioning the central part of the reflex arc. This is confirmed by the results obtained when comparing the atypical reactions in the dogs of the second and third groups. In contrast to the results which were obtained with the animals of the first group, the development of the atypical reactions which characterize the ability for functional reorganization was successful in the latter two groups. Stimulation of the tail skin and the paw led to the appearance of a paw response after a single stimulation to the tail in the first trial after 100-200 conditioning stimuli in the animals of the third group, while the animals of the second group responded in the second trial after 500-600 stimulations. After several experiments, this reaction became stable and was quite well developed.

Electrocutaneous stimulation during development of the reflex was given to dogs of the third group after two weeks and to the dogs of the second group two months after the operation when dystrophic processes had already developed in the neural pathway. However, the results of conditioning were positive. Probably, the development of the dystrophic processes was suppressed by the application of electrocutaneous stimulation. It seems likely that these play a particularly important role in preventing the development of dystrophy due to inactivity.

Verification of the above hypothesis was obtained in experiments where the stability of the evoked reactions was shown during the application of repeated stimuli by movement of the paw in response to stimulation of the tail. The latter were applied to the tip of the tail at a frequency of 1 per sec, with an intensity of 1.5 × threshold in groups of five with an interval of 1 min between the groups.

It was found that the atypical reaction of the paw had been abolished with the application of the second group of stimuli in dogs of the first group. The tail response was weakened with the application of the third group and an interval of 10 min between groups stopped both responses (Fig. 12A).

Repeated stimulation of the tail alone partially abolished the atypical reaction in the dogs of the second group and weakened the response of the tail (the organ receiving the stimulation). However, to obtain this result it was

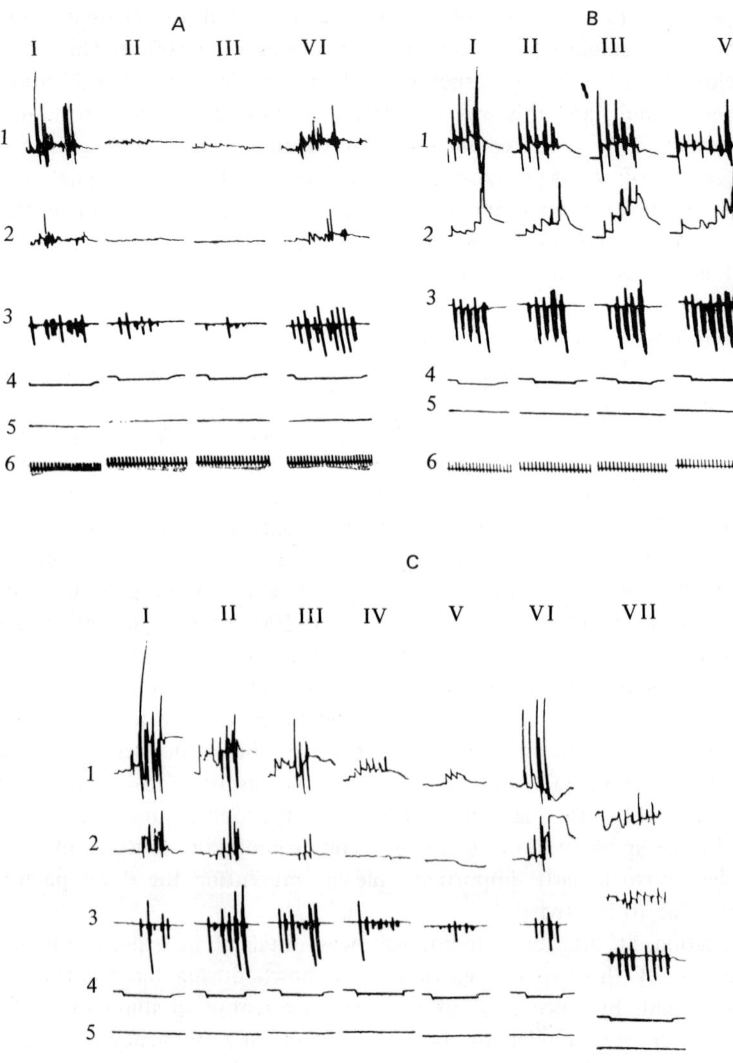

FIG. 12. Stability of the atypical reactions in dogs of different groups.

A–dogs of the first group; B–dogs of the second group; C–dogs of the third group.

Columns: I-V–response reaction to rhythmic stimulation of the tail skin; VI and VII–response reaction to stimulation of another part of skin; 1–movements of the right paw; 2–left paw; 3–tail; 4 and 5–lines showing the marks of scratching; 6–time (in sec).

necessary to repeat the application of a group of stimuli 5–6 times. After 10 min, the response of the tail and paw again reappeared. The lack of muscular exhaustion during the absence of the response was confirmed in this particular case by the appearance of a good reflex response of the tail when stimuli were applied to another tail area (Fig. 12B).

The application of repeated groups of stimuli without other treatment to the dogs of the third group neither weakened the atypical reflex reaction nor caused its disappearance (Fig. 12C). As with the tail movement, the atypical reaction of the hind paws in response to stimulation of the skin of the tail was also well developed and stable. Conduction of the reflex along the newly formed reflex arc was consistently observed with the participation of not less than two internuncial neurons.

The Development of the Mono- and Polysynaptic Motor Reflexes During the Presence or Absence of Treatment Two to Four Years After the Operation

It was interesting to follow the effect of transection of the spinal cord on the motor reflexes in dogs after a prolonged period following operation. Was there loss of the inborn motor reflexes as a result of the development of dystrophy and was it possible to inhibit the development of dystrophic processes for a long period by application of systematic treatment? The following observations were made on eight spinal dogs (lesion T_{10}–T_{11}), after postoperative period of 2–4 years. In four dogs, the treatment was started on the seventh day after operation while the other four dogs did not receive any treatment. The weight-bearing and locomotor functions of the muscles and their joints were as follows: Two of the treated animals possessed (1) normal tone in the extensor muscles of the hind legs, (2) the muscles were comparatively well developed, (3) the joints were normal, and (4) they were able to stand and take two or three steps without falling (Fig. 13A). In the two other treated dogs, the flexor tone predominated in the muscles of the hind legs which were unable to support the weight. During forward movement they could take only two to three steps with the help of their partially flexed hind legs. The muscles were found by gross examination to be in a good condition and the joints were normal (Fig. 13B).

Two of the untreated dogs had decreased extensor tone and were unable to stand or rise. When moving, they dragged their hind legs passively. Atrophic changes in the muscles were very pronounced and the joints were very much deformed (Fig. 13C). The two other untreated dogs had increased extensor tone and often remained standing, supported by the hind legs. The muscles of the hind legs were found to be in a relatively good condition but the joints were slightly deformed (Fig. 13D).

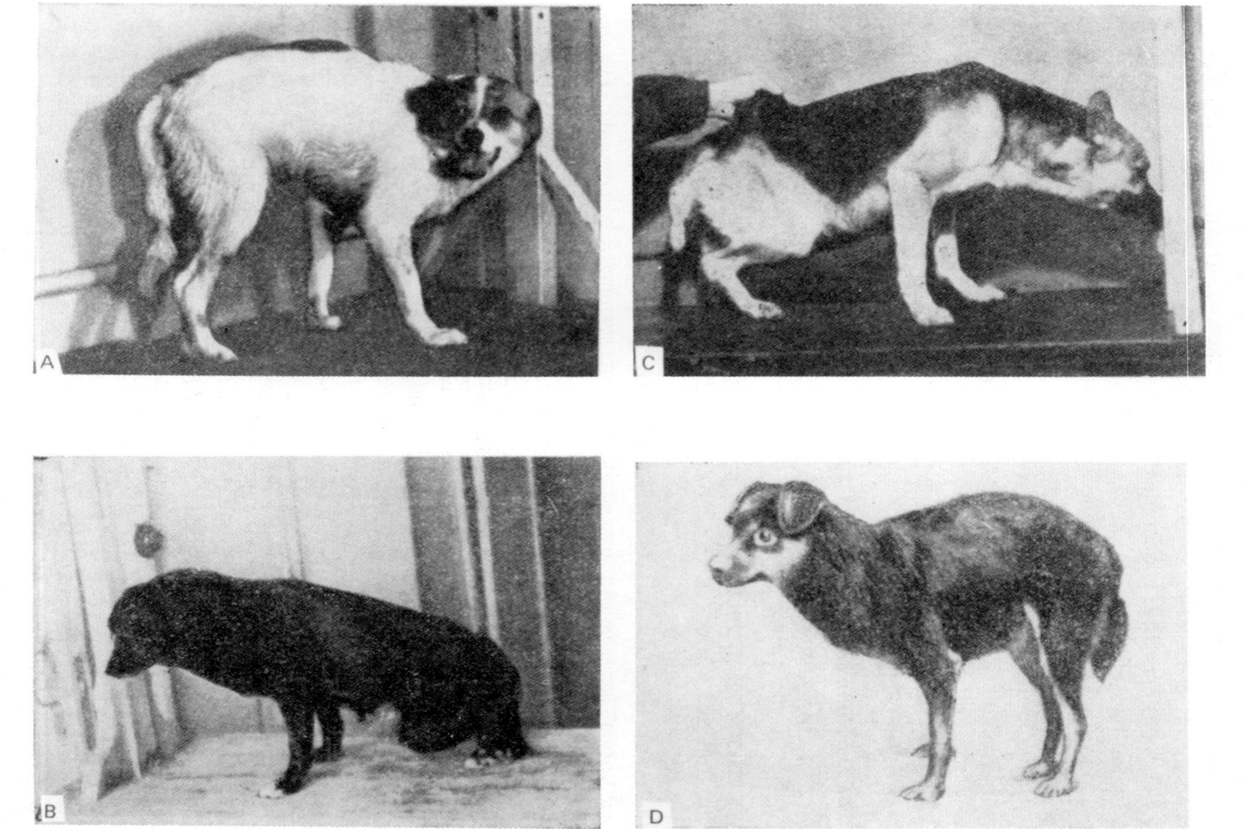

FIG. 13. Spinal treated (A, B) and untreated (C, D) dogs.

A–tone of the extensor muscles was prominent; B–tone of the extensor muscle was absent; C–tone of the extensor muscle was absent; D–tone of the extensor muscle was prominent.

Based on the hypothesis that the absence of treatment affects the interneurons and motoneurons in various ways, an investigation was made to study the condition of mono- and polysynaptic motor reflexes in the dogs of different groups. The patellar reflex was selected from the monosynaptic reflexes since it is easily obtained in animals. Of the polysynaptic reflexes, the flexor, the crossed extensor and the scratch reflexes were selected. As demonstrated from the above experiments, all the reflexes investigated were well developed and stable in the treated dogs (Figs. 14A, 15A, 16A, 17A). In the untreated animals, the scratch reflex was absent as a rule, and the flexor reflex was irregular (Fig. 15B, 16B). This can probably be explained by the unusual increase in the threshold of stimulation since 53 volts (the maximum voltage available with the stimulator) was insufficient to excite, even when the duration of the stimulus was increased up to 20 msec or the frequency was raised to 20 per sec. In the treated dogs, the flexor reflex was usually obtained in response to a stimulating impulse lasting 2-3 msec with an intensity of 30-40 volts at a frequency of 2-3 per sec.

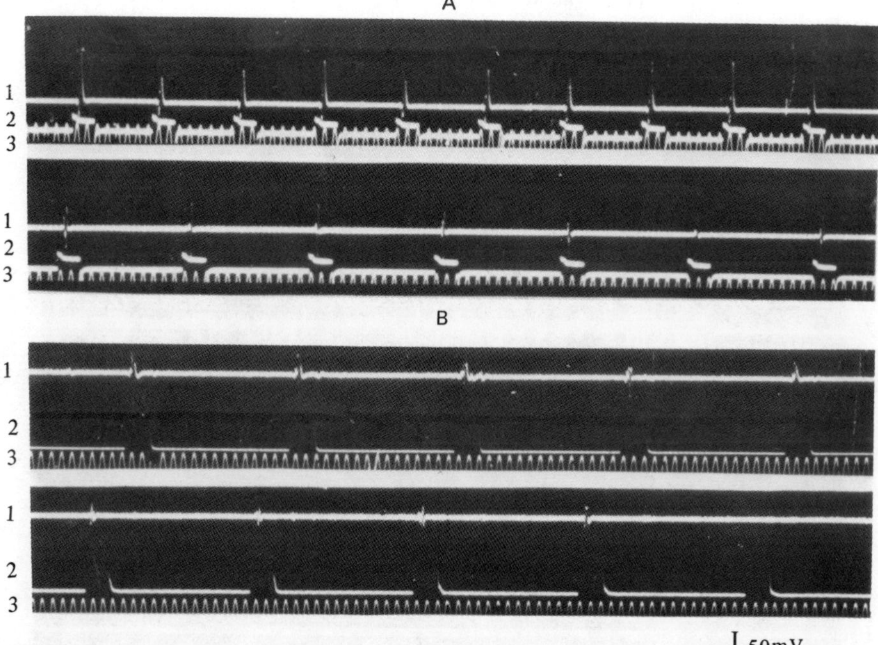

FIG. 14. Knee reflex in treated (A) and in untreated (B) dogs.

Beam of light from the top to bottom: 1–activity in the m. rectus femoris; 2–stimulation mark; 3–time, 20 msec.

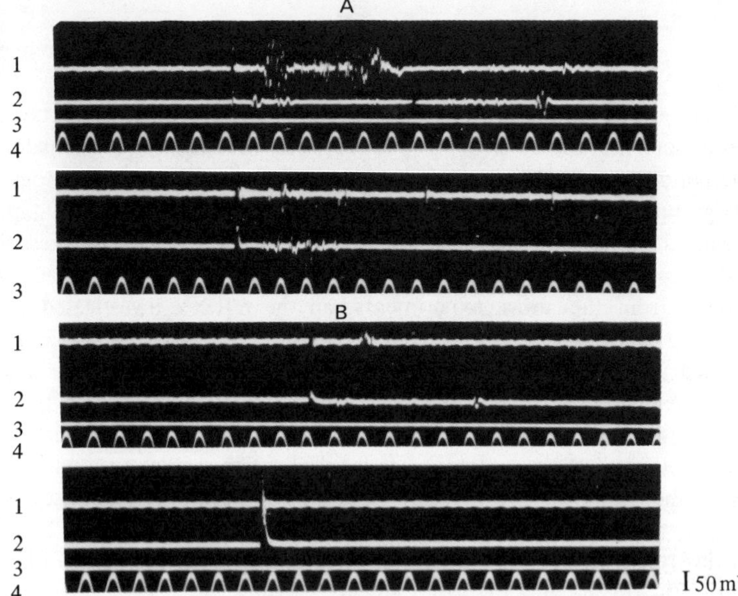

FIG. 15. Flexor reflex in treated (A) and untreated (B) dogs.

1–activity in m. bic. fem.; 2–m. tib. anterior of the ipsilateral extremity; 4–time, 20 msec.

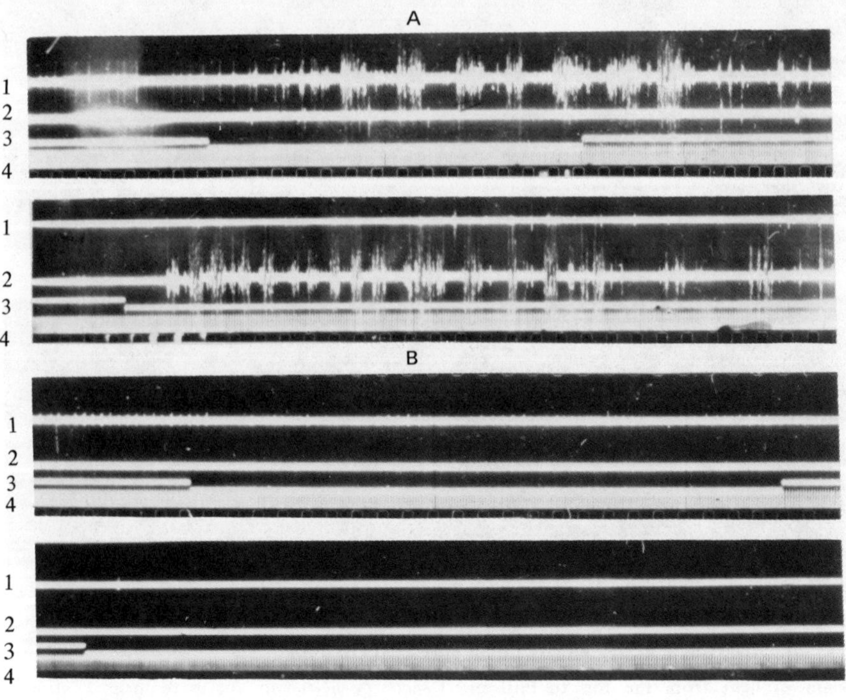

FIG. 16. Scratch reflex in treated (A) and untreated (B) dogs.

1–activity in m. bic. fem.; 2–m. tib. and ipsilateral extremity; 3–mark of stimulation.

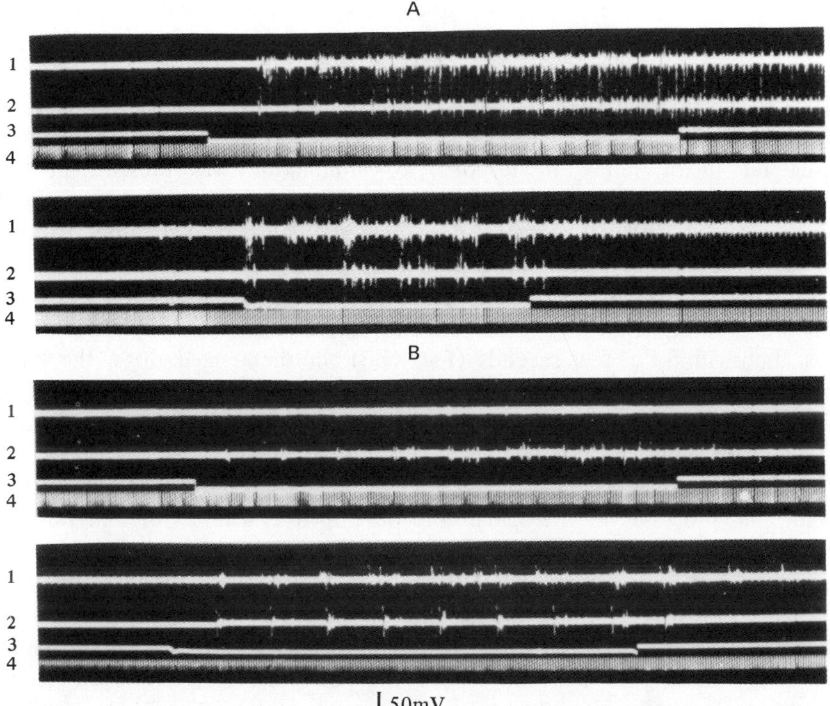

FIG. 17. Reciprocal extensor reflex in treated (A) and untreated (B) dogs.

1–activity in m. gastrocnemius of the contralateral extremity; 2–activity in m. bic. femoris of the ipsilateral extremity; 3–mark of stimulation; 4–time, 20 msec.

The crossed extensor reflex evoked by electrical stimulation of the contralateral paw was well developed in treated dogs and action potentials were recorded in the m. gastrocnemius. Likewise, the activity of the m. biceps femoris of the ipsilateral extremity was of importance (Fig. 17A). In untreated animals, examination of this reflex was made during the period when the flexor reflex was relatively well developed, about 1-1½ years after the operation. The results showed that in the two untreated animals which were unable to stand, contractile activity was not recorded in the m. gastrocnemius of the contralateral extremity. Twitching of the muscles was not observed, but flexion of the ipsilateral extremity and action potentials in its flexor were present (Fig. 17B). Disordered movements were observed in the left extremity in response to the flexion of the right extremity in the two other untreated dogs who were able to stand. The recordings showed that action potentials appeared in the m. gastrocnemius. However, they were irregular and the bursts of activity did not always correspond to a stimulus. Action potentials were recorded from the flexor of the ipsilateral extremity (Fig. 17B, bottom). Likewise, in the untreated dogs this crossed extensor reflex in which more than two interneurons participated was well developed. However, in the untreated dogs it was either absent or changed, though the ipsilateral flexor reflex in response to stimulation was present. In the untreated dogs, only the knee reflex remained constant and was fully developed (Fig. 14B). It was well developed and constant in the dogs of both groups in conditions where the stimuli were given with a frequency no higher than 3 per sec. When the frequency was increased, the muscles did not have time to recover, the tone of the extensor muscles increased, and the reflex was abolished for a few seconds (Fig. 18B). In the treated dogs, the knee reflex was evoked, even at a frequency of 50 impulses per sec. This was true, though, only after a special modification in the experiments where systematic stimuli were applied at this frequency (Fig. 18A).

These experiments confirmed our previous observations that when the dystrophic processes in the spinal cord developed as a result of inactivation, the polysynaptic reflexes were the first affected. They became unstable and disappeared in several cases, while the monosynaptic stretch reflexes remained unchanged. Kozak and Westerman (1966), investigating the after-effects of transection of the spinal cord in cats, demonstrated that treatment improved the weight-bearing to such an extent that the hind legs developed stable weight-bearing and were able to follow the front legs. They believed that during inactivity the cognitive and defensive reflexes suffer, but during the application of electrocutaneous stimulation they are reinforced–particularly those which are not subjected to dystrophic changes and which are abolished during repeated stimulation.

Judging from our results, the main difference in the degree of damage to the reflexes during inactivity depends on the degree of participation of the interneurons. The polysynaptic reflexes suffer, but a difference in stability is noticed in some of the individual reflexes. Such reflexes as the scratch reflex and atypical reactions suffer to a greater extent in comparison to the reflexes connected with weight-bearing and locomotion, extensor thrust, or the flexor reflex which, nevertheless, are seen even in untreated dogs. It is possible that the polysynaptic reflexes connected with weight-bearing and locomotion undergo self-treatment in a number of animals, hence their disturbance is less pronounced.

In our experiments, the monosynaptic reflexes–the ankle and the knee–remained unaltered in all conditions. However, inhibition of a reflex due to inactivity depends on the development of dystrophic processes, and should not be confused with the "adaptation" which appeared during application of weak stimuli of a different type.

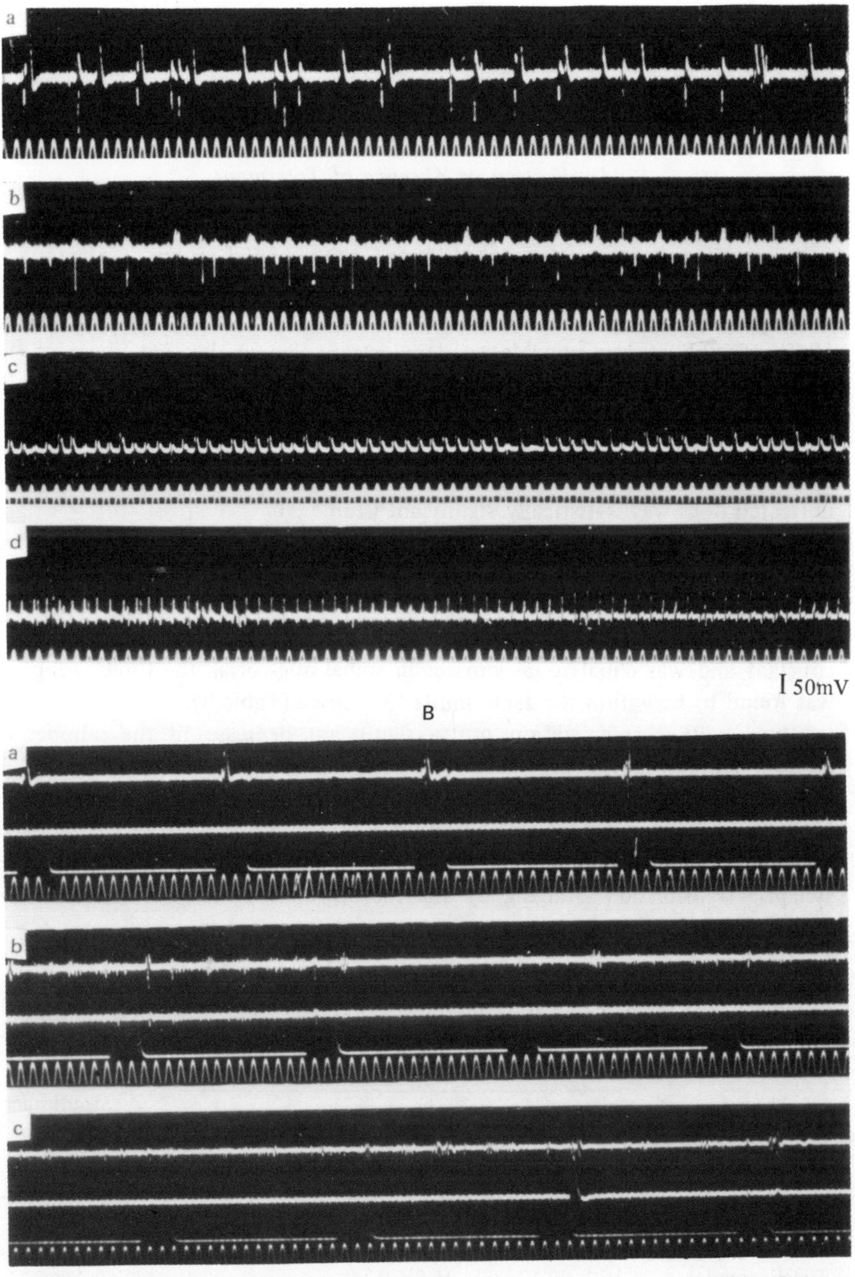

FIG. 18. Knee reflex (activity in m. rectus fem).

A—application of stimulii at the frequency of 50/sec in treated dogs: a—first experiment (20,000); b—second experiment (50,000); c—fourth experiment (100,000); d—sixth experiment (200,000). The figures in parentheses represent the number of stimulii after which the records were made. B—application of stimulii at a frequency of 3/sec in untreated dogs: a—beginning of stimulations; b—after 10 min (800 stimulations); c—after 13 min (2,500 stimulations). Time—20 msec.

The Latent Period and the Stimulation Threshold of Different Motor Reflexes in Dogs During the Application or Absence of Treatment

In order to completely characterize the reflex arcs of the mono- and polysynaptic reflexes in dogs of different experimental groups, we measured the latent period and stimulation threshold of the flexor and patella reflexes. These were compared with the results obtained in intact dogs (Nesmeyanova, 1967, 1968b). It was possible to demonstrate that in the first phase of the flexor reflex (muscular twitching in response to threshold stimulation), the latent period was unchanged both in intact and spinal treated dogs. When the reflex was present in the untreated dogs, its latency was considerably longer. This difference in the latent period of the flexor reflex in treated and untreated dogs was statistically significant (Table 2).

Very different results were obtained when the latent period of patellar reflex was measured by striking the tendon of m. quadriceps with a mechanical hammer and recording from two of its heads–m. rectus femoris and m. vastus lateralis. In intact dogs, the latent period of this reflex was constant and was equal to 5-7 msec. In spinal dogs of all the three groups, it was found to be within the same limits–5-7 msec (Table 3).

Thus, neither spinalization nor a significant decrease in the number of afferent stimuli to the central nervous system changed the latent period of this reflex which was produced by an arc with two neurons. The delay in propagation of impulses along the polysynaptic reflex arc of a flexor reflex in untreated spinal dogs definitely shows that there were severe disturbances in synaptic transmission. Judging by the fact that there was no change in the

TABLE 2. The Latent Period of the Flexor Reflex in Intact and in Spinal Dogs (in msec)

Muscles	Mean ± S.E. ($X + m$) Intact dogs	Spinal dogs Treated	Spinal dogs Untreated	Significance P values
Biceps femoris	14.9 ± 0.37	14.9 ± 0.11	–	No difference
Tibialis anterior	16.1 ± 0.17	16.3 ± 0.14	–	Same
Biceps femoris	–	14.9 ± 0.11	19.7 ± 0.77	0.001
Tibialis anterior	–	16.3 ± 0.14	20.3 ± 0.46	0.001
Rectus femoris	No activity	16.6 ± 0.20	No activity	–
Gastrocnemius	Same	16.3 ± 0.14	Same	–

TABLE 3. The Latent Period of the Knee Jerk in Intact and in Spinal Dogs (in msec)

Muscles	Intact dogs	Spinal dogs	
		Treated	Untreated
Rectus femoris	5–7	5–7	5–7
Vastus lateralis	5–7	5–7	5–7
Biceps femoris	No activity	16	No activity
Gastrocnemius	Same	16	Same
Rectus femoris Contralateral extremity	Same	20	Same

time of propagation of the monosynaptic reflex, these disturbances or changes should be related to the synaptic delay in the afferent segment of the arc, particularly in the interneurons.

Measurement of the threshold of stimulation was done with an electronic stimulator using the maximum current output. The stimuli were either single pulses lasting for 2 msec or a series of rhythmic impulses having a frequency of 2–3 impulses/sec. When necessary, these parameters were changed. As usual, two silver plates with a diameter of 3.5 mm and placed 8 mm apart served as stimulating electrodes. They were fixed to the paw with straps after clipping the hair and cleaning the surface of the skin. Pieces of cotten soaked with physiological saline prevented drying of the skin under the electrodes.

The resistance of the high frequency adapter situated in the output of the stimulator was equal to 4 kilo-ohms. The amplitude of stimulation during the course of the experiment was also constant.

The measurements were obtained at the beginning of the experiment and after a rest of 20–30 sec following the first measurement. The next procedures consisted of stimulating the skin of the paw with an electric current having an intensity above threshold, at a frequency of 2-impulses/sec for 15 min. The final measurement of threshold was made several minutes after completion of the above procedures. The results of these experiments are presented in Table 4, where it can be seen that in treated dogs the threshold of stimulation was comparatively constant. They showed little variation, either after the first application of current or after prolonged stimulation. But in the untreated dogs, the thresholds were higher and generally less stable. In a number of experiments, it was impossible to obtain measurements since the threshold exceeded the maximum output of voltage of the stimulator, which was equal to 53 volts. Similar results were also observed after prolonged stimulation. In other similar experiments, the thresholds were fairly low at the beginning but soon after the first application of current, they increased significantly.

TABLE 4. Stimulation Thresholds of the Flexor Reflex in Spinal Dogs (in volts)

Treated dogs					Untreated dogs				
		Threshold values					Threshold values		
No. of experiment	Name of dog	at beginning of experiment	after 20–30 sec	at end of experiment	No. of experiment	Name of dog	at beginning of experiment	after 20–30 sec	at end of experiment
1	Gana	33	33	42	1	Tema	>53	>53	>53
2	”	48	48	46	2	”	>53	50	>53
3	Klo	30	30	30	3	”	12	50	>53
4	”	45	45	45	4	”	53	53	>53
5	”	39	39	39	5	”	34	40	53
6	”	50	50	53	6	Okhra	30	53	53
7	”	42	42	42	7	”	50	>53	>53
8	”	53	30	40	8	”	27	49	50
9	”	47	47	49	9	”	47	53	53

Stimulation for 15 min in all cases produced a rise of threshold to 50–53 volts or higher, i.e., it exceeded the limits of measurement.

These results indicate that the condition of the sensory apparatus and the ability to propagate impulses along the central segment of a reflex arc in treated dogs differed distinctly from that of the untreated dogs. The rise in the threshold after a single stimulus, observed in the latter, indicates a rapid exhaustion of the mediator in the synaptic apparatus of the neurons participating in that particular reflex.

It was interesting to compare the morphologic changes observed in brains of animals treated in this way with the dystrophic changes which developed in transected spinal cords, as a result of inadequate afferent stimuli and in the absence of supra spinal impulses. We also examined the effect of treatment on the condition of reflex activity in a transected spinal cord.

The Condition of Neurons in the Distal Part of the Transected Spinal Cord Depending on Its Functional Activity

Morphologic investigation of the spinal cord was conducted on dogs from 14 days to 12 months after transection (Brazovskaya et al., 1966). Sections from the lumbo-sacral region of the spinal cord were stained according to Nissl, and impregnated with silver by various methods. The diameter of the neurons and synapses in the lateral group of nuclei of the ventral horn (motoneurons) were examined. Similar studies were made of the central and ventro-medial part (interneurons) and in the nucleus of Cajal of the intermediate zone. All the measurements were made on cells of the seventh lumbar segment.

Treatment of the animals (by cutaneous stimulation: see p. 47) was started on the third day after operation and was carried out daily. In some dogs, where observations were made for a prolonged period, treatment was started on the tenth day after operation. Except for the treatment, the rest of the experimental conditions were the same for all animals.

The results of the morphological investigations on the brain of these animals, 6–12 months after operation, represent the mean values for each group of animals (Table 5).

A marked difference in the sizes of the neurons and synapses was observed in the animals of different groups, which was highly significant.

These results present evidence on the question of how quickly atrophic changes are developed in the neural structures of the spinal cord and whether they can be prevented by modifying the afferent stimuli as early as the third day after operation. Experiments were conducted in which the diameter of the neuronal cell body was observed, 14 days after operation. The results of these experiments are presented in Table 6.

TABLE 5. Diameter of the Nerve Cells in Treated and Untreated Dogs, 6–12 Months after Operation (in microns)

Type of cell	Mean diameter ± S.E. ($X + m$)			Difference %	Significance P values
	Normal	Untreated	Treated		
Motoneurons	65 ± 0.60	56 ± 0.66	65 ± 0.82	13.8	0.001
Interneurons	50 ± 0.63	29 ± 0.60	37 ± 0.60	21.6	0.001
Synaptic terminals	–	1.3 ± 0.064	2.0 ± 0.054	35.0	0.001

It is clear from Table 6 that the atrophic process had already started within this period of 14 days, but it was less prominent than that observed after 6–12 months. At 14 days, the diameter of the motoneurons in the untreated animals was 6.1% smaller compared with the treated ones (instead of 13.8% at 6–12 months). The diameter of the motoneurons in the treated animals was within normal limits.

Table 6 also shows a considerable change from normal in the diameter of the interneurons at this time. Even in the treated animals this was 35 μm; or, in other words, their diameter was less than normal. In untreated animals this was even less (by 8.5%). At this time, the diameter of the synapses in treated animals was found to be within normal limits and in untreated ones was reduced by 30%.

After 6–12 months, the diameter of the motoneurons in the untreated dogs was reduced by 13.8% in comparison to those of the treated ones. However, the mean diameter of the motoneurons in these latter animals was 65 μm, which was within normal limits for unoperated controls.

As is well known, the central part of the ventral horn is the site of synaptic connection between the long propriospinal pathways which produce inhibition and excitation of the internuncial cells (Eccles, 1959; Szentagothai, 1951). In order to establish whether there was any difference in the degree of

TABLE 6. The Diameter of Neurons and Synapses in Treated and Untreated Animals 14 Days after Operation

Type of cells	Mean diameter ± S.E. ($X + m$) (μm)			Difference between treated and untreated % of treated	Significance P values
	Normal	Untreated	Treated		
Motoneurons	65 ± 0.60	61 ± 1.20	65 ± 1.22	6.1	0.001
Interneurons	40 ± 0.63	32 ± 0.68	35 ± 0.67	8.5	0.001
Synaptic terminals	–	1.4 ± 0.0047	2.0 ± 0.0062	30.0	0.001

development of the dystrophic processes in the excitatory and inhibitory neurons, measurement of the cells of the intermediate nucleus of Cajal was obtained in identical preparations having a direct inhibition path leading to an antagonist (Eccles, 1959). Measurements were also made on those cells which were identified by these authors as being inhibitory Renshaw cells. This was confirmed by morphological investigation (Schimert, 1939; Szentagothai, 1961).

The mean diameter of the cells in the nucleus of Cajal was 28 μm in treated animals and 33 μm in control. However, in the untreated group the mean diameter was only 22 μm, i.e., the difference between them was 21.48%. Approximately the same type of correlation was also obtained for the Renshaw cells. Their mean diameter in treated animals was equal to 25 μm and in control 30 μm, but in untreated animals it was 20 μm. The difference was about 20%.

Thus, atrophy of interneurons of animals in different conditions remained within the limits of 20–21%, but no atrophy was found in the excitatory or inhibitory units.

Clear differences were observed when studying the neuro-fibrillar apparatus in treated and in untreated animals. In the former, as well as in normal animals, a dense network of fine neurofibrils could be seen uniformly covering the cell body and dendrites of the ventral horn cells, thus forming a moderate condensation around the nucleus. In untreated animals, the neurofibrils were not impregnated with silver in a substantial proportion of the cells and were not identified in many places. These results characterize the condition of the neuronal apparatus after a prolonged interval, when the atrophic process had already stabilized following the operation.

From this data, it can be seen that the nature of changes in the diameter of different types of nerve cells in untreated animals, 14 days after operation, was similar to that observed 6–12 months later, i.e., the interneurons suffered to the greatest extent while the motoneurons were the least affected. Thus, the treatment using cutaneous stimulation prevented the development of atrophic processes in the motoneurons and synapses while it partially protects the interneurons.

In particular, the results which were obtained in the animals after temporary asphyxia of the spinal cord convincingly demonstrate the difference in sensitivity of the different types of neurons to an unfavorable situation. Thus, after temporary occlusion of the thoracic aorta, 75% of the interneurons died while, at the same time, almost all the motoneurons remained intact (Gelfan, 1963; Gelfan & Tarlov, 1963). The spinal interneurons have an extensive integrative function; therefore their death severely jeopardizes the spinal reflexes (Gelfan, 1963). In dogs with experimental hind limb rigidity, the density of axosomatic synapses was significantly reduced to about 15% of normal, while the density of axodentritic synapses was 35% of normal (Gelfan & Rapisarda, 1964). In asphyxia produced by increasing the pressure in the subdural space of the spinal cord for 25 min, 90% of the interneurons and about 80% of the big motoneurons died (Van Harreveld, 1962; Van Harreveld & Shade, 1962).

These observations indicate that an important cause of structural and functional changes in the neural connections of the distal part of a transected spinal cord is an inadequate blood supply due to stasis produced as a result of inactivity.

Dystrophic processes in the spinal cord developed quickly in the absence of supraspinal influences and afferent input. These mainly affect elements in the afferent part of the reflex arc–the interneurons and synapses on the motoneurons, i.e., mainly forming connections with these intervening neurons.

The decrease in diameter of the neurons in our experiments was uniformly observed in the interneural cells in different nuclear groups, independent of their physiological characteristics. For example, the changes were similar in anterior horn cells where the intersegmental fibers terminate on Renshaw cells and in Cajal's nucleus.

The involvement of the above processes in the various groups of interneurons and the similar type of observed change indicate that these cells belong to pathways which are very similar and which are responsible for a uniform reaction in response to a change in the functional activity of the spinal cord. Moreover, interneurons are more susceptible to this change when compared to motoneurons.

The treatment which was applied systematically beginning from the fourth to the tenth day after operation prevented the development of the dystrophic processes in the distal part of the transected spinal cord. This was due to the activity of all the structural elements of the neural connections in the spinal cord: the nerve cells, the synapses on them, and also the peripheral receptors of the muscles and joints. Increased circulation appeared to be an important factor for the recovery of normal spinal function, which was achieved by the application of different types of treatment.

The significant difference we observed in the condition of the reflexes and neural structures in the spinal cord of treated and untreated dogs prompted us to start investigating the activity of motor units which determine the tension, in order to reveal the exact changes resulting from inactivity.

The Activity of Motor Units in Spinal Dogs

The activity of motor units has been studied for a long time. Adrian and Bronk (1928) first demonstrated that this activity reflects the action of motoneurons recorded from a nerve trunk. A motor unit is composed of a motoneuron and the muscle fibers innervated by it. It is a single entity; an impulse transmitted by a motoneuron usually reaches all the muscle fibers of that particular motor unit. The degree of muscular contraction has been shown to be dependent on the number of motoneurons excited and, to some extent, on the frequency of their discharge (Person, 1969). The correlation between these parameters differs in different muscles and in individual motor units. In moderate muscle tension, the frequency of discharge from individual motor units reaches 20-35 impulses/sec. Increasing the tension of the muscle may increase this to 50 impulses/sec (Bigland & Lipold, 1954). It is not possible to record the activity of motor units during voluntary relaxation of the muscle under normal conditions. With the application of mild tension or during postural activity, impulse frequency may reach 7-10 impulses/sec and is easily recorded.

The activity of several motor units is characterized by dissynchronization in the rhythm of their discharges, which helps to maintain the continuous normal tone of the muscle (Gelfan, 1963). We will not describe the morphologic and physiological action of motor units as it is beyond our investigation. Those who are interested in this question may go through the monograph of Person (1969), where this has been reviewed in detail.

We studied the activity of motor units (Nesmeyanova, Pyatetskii-Shapiro, & Shik, 1964, 1965) in m. gastrocnemius in spinal and in intact dogs. This is an antigravity muscle which ensures the erect posture of man and corresponding balance of dog. The activity was recorded with the help of needle-shaped electrodes manufactured by "Diza." Recording of potentials in muscles of paralyzed extremities is somewhat difficult, as can be judged from the results presented above.

A big motor unit has a diameter of 5-10 mm (Buchthal, Guld, & Rosenfalck, 1957b). The tip diameter of the needle-shaped electrode manufactured by "Diza" was 0.1 mm, inserted in a Cannula–0.45 mm; accordingly, the conducting surface was equal to 0.04 mm^2. These electrodes simultaneously recorded the potentials of several motor units due to the fact that the fibers of different units are intermingled (Buchthal, Guld, & Rosenfalck, 1975a) and this somewhat simplified the recording.

In intact animals, stable activity of several motor units was recorded simply by placing the hind legs of the dog on the floor. In spinal dogs, particularly in untreated ones, we pressed the ipsi- or the contralateral thigh which produced tension in m. gastrocnemius, lasting for 10-20 sec, and recorded the appearance of potentials from the motor units. This interval was sufficient to allow recording the activity. These action potentials from the motor units were fed through an amplifier UBP 1-01 to the input of an oscillograph N_{102} and were photographically recorded at a film speed of 250 mm/sec. The measured intervals between individual impulses and the trains of potentials were analyzed by a digital counter.

The mean interval between the discharges of individual motor units in spinal and intact dogs during normal postural activity was constant and corresponded to approximately 10 impulses/sec, which was within the usual limits of discharge frequency of these units. The absence of supraspinal influences was not reflected in the frequency of impulses of the motor units.

It was interesting to compare the constancy of the intervals between discharges of individual motor units in intact and in spinal animals. This might identify the character of spinal transection or, more precisely, the activity of the motoneurons. The distribution of interval duration was presented in histograms where the intervals were plotted for a duration of 0.2 msec in both sides of the average, against the number of cases in percentage. The histogram showing the duration of intervals for intact dogs has a single peak, narrow and symmetrical, which shows the definite constancy of the intervals (Fig. 19A).

In spinal dogs the histograms as a whole are consistantly symmetrical and have a single peak (Fig. 19B). The uniform distribution of intervals in all the dogs suggests that the mechanism which determines the activity of motoneurons in resting conditions is, to some extent, automatic and is carried out by the segmental apparatus of the spinal cord.

However, in individual spinal dogs, the nature of the histogram was different. The histograms were usually irregular in untreated dogs who were capable of little movement and who were unable to stand due to the absence of extensor tone. On the other hand, in treated animals, the histogram peak was very sharp. A histogram with a very sharp peak was also obtained in a

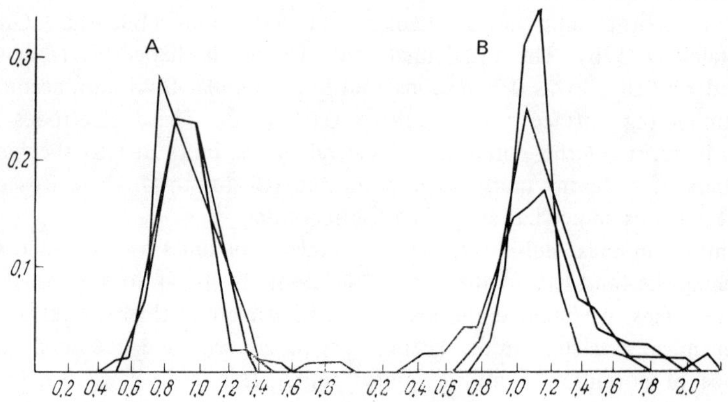

FIG. 19. The distribution of the duration of intervals in intact (A) and in spinal (B) dogs.

Abscissa—interval length in relation to mean; ordinate—frequency noted in respective interval length.

The distribution for each of three animals is represented in each graph.

dog having an increased extensor tone, though it was untreated. Probably, the presence of the tone of the extensor muscles was an important factor for the stability of the intervals and was present in some spinal dogs and increased with treatment. Treatment in muscular work was shown to increase the constancy of intervals between the spike potentials (Kawakami, 1955).

Changes in the stability of impulse intervals of motoneurons in the muscles of untreated spinal dogs might not be due to dystrophic processes in the motoneurons themselves, but to some changes in the interneurons. Gelfan and Tarlov (1963) suggested that increased fluctuation in internals might be due to a change in the function of the inhibitory interneurons, particularly in the Renshaw cells. It is quite possible that treatment helps in normalizing the interaction between the α- and γ-systems at the segmental level, which is significant for the maintenance of muscle tone (Granit, 1957).

In order to explain the causes which might favor the development of normal muscle tone after transection of the spinal cord, it is essential to examine the factors which maintain it and the causes for the development of pathological muscle tone (spasticity) which is a symptom of several disorders of the central nervous system.

Pathologic Muscle Tone

By the term muscle tone, we understand the resting tension of a muscle which results because the distance between the joints is somewhat more than the resting length of the muscle itself (Gurfinkel' et al., 1965). In the resting condition, the tension of the muscle is represented solely by its elastic properties, but in the conditions required for maintaining posture when the subject is standing, activity is observed in the antigravity muscles, particularly those of the leg.

So far, our interest has been focussed on the postural tone of those muscles, which maintain erect posture; let us now see what is known about the neural mechanisms which supply them.

To obtain normal muscle tone, it is necessary to have continuous descending activity impinging on the motoneurons of higher segments acting on the α and γ system at the segmental level (Granit, 1956; Granit & Holmgren, 1955; Granit, Lob, & Kaada, 1952). A schematic diagram of this is represented in Fig. 20, for a better visual concept of the interaction of the α- and γ-motoneurons at the segmental level. The activity of the muscle spindles plays an important part in the formation of muscle tone which maintains the tonic activity provided by the γ-motoneurons (Hunt, 1951). The characteristic feature of the γ-motoneurons is the high degree of their excitability; thus, the stimulation threshold of γ-motoneurons is considerably lower than α-motoneurons (Hunt, 1951). In response to a single afferent volley, they often gave repetitive responses at high frequency (Hunt & Paintal, 1958).

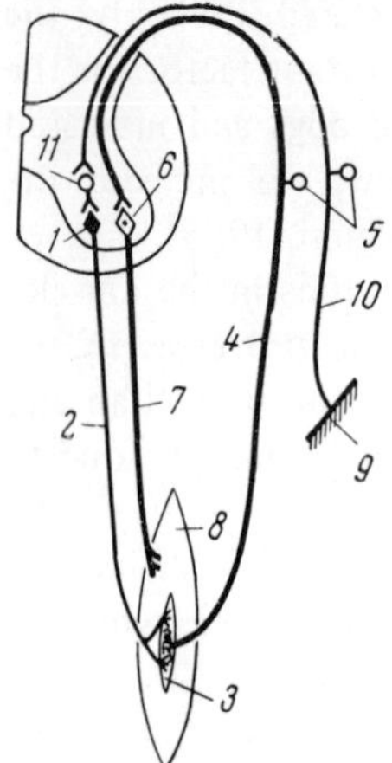

FIG. 20. The schematic representation of the interaction between the α- and γ- motoneurons in the segmental level.

1. γ-motoneuron; 2. γ-efferent fiber; 3. muscle spindle; 4. afferent nerve fiber of group 1a; 5. cells of a spinal ganglion; 6. α-motoneuron; 7. motor nerve fiber; 8. muscle; 9. skin; 10. cutaneous nerve; 11. interneuron.

There are reports showing significantly higher sensitivity of the γ-motoneurons even to weak cutaneous stimulation (Eldred & Hagbarth, 1954). Subsequently the muscle spindles can remain active after stopping the γ-fiber stimulation. This after-effect may be observed for 7 sec after a stimulation of 1-2 sec, at a frequency of 20 per sec (Hunt & Kuffler, 1951).

Owing to these characteristics, the γ-system not only assists in the effective operation of the stretch receptor but may also be utilized as a firing mechanism for the initiation of movement and for the maintenance of tone (Granit, 1957).

In several disorders of the central nervous system, pathologic muscle tone is increased–such rigidity may be represented by a resistance of the extremity to passive displacement of the joint. The causes of rigidity and the mechanisms of its appearance may be different. Granit has described two types of rigidity: (1) decerebrate type–decreased by deafferentiation of the extremity, and (2) ischemic type–where deafferentation has no effect. The first type of rigidity was initially described by Sherrington (1898) in experiments involving transection of the mid brain. He characterized it as an exaggeration of posture. Moreover, this rigidity was noticed in all the muscles of an extremity, in both the extensors and also the flexors. It was not eliminated by denervating the skin, but was absent in the deafferented animal, from which it was concluded that this type of rigidity is dependent on the propioceptive reflex, the receptors for which are found in the muscle itself. Granit reported that this rigidity is due to the activation of γ-motoneurons. The second type of rigidity, appearing after ischemic decerebration, is exclusively due to activation of the α-motoneurons as deafferentation has no effect on it (Pollock & Davis, 1930, 1931).

Rigidity becomes very apparent as a result of temporary asphyxia of the spinal cord. The causes of its appearance are variously explained by different authors. Gelfan and Tarlov (1959) considered that, as a result of dystrophic processes mainly affecting the interneurons, the motoneurons are freed from their normal inhibitory influences and their activity increases very rapidly, causing the development of rigidity which appears within 24 hr after asphyxia. However, destruction of the interneurons should inevitably damage the γ-loop, and, as a result, this system cannot be responsible for the appearance of rigidity. When they are subjected to increased excitability, the α-motoneurons are particularly liable to produce rigidity (Gelfan, 1964; Tarlov, 1967).

A similar view was held by Lebedev (1959a, 1959b, 1963) who considered that during the development of hyper-reflexia, following spinal cord asphyxia, the increased activity from the side affected by the dystrophic interneurons is of greater importance since it is responsible for producing increased activity in the motoneurons.

Van Harreveld (1962, 1964) suggested that the main cause for the development of rigidity was activation of the myotatic reflex associated with an enhanced activity of the γ-motoneurons and the ability of the α-motoneurons to respond to high frequency afferent impulses (Van Harreveld & Spinelli, 1965). This statement was based on experiments with de-afferentiated animals in which rigidity did not appear after temporary asphyxia of the spinal cord.

The possibility of evoking rigidity by activation of α-motoneurons, independent of the activation of muscle spindles, was reported by Hnik (1960), who observed an increase in the tone of the extensor muscles of the hind legs in rats and cats, 7-10 days after the deafferentation. He explained this phenomenon, including the spontaneous increased excitability of the extensor-motoneurons, as a result of deafferentation, which corresponds to the hypothesis suggested by Cannon and Rosenblueth (1951). Experiments involving antidromic inhibition failed to corroborate the view that rigidity in chronic spinal animals, following asphyxia, was due to destruction of Renshaw cells (Gelfan, 1966).

After the transection of the spinal cord at the level of mid and lower thoracic segments in our experiments, there was a prevalence of flexor tone in the muscles of the hind legs. However, in some dogs, the tone of the extensor muscles increased after 1-1½ years. The limb became firm and was not flexed; however, this might be followed by a sudden, complete relaxation. These animals experienced an extension reaction, as reported by Sherrington (1909, 1913). This relaxation was due to a sudden inhibition of afferent discharge to the motoneurons when, in the process of stretching, the muscles were subjected to a discharge from tendon receptors (Eldred et al., 1953). This suggests that the γ-system plays an important role in the development of the extensor tone in the muscles of the animals' hind legs, after transection of the spinal cord. This hypothesis has been confirmed by a number of observations.

In order to understand this process, let us examine the functions of the individual elements of the γ-system. The muscle spindles are composed of two types of intrafusal fibers having different afferent and γ-efferent innervations: These are γ_1 and γ_2 fibers. Correspondingly, in a reflex, stretching can be divided into two components–the phasic and tonic–which, according to Rushworth (1964), have different central mechanisms. The phasic component of the reflex is connected with the phasic α-motoneurons and the tonic with the tonic α-motoneurons.

Electromyographic investigation of clinical spasticity has demonstrated that both these components are involved in the development of spasticity (Yusevich, 1970). In mild spasticity, there is excitation of the phasic component of the reflex: the stretching presumably associated with an increased activity of the γ_1-system and in severe spasticity–γ_2-system (Rushworth, 1964). Along with these facts, there are many reports showing that spasticity can develop without the participation of γ-system. In fact, if the γ-motoneurons are responsible for increased muscular tone, then their basal activity should rise in comparison to normal. Meanwhile, there are reports of significant lowering and even stoppage of basal activity of the γ-motoneurons after spinal transection (Barnes, 1964; Diete-Spiff, Dodsworth, & Pascos, 1962). In an isolated segment of the spinal cord of cats, the basal activity was absent in the majority of the γ-motoneurons 5-6 months after operation (Maksimova & Afelt, 1970). In particular, there was an appreciable lowering of the basal discharge of the γ-motoneurons regulating the tonic sensitivity of the afferent terminals (Alnaes, Yansen, & Rudjord, 1965).

The possibility of ensuring increased muscle tone (spasticity) in spinal trauma with the α-system alone is confirmed with Tarlov's experiment (1967), in which flexor tone was developed significantly in a patient with a spinal cord injury. It was not reduced either by transection of the dorsal roots which destroyed the γ-loop, or by spinal transection; it was abolished as a result of transection of the ventral roots which interrupted the motor reflex provided by the α-system.

These reports contradict each other on the mechanism of formation of muscular hypertonicity during spinal cord transection. This might suggest that, as in decerebration, there is a possibility of development of two types of rigidity–one appearing with the participation of the γ-system and the other without its participation.

The factor which is responsible for the development of the dystrophic process in the distal part of the transected spinal cord is basically related to the appearance of increased muscular tone. It is impossible to control this serious condition, which is associated with spinal trauma, without understanding its causes. In our opinion, the principal factor responsible for its development is the dystrophic processes involving the interneurons and the γ-motoneurons. The coordination between the α- and γ-system which is necessary for the maintenance of normal muscle tone has been altered. The development of the dystrophic processes in the γ-motoneurons is supported indirectly by observations of the significant lowering of their basal activity which has been shown in an isolated segment of spinal cord in cats (Maksimova & Afelt, 1970).

What preventive measures can be adopted to control the development of pathological hypertonicity in the muscles of the extremities in spinal animals?

If the dystrophic processes in the neural elements are responsible for the development of pathological hypertonicity, the application of treatment and additional afferent stimulation should prevent this and should be able to eliminate it. Observations on experimental spinal dogs demonstrated that without treatment there is more frequent development of pronounced hypertonicity in the muscles of the extremities as compared to those which received treatment. In the majority of animals, the flexor tone was more prominent, but in some the extensor tone was greater. In the treated dogs, extensor or flexor tone was similarly prevalent, but in a very mild form. The extensor tone did not prevent bending the legs, but the flexor tone only allowed standing with the partially flexed legs. Thus, the signficant decrease in the dystrophic processes which would be expected with treatment normalized the muscle tone to some extent. In order to confirm the significance of treatment in the development of motor function, the locomotor ability was examined in different dogs. The animals were characterized according to the degree and nature of their muscle tone, depending on the condition of the neural connections in the spinal cord, and, at a later stage, depending on the condition of their motor reflexes.

The Walking Capacity of the Treated and Untreated Dogs in the Presence of Strychnine

How can one explain the ability to walk in the absence of a stable, weight-bearing restraining movement? The degree of muscle tone can be measured by observing the activity of the motor units (Gurfinkel' et al., 1965). Owen and Sherrington (1911) demonstrated that in a decerebrate dog, the activity in the m. gastrocnemius significantly increased with strychnine, but the tone of the muscles also increased. We expected that in a spinal dog a subconvulsive dose of strychnine would produce activity in the m. gastrocnemius, with increase of extensor tone, and the dog would be able to stand on its legs.

In order to compare the locomotor ability in dogs of different groups, we repeated the experiment of Owen and Sherrington under different conditions. The activity from the m. gastrocnemius was obtained with an ordinary needle electrode covered with varnish and the potentials recorded through an amplifier (UBP1-01) were fed to an integrator which summed their area (the amplitude and the frequency of the impulse) by a digital counter. The impulses were counted by the integrator for a period of 10 sec (multiple) with a calibration of 20 mV = 300 impulses per 10 sec).

In all the experiments on dogs in a resting condition, when hind legs were suspended in straps but not touching the floor, the initial activity in the m. gastrocnemius was zero. After an interval of 5–30 min following the administration of 1% solution of strychnine at a dose of 0.01 mg/kg body weight, the muscular activity started increasing abruptly and in about 30–60 min reached a maximum. This was observed in all the dogs independent of treatment (Fig. 21).

If the dog was lowered to the floor, between 30–60 min after administration, it was able to move through the use of its hind legs. Analysis of the character of this movement showed that, though the extensor tone was uniformly good in all the four dogs undergoing the test, the ability for movement in untreated dogs differed considerably from that of the treated ones. The two treated dogs ran by flexing and stepping with the hind legs in a manner which was difficult to differentiate from the movements of intact animals. In contrast, both the untreated dogs used their hind legs continuously but they were unable to place them: Flexing them intermittently, they jumped mechanically, operating both legs simultaneously.

In this experiment, although all the animals were eventually able to achieve an equal degree of movement of their hind legs, the beneficial effect of

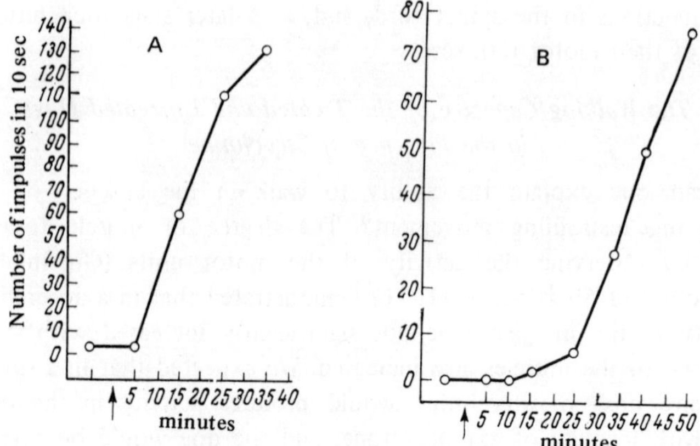

FIG. 21. The change of activity in the m. gastrocnemius under the influence of strychnine in treated (A) and in untreated (B) dogs.

Abscissa–time (in min); ordinate–number of impulses for 10 sec at a calibration of 20 mv–300 impulses for 10 sec. Arrow–administration of strychnine.

treatment could be seen, as it enhanced the ability of the peripheral apparatus (joints and muscles) to carry out movements in a normal pattern. By contrast, absence of treatment resulted in deformed joints and flabby muscles which were unable to provide natural walking. However, the main difference caused by treatment probably depended on the condition of the interneurons in a spinal cord. In the first case, the alternate flexion and extension were carried out by the transmission of impulses along a multineuronal reflex arc, but in the second case these connections were disturbed.

It may be thought that if it was possible to increase the tone of the extensor muscles in spinal dogs, they might be able to support their body and ensure locomotion. It is possible that more intensive treatment in a more effective direction than that which was used in our experiments should completely normalize the activity of γ-motoneurons in spinal animals. The restoration of a normal relation between the α- and γ-motoneurons would favor the development of normal tone of the antigravity muscles.

In conclusion, we feel that under the conditions of treatment which we adopted, the dystrophic processes in the spinal cord were practically absent. This resulted in the restoration of motor function in our spinal animals being more complete. The pathologic muscle tone was not at all pronounced, and there was no a-reflexia, preventing the appearance of motor activity and the development of new reflexes. There was no atrophy of the muscles nor were the joints deformed. There were no pronounced atrophic changes in the spinal interneurons.

The absence of these damaging factors led to activation of the reflex activity which later helped in the development of the restorative processes.

CHAPTER III

REGENERATION OF INTRASPINAL AXONS IN MAMMALS

Problem of Regeneration

The Influence of Traumatic Degenerative Processes on the Regeneration of Animal Tissues and Organs

Physiological regeneration, i.e., the replacement of cells and tissues in an organism, goes on constantly throughout life in all types of animals. However, the situation is different in the case of reparative regeneration, i.e., the restoration of an *organ* after its removal, where the decisive factor is the type of animal. Many lower vertebrates possess a great capacity for regeneration, such that their lost limb or tail may be easily restored. On the other hand, higher mammals are not capable of restoring lost organs, since the capacity for regeneration is reduced or lost to a significant degree in the process of phylogenetic development. This is in agreement with the law formulated by Darwin (1868): "The higher the level of phylogenetic development of an animal, the less is its regenerating capacity."

However, when studying the process of regeneration, some forms have been found which failed to conform to the above rule. A number of internal organs in mammals regenerate nicely by the multiplication of intact cells without modifying the shape of the organ itself. This type of regeneration is known as compensatory hypertrophy (Liozner, 1956, 1957, 1961, 1962; Vorontsova, 1949, 1953; Vorontsova & Liozner, 1955). These authors consider that in all animals such cellular proliferation will appear under specific demands, such as the rate of their metabolic processes, independent of the overall development of the regenerating capacity of these organs.

Studitskii (1954) believes that the capacity for reparative regeneration is higher in mammals than in lower vertebrates, due to their more active metabolism. The peripheral nerve of a rat regenerates more rapidly than that of the axolotl (Zelikina, 1954). Mammalian muscle may successfully restore its own structure and function after degeneration (Studitskii, Zhenevskaya, & Rumyantseva, 1956). The healing reaction of muscle after an injection goes on slowly in the axolotl and continues for 45 days; but in rats, healing is completed by the seventh day after similar injections, (Gilev, 1954). A series of experiments studying the regeneration of the long bones and plantar tubercles in chicken and in axolotl showed that restoration of many tissues in higher vertebrates can proceed in the same way as in lower vertebrates. The rate of replacement of tissues and the frequency of their traumatization play an important role in successful regeneration (Studiskii & Striganova, 1951). The higher phylogenetic development of an organism provides better internal organization for adaptive reactions on which regeneration is dependent, according to Studitskii (1966).

Polezhaev holds a somewhat different view about the regenerating capacity of animals. In his opinion, the failure of reparative regeneration to take place in higher vertebrates is due to the fact that highly differentiated tissues are poorly dedifferentiated when damaged (they fail to lose their specialized characteristics). In order to recover the regenerating capacity, it is essential to induce disintegration artifically and this will produce subsequent dedifferentiation of these tissues, which favors regeneration.

This author's view was supported by the experiments in which he tried to produce regeneration in the amputated stump of a tadpole limb by systematically traumatizing it. This intensified disintegration of the tissues, and as a result, the traumatized limb, was regenerated but the control (untraumatized) limb remained unchanged (Polezhaev, 1933b). Histological investigation demonstrated that there was an intense dedifferentiation of the mesodermal tissues of the remnant organ in the stump and the quick formation of blastema (Polezhaev, 1935). A similar dependence of regeneration on the degree of traumatization of tissue up to the point of complete degeneration (by keeping the nerve and the blood supply intact) was also demonstrated in axolotl (Polezhaev, 1933a, 1934).

Loss of regenerating capacity is also connected with the degree of tissue differentiation in an organism during ontogenetic development. In some cases, this may be restored by the disintegration and dedifferentiation of the tissues.

On the basis of investigation over several years, the main factors governing the process of regeneration were identified by Polezhaev (1958, 1972) who concluded that the regenerative capacity of an organism could be changed by influencing its metabolism or by changing the conditions of its development.

Description of the factors regulating the regeneration of organs and tissues in animals can be found in the reviews by Needham (1952) and Urbani (1965). The processes governing the loss and restoration of regenerative capacity of organs in different types of animals were summarized by Polezhaev (1968, 1972).*

Let us examine what we know about the role of tissue disintegration in relation to the processes of regeneration. The first indications of the importance of tissue disintegration are met in the works of Bier (1917-19, 1923) and Haberland (1922). Carrel and Ebeling (1923, 1924) found that during the process of resorption in the initial stages of regeneration, there appeared nutritive and stimulating substances, i.e., trephones, derived from the products of protein breakdown. The necessity of cell destruction to provide better regeneration was reported by Morozov (1935).

Significant progress in the study of the role of disintegration products in regeneration was made in Nasonov's work (1935, 1936a, 1936b). He thought that disintegration products were extremely important for organ formation, and supported his concept in several different types of experiments. The implantation of cartilage from a limb of axolotl below its skin led to the development of an additional paw. However, if the same cartilage were dried or preserved in alcohol and ether, this phenomenon did not occur. Nasanov suggested that cartilage undergoing disintegration was converted into proteoses which were responsible for organizing the process of regeneration. Zelinskii and Silaev subjected cartilage to a mild hydrolysis in 1% HCl lasting more than two years, so that the tissue was only degraded up to the level of proteoses. The hydrolyzate, later tested on axolotl, gave active and complete growth of an additional limb (Nasonov, 1941; Zelinskii, 1946). Nasonov's findings were confirmed and developed by Fedotov (1943). Zelinskii and Fedotov (1941) and Zelinskii (1946) confirmed the phenomenon discovered by Nasonov and extended the analyses. They concluded that disintegration of tissues helps the formation of non-nitrogenous derivatives of amino acids which act as catalysts during the hydrolysis of proteins which are essential for the reconstruction of new tissues.

Bromlei and Orekhovich (1934c) were convinced that in the residual parts

*Editor's note: Polezhaev's extensive experimental and theoretical studies can be found in his monograph (1972) translated into English.

of an amputated organ the process of disintegration was more intense than in normal tissue and suggested that this was due to the proteolytic activity of the tissues in the regenerated part. In fact, they found that the enzyme cathepsin was more active in regenerated tissue and in the periphery bounded by the surrounding organ than the cathepsin found in normal tissues (Bromlei & Orekhovich, 1934b, 1934a; Orekhovich, 1937). This is also true of mammalian tissues (Orekhovich, 1938). The amount of reduced glutathione in the blast cells of regenerated tissue is increased significantly above normal and produces conditions which were favorable for stimulation of the activity of proteolytic enzymes.

Later, it was shown that the rise of cathepsin activity in regenerated tissues is only observed during the period of tissue dedifferentiation. Once the growth and differentiation have started, enzyme activity even falls short of its initial level (Ryvkina & Striganova, 1939a, 1939b).

Skorobogatova (1951a, 1951b) compared the proteolytic activity of the tissues in the stump of an amputated extremity and the degradation of proteins in rats and mice, with these processes in axolotl, and noticed a significant difference in their intensity and duration, depending on the type of animal. In rats and mice, the processes were less pronounced and completed more quickly, but in axolotl they were much more prolonged. She suggested that prolonged availability of disintegration products of the tissues in the area of growth had a favorable effect on the progress of regeneration. In fact, it was found that the amount of RNA in the leg-stumps of axolotl and amphibian tadpoles during the process of regeneration was considerably increased in specific phases of blastema development (Barakina, 1951a, 1952a). The reinnervation of axolotl limbs has been described by Cass and Mark (1975). In mice, no increase in the concentration of RNA was observed after such an operation (Barakina, 1952b). However, when the mucous membrane of the mouth or tongue was damaged, the concentration of RNA was considerably increased (Yüan Li-young, 1959; Dmitrieva, 1954). An increase in the concentration of RNA in the process of disintegration of the tissue in lower vertebrates was similarly reported by Urbani (1965).

At the time of regeneration, quantitative as well as qualitative changes occur in nucleic acids. The change of the cell's inherent metabolism produces changes of the molecular structure of the nucleoproteins (Howe & Bodian, 1941). In the cell body of a regenerating axon, the RNA is transformed to a more active form (Brattgard, Hydén, & Sjostrand, 1958).

The use of methods for restoration of regenerative capacity, based on the stimulation of the processes of disintegration and the dedifferentiation of tissues in mammals, has been found to be successful. Polezhaev and his colleagues obtained good results in experiments on the regeneration of damaged skull bones (Gintsburg, 1952, 1954; Matveeva, 1958; Polezhaev,

1951, 1957; Polezhaev, Matveeva, & Zakharova, 1957), in dental tissues (Polezhaev, 1958), and similarly in investigations of healing experimental damage to cardiac musculature (Polezhaev, Akhabadze, Zakharova, & Mant'eva, 1958, 1959; Polezhaev, Akhabadze, Muzlaeva, & Yavich, 1965). The work of these investigators has been reported in a monograph written by Polezhaev (1968). [English translation, 1972]

Along with the disintegration and the dedifferentiation of tissues, the reinnervation of the regenerated organ is also important for effective regeneration, as has been reported by a number of investigators (Inoue, 1958; Kudokotsev, 1960, 1966; Schotte, 1926; Singer, 1952, 1959a, 1963; Weiss, 1925). The role of innervation in the process of regeneration is connected with an increase of the quantity of acetylcholine in a regenerated part during a particular stage of its development (Singer). If the denervation of an organ fails to produce an increase in the quantity of acetylcholine, regeneration will not succeed.

It may be concluded that the disintegration of tissues produced as a result of the activation of proteolytic enzymes, favors the development of a new process, stimulating the formation of RNA and transforming it to a more active stage. Favorable conditions are thus produced for the synthesis of protein, the basic material for the formation of tissues in a regenerating organ. A review of neuronal degeneration and regeneration has been presented by Clemente (1972).

Regeneration of Peripheral Nerve in Mammals and Spinal Axons in Lower Vertebrates

Regeneration of axons capable of normal conduction is a problem in itself. This differs from regeneration of an organ which requires a number of intricate processes, particularly the division of cells in different tissues, their growth and the organization of the new organ. Regeneration of nerve would appear to consist in the simple growth of transected axons sprouting from intact nerve cells. In fact, the regeneration of a *peripheral* nerve progresses rapidly and, as a rule, is successful (Guth, 1956; Gutmann, 1958; Lee, 1929). Protein synthesis is carried out in the neural perikaryon and the protoplasm is transported along the axon to the region of transection (Lubinska, 1956a, 1956b; Miani, 1960; Weiss & Hiscoe, 1948; Young, 1945) where the oozing drop of protoplasm is thickened, forming an elongation of the axon (Weiss, 1955a, 1955b; Weiss, Taylor, & Pillai, 1962). Droz and his associates (Droz, 1963; Droz & Leblond, 1962) observed that protoplasmic protein can be transferred from the cell body to the end of its axon in 16 days. Only the mobile fraction of the protein is moved and the other stable fraction is left inside the body of the cell. Besides protein, a flow of enzymes has been demonstrated to accompany that of protoplasm (Friede & Knoller, 1964);

acetylcholine esterase activity has been observed in both the proximal and distal parts of a severed axon while the appearance of previously labeled material in both places shows the movement of the enzyme in two directions (Zelena & Lubinska, 1962). The latter observation indicates a differential movement of individual components of axoplasm (Lubinska, Niemierko, Oderfeld, Szawara, & Zelena, 1963; Lubinska, Niemierko, & Zelena, 1963). The cell body provides the nutrition for the axon through a neuro-secretion which is the principal manifestation of trophic function (Gutmann, 1962). Acetylcholine is believed to be one of the agents which are partially responsible for the process of regeneration (Singer, 1959a, 1965).

The essential factor for successful regeneration of a peripheral nerve is the secondary or Wallerian degeneration, developing in the distal part of a transected nerve after separation from the body of its nerve cell. The products of protein disintegration appear along the course of a nerve as a result of this degeneration and may be utilized for reconstruction of the axon. Schwann cells, which are found in large numbers in the membrane surrounding an axon, are involved in the process of regeneration—as well as the growth of an axon, its maturation and later on the conduction of a nerve impulse (Held, Ghang, & Tasaki, 1958; Heller, & Hesse, 1961a, 1961b; Marinesco & Minea, 1919; Schmitt, 1957). After the transection of a nerve, the number and size of the Schwann cells increases and they form Bungener's bands synthesizing more of the enzymes which are responsible for the disintegration and later the reconstruction of the axon. Owing to this increased metabolic activity, the Schwann cells may help in the movement of protoplasm along an axon (Lubinska, 1961, 1964, 1965).

The fact that Schwann cells continuously synthesize protein is also important. During experimental inhibition of Schwann cell proliferation, nerve regeneration was arrested (Edds, 1955). This might be explained by the fact that the newly synthesized intrinsic protein molecules are not enough for reconstruction of the axon. According to Krentzberg's finding (1967), obtained by using autoradiography, the synthesis of protein is considerably increased during nerve regeneration, particularly in the Schwann cells.

Full-fledged tropism in a growing axon is maintained by a number of conditions. For example, an optimal temperature causes the highest rate of growth of peripheral nerve, which is about 4.4 mm in 24 hr after a compression lesion in rabbit and 3.5 mm after transection (Guttman, Guttman, Medawar, & Young, 1942). The rate of growth of a nerve in man can reach 2 mm per day (Sunderland, 1947).

Does axonal growth occur after transection of the spinal cord in lower animals, and if so, to what extent? This question cannot be answered in a single sentence. A number of experimental investigations studying the main factors responsible for successful regeneration have demonstrated that regeneration is not solely dependent on the position of an animal in the phylogenetic order of vertebrates. Thus, there is complete regeneration of spinal cord in tailed amphibians (Hooker, 1915, 1917, 1925; Lorento de No, 1921; McGreight, 1924; Tuge & Hanzowa, 1937) but, in comparison, regeneration does not take place in tailless adult amphibians (Jankovska & Afelt, 1964; Piatt, 1955). In bony fish, which stand at a higher level of phylogenetic development, anatomical and functional regeneration generally takes place in the spinal cord (Koppani, 1955) as well as in the auditory and optic nerves (Westerman, 1964). This may be due to the fact that in tailed amphibians and in bony fish the ependymal cells of the central canal (even in adults) have an embryonic character and so they never lose the ability to proliferate and form new ganglion cells which promote the active growth of axons (Kirsche, 1960). The characteristic feature of the tailless amphibians is their extraordinary susceptibility to infection, as a result of which, according to Nasonov (1941) they developed the ability of quickly healing the stump of an excised organ which is very vital for the preservation of life.

Along with this, success in the regeneration of axons in the central nervous system in lower vertebrates is ensured by the same conditions which promote the regeneration of the peripheral nerve. For example, in a salamander the upper motor neuron axons form a part of the ventral roots in several segments inside the spinal cord and the results of their transection is analogous to the transection of peripheral nerves (Holtzer, 1955).

Several Causes for the Abortive Regeneration of Intraspinal Axons in Mammals

A different picture is found during the regeneration of intraspinal axons of mammals. Earlier investigators, using the silver impregnation method in rabbits demonstrated that axons inside the spinal cord grow slowly and, following injury, solitary fibers, following the course of blood vessels, may occasionally, penetrate the scar formed at the lesion (Cajal, 1928; Samarin, 1926, 1929). They concluded that the growth potential of the nerve fibers was rather slow and the scar was an insurmountable barrier.*

Due to the development of modern histologic techniques in the second quarter of the 20th century, interest increased in the problem of regeneration of axons in the central nervous system. The question was raised whether regeneration occurred in either the embryonic period or in the first few days of the postnatal life of mammals, when the tissues were still in their embryonic stage and not differentiated. The results obtained by different workers were contradictory. Some of them obtained negative results after

*The recovery of conduction in efferent and afferent fibers of the injured spinal cord has been evaluated by neurophysiological techniques (Deekcke & Tator, 1973).

transecting the spinal cord of fetal guinea pigs and rats (Hess, 1955, 1956; Hooker & Nicholas, 1927, 1930), and they concluded that regeneration is arrested due to failure of circulation. Other investigators reported restoration of motor functions in a small percentage of cases during similar experiments (Gerard & Crinker, 1931; Gerard & Kappani, 1926; Migliavacca, 1931). After transecting the spinal cord of 4-day-old puppies, Freeman (1952a) left them with mothers who reared them. The weight-bearing and the locomotor-functions were considerably restored in four of the puppies which survived. Windle (1956) summed up the results of experiments on regeneration in fetuses and newborn and concluded that this result was due to the mitosis of neuroblasts which continues in rats for 20–22 days of postnatal life. Chambers (1955) considered that another important factor was the development of a less dense scar tissue. Thus, reparative regeneration in young animals basically takes place from the undifferentiated neuroblasts (of an embryonic type), and occurs in the same way as in lower vertebrates.

Attempts to induce regeneration of the spinal cord in adult mammals produced different results. Hess (1954a, 1954b) and Davidoff and Ransohoff (1948) repeated the experiments of Ramon y Cajal and of Samarina but got negative results. Sugar and Gerard (1940) obtained the growth of fibers either singly or in groups through the scar in 4 out of 13 young rats following complete transection of the spinal cord; part of these fibers were intraspinal. They observed a significant restoration of function in these rats. In the experiments by Freeman and his group (Freeman, 1952a, 1952b, 1954, 1955; Freeman, Finneran, & Schlegel, 1949), where about 1,000 rats were used, a small percentage of cases showed a partial restoration of their coordinating movements and growth of nerve fibers in groups across the line of cleavage. However, there is doubt about the results of these experiments, as it has been suggested that the cause of restoration was either an incomplete transection of the spinal cord (Barnard & Carpenter, 1950) or the liberation of an autogenous pyrogen (Windle, 1955).

Several investigators observed the regeneration of nerve fibers after the hemisection of the spinal cord in cats and dogs (McCouch, Austin, & Liu, 1955; Zemlyanskaya, 1940). One cause of successful regeneration of axons in a spinal cord during its hemisection may be the absence of a gap between the spinal stumps which subsequently leads to the formation of a weak scar and thus favors the growth of nerve fibers from one stump to another.

The attempts to induce regeneration of conducting fibers in an adult mammalian spinal cord failed to produce uniform results. One of the reasons for failure in these experiments was the appearance of a pia-glial scar barrier in the area of cleavage. This was reported even by earlier investigators. The extent of scarring and the degree of obstruction depended in individual experiments on the type of animal which was used (Arend, 1972). The completeness of the section as well as the nature of the cleavage influenced the results and some of the reported contradictions could have been due to these factors. Several investigators studied the formation of a spinal scar. Yakeovleva (1951, 1956), working with rats, observed the accumulation of glial cells in the area of the lesion within the first few days after cord transection. According to her findings, development of a collageneous scar had already started on the third day but the growth of nerve fibers could only be seen following the seventh day after operation, in which case, the growing fibers would be expected to meet a developed scar obstructing their course. The rapid development of a collageneous scar is an insurmountable obstacle to the growth of axons, and this has also been reported by other investigators (Brown & McCouch, 1947; Gorodinskaya & Minut-Sorokhtina, 1948). Windle and his colleagues investigated the possibility of regeneration of intraspinal axons in mammals and came to the conclusion that its abortive nature could be explained by the formation of the insuperable pia-glial barrier; whereas in its absence, growth of nerve fibers can take place (Windle & Chambers, 1950; Windle, Clemente, & Chambers, 1952). Thus, a new trend in investigation appeared–the search for methods which could prevent the growth of scar tissue in a transected cord.

Scar Prevention and Substances Inhibiting Scarring

In order to exclude the growth of connective tissue between the ends of a transected cord, Davidoff and his colleague (Davidoff, 1951; Davidoff & Ransohoff, 1948) wrapped the stumps with a gall bladder or put them in gelatin capsules. However, under these conditions Davidoff and Ransohoff failed to notice growth of axons in cats. They concluded that poor growth potential of the intraspinal nerve fibers is the main cause of the failure of regeneration.

Another group of investigators wrapped the spinal stumps during transection with porous "Millipore" nylon membrane which allowed the flow of axoplasm but hindered the growth of scar elements. In experiments on cats and monkeys, this helped to give proper orientation of the growing fibers and the latter grew a few millimeters beyond the region of cleavage in cats. However, growth was limited when this procedure was used in monkeys. Restoration of function in these animals was not observed (Bassett & Campbell, 1962; Bassett, Campbell, & Husby, 1959; Campbell, Bassett, Husby, & Noback, 1957a; Campbell, Bassett, & Noback, 1957b; Campbell & Windle, 1960; Noback, Bassett, & Campbell, 1958).

Realizing the difficulty of inducing regeneration of normal axons and the necessity of helping hospitalized patients, neurosurgeons have been prompted to search for other methods of making connections between the separated spinal stumps. Thus, they tried to establish artificial anastomosis between nerves in the separated stumps of the spinal cord (Finikov, 1921). Efforts were also made to connect nerves supplying the posterior extremity with those originating from the proximal stump of a spinal cord (Bénes, 1958) and thus to innervate the femoral nerve from the intercostal nerve in experiments with dogs. These operations did not restore the function of the paralyzed limbs, probably due to the great technical difficulties associated with such an operation. Turbes and Freeman (1958) also used intercostal nerves for an anastomosis, taking them from above the level of transection and implanting them 2 cm below it. In 25 out of 30 operated dogs, 10–14 days after the implantation, there was restoration of the weight-bearing and the locomotor functions. Five dogs in this group were subjected to a transection of the implated nerve, as a result of which the restored functions were lost. Histologically nerve fibers and Schwann cells extended from the end of the implanted peripheral nerve to the distal segment of the spinal cord. In other experiments on cats, the tenth thoracic nerve was implanted into a proximal segment of the spinal cord. Though the results were not uniform, in some cats there was a restoration of function and histologically, a nice growth of fibers was noticed in both directions (Perkins, Babbine, & Freeman, 1964). These authors considered that there was a possibility of formation of neuronal connections in the spinal cord by the implantation of a peripheral nerve (Jacoby, Turbes, & Freeman, 1960).

From the experiments reported above, it is clear that there are two main problems in the regeneration of conducting axons in the adult mammalian central nervous system; first, the rapid formation of a dense spinal scar and second, the lack of growth potential of the CNS axons. What is the principle cause of the absence of regeneration? In order to answer this question, it is necessary to discover methods which will prevent the rapid formation of a dense spinal scar and then study the degree of regeneration which can be obtained in these conditions. Investigations aimed at these objectives were made both in the Soviet Union as well as in other countries.

Piromen

The appearance of pyrogens—the substances retarding the formation of a dense spinal scar—placed the problem in a new light. A great contribution in this direction was made by the work of a group of American investigators, headed by Windle. They conducted a series of experiments in which a bacterial polysaccharide Piromen, was used as a substance inhibiting the development of spinal scar formation, based on the idea that intraspinal axons are capable of growing but the pia-glia membrane is a serious physical obstacle to this growth. Even in the first experiments of Windle and Chambers, the results were very encouraging. In four out of the nine cats receiving Piromen, the pia-glial barrier was absent and instead they found a loose parenchymatous tissue through which the nerve fibers could grow. In one case, when the stumps of the transected cord were not separated during operation, the nerves and the root fibers grew through the area of the lesion. However, they did not report the restoration of function (Windle & Chambers, 1950, 1951; Windle et al., 1952; Clemente, Chambers, Greene, Mitchell, & Windle, 1951). Later, in an experiment on 18 monkeys, restoration of the foot movement was obtained in one of them (Windle, Litrell, Smart, & Joralemon, 1956). Clemente and Windle (1954) came to the conclusion that Piromen removes a major obstacle by preventing the rapid formation of a glial scar and fibroblastic proliferation and, thus, the intraspinal fibers have an opportunity to grow through the lesion area. These studies were restricted to the study of the morphologic picture of the damaged area. Though there was a significant difference in the nature of the scar formation in the animals receiving Piromen and in the controls, the growth of the fibers in the experimental animals was limited. Occasionally, individual fibers or a small bundle grew through the scar, but these may have originated from a root.

Electrophysiological experiments were conducted by Scott and his associate (Scott, 1955; Scott & Clemente, 1951, 1952a, 1955) with the idea of identifying the newly grown fibers. The possibility of nerve impulse conduction through the lesion was studied in animals whose spinal cord had been transected and was later subjected to histologic investigation. The experiments involved five out of eight treated cats, using fine electrodes having a tip diameter of 125 μ. Ascending fibers in the lateral column of the cord were stimulated 43 mm above the transection and it was possible to record action potential 30 mm below the level of transection. The amplitude of these potentials varied from 6–21% of normal but the rate of conduction was fully comparable with that in the proximal part of a cord. In isolated cases, stimulation of nerve bundles in the caudal segment of the spinal cord led to the appearance of action potentials in the cranial segment. They concluded that the central neurons could regenerate and regain the ability to conduct normal impulses. In one of their reports, Scott and Clemente (1952a) even made highly optimistic conclusions; they suggested that the use of Piromen and the proper realignment of the ends of a transected cord were essential requirements for regeneration of nerve pathways in the spinal cord. When summarizing his own extensive work on rats, Freeman (1955) similarly concluded that the administration of Piromen favors the growth of nerve fibers as it retards the development of a collagenous scar. Some of his experimental rats, which survived for a period of 216 days, possessed good coordinating movements which were abolished irreversibly after a second transection of the spinal cord.

Thus, the results of the American investigators on the regenerating characteristics of the spinal neurons using various approaches gave very hopeful results. However, Lance (1954) examined animals for a period of up to 173 days after transecting the pyramidal tract in the region of the brain stem in cats and subsequently administered Piromen but failed to notice conduction of impulses through the area of transection. Arteta (1956), on the other hand, confirmed the effect of Piromen on the formation of scars but noticed only an abortive growth of fibers through the lesion area during its use following hemisection of a spinal cord in cats. Thus, the question of the possibility of facilitating the regeneration of nerve fibers by the use of pyrogenic substances remained open to question.

Considering the important role of regeneration for the restoration of function after transection of the spinal cord, we also started working on this problem. In 1954, the work was started by Prof. Planel'es and P. Z. Budnitskaya of the Gamaleya Institute of the USSR Academy of Medical Sciences, on a suggestion of academician L. A. Orbeli. Subsequently, a bacterial lipopolysaccharide, Pyrogenal, was isolated which provided the possibility of actually investigating the problems of spinal regeneration.

Pyrogenal

Pyrogenal is a bacterial lipopolysaccharide isolated from the gram-negative cultures of *P. aeruginosa* or *S. typhossa,* by enzymatic hydrolysis of the microbial mass, followed by purification of the lipoplysaccharide with organic solvents (Budnitskaya, 1960, 1961, 1962). It is an active, protein-free pyrogen similar to Piromen and chemically it is related to dicarbonyl diphospho-serala lipopolysaccharide. Pyrogenal is nontoxic in clinically useful doses (Budnitskaya, 1965).

The bacterial lipoplysaccharides consist of a group of substances known as pyrogens because the pyrogenic response was the first of various biological reactions to be observed. At present, this group of substances is characterized, not only by their pyrogenic reaction but also by their reactions with white blood corpuscles.

The administration of lipoplysaccharides to an organism produces leukopenia, which is followed by leukocytosis. Subfebrile doses of pyrogens will not produce leukopenia but only leukocytosis, which is characteristic of the activity of such substances at this dose level (Budnitskaya, 1963).

The sensitivity of different types of animals to Pyrogenal varies, and to a certain extent it depends on the position of an animal in the phylogenetic order. Thus, man is more sensitive than horse, dog, and rabbit while rats are least sensitive.

The febrile reaction depends on the susceptibility of an individual animal; cases have been recorded where the febrile reaction was absent during administration of a very high dose (Budnitskaya, 1963). Since we were interested in the specific action of Pyrogenal, namely, its effect on the formation of a spinal scar, we will not discuss the pyrogenic response of pyrogens but mainly the similarities between them, which initially appeared in leukocytosis. The pyrogenic action of Pyrogenal was reviewed by Veselkin (1957).

Mechanism of Action of Pyrogens

It was demonstrated by Windle (1950) and Windle, Wilcox, Rhines and Clemente (1950) that prolonged administration of pyrogens stimulates extramedullary hematopoiesis. This effect involves the hypophysis, since the adrenal system of an organism when activated by pyrogens is responsible for the changes in white blood corpuscles (Braude, Vaisberg, Afanas'eva, & Givental', 1961; Eic-Nes, Demertion, Mayne, & Jones, 1957; Dzheksenbaev & Ozeretskovskii, 1964b; Engel, Brichant, Delmer, Vernet, & Rindel, 1957; Kinderling, Wöhler, & Westphal, 1953; Kirkendall, Hodges, & Jannary, 1951; Wexler, 1963; Wexler, Dolgin, & Tryczinsky, 1957; Windle, 1952). The removal of suprarenals lowers the leukocytic reaction which appears during the administration of pyrogens to a considerable extent (Mitchell, 1952; Mitchell & Stuart, 1951), and this reaction can be restored only after the transplantation of suprarenal tissue (Stuart, 1955). Hypophysectomy or the removal of other endocrine glands also produces some change in this reaction–reducing and delaying it for some time (Stuart, 1952). Thus, removal of the thyroid gland in rabbits failed to raise the body temperature which is partially due to a restriction of heat radiation during the administration of Pyrogenal (Dzheksenbaev, 1959). Histologic changes of the suprarenal glands were observed in all the animals receiving the lipoplysaccharide complex (Windle, 1950; Windle, Chambers, Ricker, Cinger, & Koenig, 1950; Windle, Wilcox, Rhines, & Clemente, 1950). Determination of the change in concentration of oxycorticosteroids during administration of lipopolysaccharide at a dose of 0.2 μg in man showed that this produced a rise in the level of oxycorticosteroids by 21 μg per 1000 ml of plasma (Brichant, Engel, Demanet, & Riondel, 1960). Administration of Pyrogenal alone to guinea pigs led to a rise of 17-free oxycorticosteroids which in duration and actions corresponded with the change which appears in response to administration of ACTH. However, this reaction was only noticed during the appearance of a febrile reaction to the Pyrogenal and accompanied changes in body temperature (Dzhedsenbaev & Ozoretskovskii, 1964a, 1964b). The results obtained by these authors to an administration of a small dose of Pyrogenal (0.1 μg/kg), in the absence of a febrile response, led them to suggest that the pyrogenic action of Pyrogenal is not a specific one but depends on the reaction to stress induced by a change of temperature. A similar view has been held by Eichenberger, Schmidhauser-Kopp, Hurni, Fricasay, and Westphal (1955a, 1955b) who reported that leukocytic changes should be considered as part of the general syndrome of "stress" reported by Selye (1950). However, other investigators think that the leukocytic change is specific in response to the stimulation of hypophysis (Wexler, 1963; Takebe, Setaishi, & Hirama, 1966). Veselkin (1965) has suggested that Pyrogenal should be considered as a specific stimulator although it has a number of other properties which are usually seen with stress-producing agents.

What changes in an organism are indicated by a significant increase in the number of leukocytes in peripheral blood? The role of leukocytes in wound healing was established long ago by the work of Carrel and Ebeling (1923, 1924); they liberate a nutritive substance—trephone. Khrushchev (1944, 1945, 1958) showed that trephone, which has a specific role in wound healing, is produced by the action of leukocytes during the breakdown of serum proteins. Developing this hypothesis, Shreder (1949) considered that the effect of trephone was associated with the acquisition of a new property depending on the ratio of products of the leucocytic enzymatic activity. The experiments, which were conducted with the idea of explaining the ability of leukocytes to participate in the synthesis of DNA, RNA, and protein, demonstrated that big and medium sized leukocytes participate in the above processes. The disintegrated lymphocytes and other agranulocytes provided the material for the above synthesis (Khrushchev, Skurskaya, & Zontak, 1966). Consequently, the leukocytes actively participate in the metabolism of nucleoproteins.

Structural changes in tissue during the formation of a scar also take place due to the continuous participation of leukocytes. Corresponding enzymes are necessary to split the mucoprotein (proteoglycons and glycosaminoglycons) of the connective tissue ground substance. The pyrogens have more affinity for the leukocytes and are quickly absorbed by them in the blood liberating some unknown substances which activate the fibrinolytic enzymes, converting the plasminogen to plasmin (Fibrinolysin). Later, the fibrin of the blood and the mucoproteins of the connective tissue ground substance are split (Eichenberger et al., 1955a, 1955b). For the formation of a more fragile connective tissue, the liberated chondroitin-sulfate should be split further into n-acetylglucosamine and hexuronic acids. This is carried out with the help of the enzyme, hyaluronidase (Garcin, 1955; Sundbland, Egelius, & Jensson, 1956).

Chondroitin-sulfate competes with heparin for hyaluronidase (Matthews & Dorfman, 1955). Decrease in the concentration of heparin allows the hyaluronidase to react with the chondroitin. The mast cells in connective tissue are the source of heparin (Asboe-Hansen, 1958; Fulton, Maynard, Riley, & West, 1957; Wichman, 1955) through disintegration of the granules, liberating heparin by the action of pyrogen; likewise the number of mast cells are also considerably reduced (Stuart, 1950). According to another opinion (Danilova, 1958), the cementing substance of connective tissue is considered as the source of heparin, to which it is bound. Hence, it could be thought that the amount of heparin is lowered by the action of pyrogens as a result of a change in the cementing substance and by a reduction in the number of mast cells. Thus, chondroitin is liberated from the bond of heparin by the effect of pyrogens and is hydrolyzed by hyaluronidase which favors the formation of a more friable connective tissue. The activation of histamine liberated from the mast cell granules, similarly, plays an important role, as it stimulates the action of hyaluronidase (Planel'es, 1965) in such a fashion that it loses its ability to act on heparin (Kaznacheev, 1960; Kaznacheev & Lozovoi, 1958) (Fig. 22). In the opinion of several investigators, heparin can inhibit enzymatic activity of cells and thus regulates their metabolism (Kaznacheev, 1965; Shurin, 1965).

If we consider that the permeability of the connective tissue ground substance increases under the action of hyaluronidase (Acadi, Dougherty, & Cohran, 1956; Kaznacheev, 1965) and if the above schematic diagram is correct, then the administration of pyrogens should increase tissue permeability. However, conflicting results have been reported. Thus, Eichenberger and his associates (1955) found that one hour after the administration of a pyrogen, the permeability increased but according to Vasil'ev and Saksonov (1957) it decreased, even within 15 min after the administration of Pyrogenal. The maximum decrease was observed after 3 hr.

Experimental Results:

Our studies (Iordanskaya & Nesmeyanova, 1960) of tissue permeability were conducted in rabbits by the use of two different xylol stains (Oivin & Monakova, 1953) and by the distribution of methylene blue (Muratov, 1960; Sergeev, 1954). We found that the capillary permeability was increased after a single administration of Pyrogenal at a dose of 10 μg/kg which produced febrile and leukocytic reactions. After an hour this increase amounted to 100 percent but within 2 hours it had started decreasing and at the end of 3–4 hours, reached a minimum which was equal to 50 percent of its initial value. After 5-6 hours and up to the first 24 hours, the capillary permeability continued to remain at a level below normal and then started rising. On the sixth day it reached a maximum which was equal to 200 percent of its initial value. The increased permeability, as indicated by methylene blue, was retained for a long time, say, for a period of 20–30 days after the administration of Pyrogenal. These observations confirmed both the results of Vasil'ev and Saksonov (1957) who noticed a decrease of permeability 3 hours after the administration of Pyrogenal and also the findings of Eichenberger and his group (1955a, 1955b) who demonstrated an early increase of

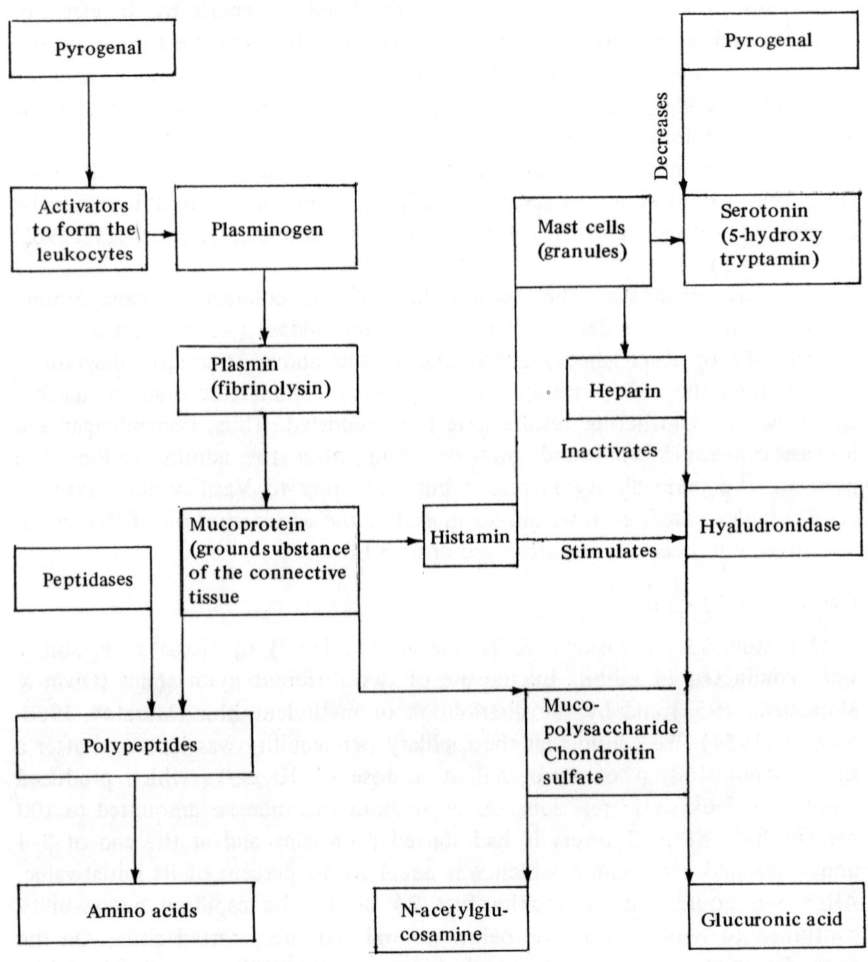

FIG. 22. A schematic diagram of the possible action of Pyrogenal on the ground substance of the connective tissue.

permeability after an hour. The uniformity of the results obtained by our two different methods permitted us to think that capillary changes did not significantly influence the results and the sequence of the changes in permeability was mainly due to the connective tissue ground substance. It seems probable that the decrease in permeability, during the first few hours after the administration of Pyrogenal, was due to the inactivation of the hyaluronidase by heparin which, as noted above, was liberated in large amounts from the disintegrated granules of the mast cells by this time. Subsequently, the significant and prolonged increase of permeability established by the methylene blue method is probably explained by a decrease in the number of mast cells (Stuart, 1952) as a consequence of their increased destruction. In this case, hyaluronidase was not inactivated by heparin and acted to split the chrondroitin-sulfate, thus causing an increase in tissue permeability. The cause of increased permeability in the first hour after the adminsitration of Pyrogenal remains unexplained; probably, some additional factors were responsible.

The activation of plasminogen, similarly, may take place by the action of other substances like trypsin, vitamins, corticosteroids, and catecholamines after their administration. An increase in the amount of corticosteroids in blood by Pyrogenal causes a depolymerization of the ground substance of the connective tissue, and a second additional chain reaction is established, changing the permeability of the tissues. Thus, the latter is changed by the action of Pyrogenal and it was found that even after a single administration of Pyrogenal, these changes were not uniform at different intervals of time, and may continue for nearly a month.

Dose of Pyrogens and the Frequency of Their Administration

The duration of the effect due a single dose of pyrogenic substance was reported by several investigators. Ginger and Windle (1952) found that hypertrophy of the thymus and lymphatic organs as well as secretion of adrenaline were continued for 2-5 days. In line with this, leukocytosis was observed up to 96 hours after large doses of pyrogenic substances (Wexler, Fachnrich, Weiss, & Grace, 1957). The results of Danilova (1958, 1961) showing the growth of fresh connective tissue in dogs, even as long as two months after the administration of a single dose of Pyrogenal, can be explained easily on the basis of the previous reports.

The duration of action of Pyrogenal may be related to the liberation of endogenous or secondary pyrogens, the presence of which was confirmed in several investigations reviewed by Sorokin (1965). It was found that contact of bacterial pyrogen with leukocytes or serum proteins leads to the formation of endogenous Pyrogenal. During the study of the action of endogenous pyrogens, it was suggested that the process of liberation of pyrogenic substances from leukocytes is an active one and enzymatic in nature. This was also confirmed by Kaiser and Wood (1962) and Sorokin (1964, 1965). However, in Planel'es opinion (1965), the prolongation of the action of Pyrogenal on tissue metabolism is provided by a bacterial pyrogen which, by itself, initiates a chain of complex reactions. The action of a large dose differs from a small one only by the rate and intensity of the reactions it initiates and not by the type of reactions. Hence, subfebrile doses may be equally effective.

There are many reports showing the beneficial effect of pyrogens in subfebrile doses. Greene and his associates (Greene, Stuart, & Joralemon, 1953) noticed a better survival of rats following hot cautery of the skin by the administration of Piromen at a dose of 0.51-0.73 μg/kg as compared to a dose of 2 μg/kg. Scott (1955) found that Piromen administered to spinal cats, at a dose of 0.6 μg/kg, led to a better regeneration of axons and restoration of function than a dose of 28 μg/kg. According to McCullough (1959), the optimum dose level of Piromen administered locally at the site of a transected rat sciatic nerve were the subfebrile doses of 0.5 μg/kg and not doses varying from 5-25 μg/kg, since the scar was more friable at the lower level. Freemen (1955) noticed a better restoration of function and survival of spinal rats after the administration of Piromen at a dose of 10 μg/kg and the worst results with administration of 15-30 μg/kg. Even a very small dose, 0.1 μg/kg, when administered to a rabbit, changed the tissue permeability after considerable delay following administration of Pyrogenal (Iordanskaya & Nesmeyanova, 1961). The good effect of subfebrile doses was attributed by the majority of investigators to the absence of associated adverse effects. It was reported that pyrogenic doses of the preparation caused accumulation of fluid in the peritoneal cavity and increased salivation, nausea, vomiting, etc. (McCullough, 1959; Selavry & Kraus, 1958). Neither the dose dependent action of pyrogens on the metabolic processes nor the question of whether an increase in the number of leukocytes is essential for initiation of the processes which may influence tissue permeability has yet been discussed. Judging from our findings (Iordanskaya & Nesmeyanova, 1961), tissue permeability may be increased without a leukocytic response, though to a lesser extent than in the presence of leukocytosis.

The greater effectiveness of subfebrile doses of Pyrogenal on the formation of a spinal scar, when compared to pyrogenic doses, was confirmed by experiments involving the administration of different doses of Pyrogenal, partially inside the area of a spinal lesion in rats (Nesmeyanova, Arnautova, Brazovskaya, & Nikityuk, 1965; Nesmeyanova, Iordanskaya, & Brazovskaya, 1963).

The relative influence of pyrogens depending on the frequency of their administration was not adequately explained. Tolerance to a pyrogen is developed slowly (Nesset, Ginger, & Byrne, 1951). Adaptation of the febrile reaction does not result from repeated application of pyrogens in high doses, but is developed quickly by the daily administration of small doses which facilitate the accumulation of large quantities of glutathiones in the operated animals and, in turn, suppressing the action of pyrogens on leukocytic metabolism (Stuart, 1955). After an interval of three weeks and with the administration of an increased dose, the febrile response can be fully restored (Beeson, 1947a, 1947b).

The action of a single dose of Pyrogenal was reflected in the condition of the subcutaneous connective tissue, two months after its administration (Danilova, 1961). The condition of scar tissue in the spinal cord of dogs receiving Pyrogenal differed considerably from that of the control animals after an interval of 6-15 months subsequent to administration (Brazovskaya, Nesmeyanova, & Iordanskaya, 1960; Nesmeyanova, Brazovskaya, & Iordanskaya, 1958). These findings corroborate the observations of other investigators (Wexler & Faehnrich et al., 1957).

Trypsin

In a number of investigations, trypsin was used as an inhibitor of the scarring process for comparison with the effect of pyrogenic preparations. Trypsin is a proteolytic enzyme which splits the denatured proteins in necrotic tissues but has no effect on living tissue. This lack of action by trypsin is due to the presence of specific inhibitors in living tissues, which suppress the action of the enzyme (Veremeenko, 1967). The high proteolytic activity of trypsin and its anti-inflammatory effect are used in the treatment of burns, thrombophlebitis, edema, and in other inflammatory processes (Golden, 1955; Klyle, Arnoldi, & Kupperman, 1957; Martin, 1955, 1957; Martin, Brendel, & Beiler, 1955; Raker, 1957; Stuteville, Lanfranchi, & Wallach, 1958). The results of work on this problem were reviewed by Veremeenko (1967). Martin is of the opinion that the ability of trypsin to reduce edema is due to its ability to depolymerize tissue by activating plasmin. However, Veremeenko doubts this and believes that the anti-inflammatory action of trypsin depends on its specific proteolytic activity.

Trypsin was used on dogs by Freeman and his associates as an inhibitor of spinal scar (Freeman, McDougall, Turbes, & Bowman, 1960) and they obtained the anticipated effect. Our preliminary experiments used rats with an injection of trypsin in doses of 0.15-2.00 μg/kg, after topical administration of the drug at the site of the spinal transections for the first ten days after operation. The observations were made during the next 2½ months. It was found that the scars of animals receiving small doses of trypsin were similar to those in animals which received Pyrogenal. They consisted of transverse fibroblastic bands with oval nuclei and a small number of thin collagen fibers between them. They contained a large number of macrophages and thin-walled blood vessels. The spinal scars of rats receiving a large dose of trypsin were rather compact (Nesmeyanova, Brazovskaya, & Arnautova, 1964a).

Hormones and Corticosteroids

Attempts to use other preparations for controlling the formation of a dense spinal scar were less successful than those with pyrogens or trypsin. Since Piromen increases the function of the suprarenal cortex in addition to its effect on the nature of scar formation, some experiments were conducted in which ACTH was used (Mitchell & Stuart, 1951; Windle, 1950, 1952; Windle & Wilcox et al., 1950). Others tried desoxycorticosterone (DOCA) which in some instances had an effect similar to that of Piromen. This suggested that it might be used as an inhibitor of the scarring process (Stuart, 1951a, 1951b). The work was conducted on cats, rabbits, and rats in which the proximal stump of a transected facial nerve was transplanted inside the brain (Clemente, 1952, 1955; Windle, Clemente, Scott, & Chambers, 1952). The purpose of these experiments was to find out whether regenerating peripheral nerves can overcome the glial barrier which is formed in damaged brain if scar inhibitors are present. The results of these experiments showed that, in animals receiving cortisone, as well as in controls, regeneration did not progress beyond the site of implantation. However, in the animals receiving Piromen and DOCA, the growing fibers extended beyond the site of implantation and grew inside the brain substance. The growth of the nerve fibers beyond the site of implantation was less prominent with ACTH alone than with administration of ACTH and Piromen together. However, the action of DOCA was not as successful as that of ACTH, since the collagen scar in the brain was found to be less permeable after 90 days, in animals which were treated with this substance, than in controls, although the pia-glial barrier was not involved (Clemente, 1958; Clemente & Windle, 1954). These findings were corroborated in the work of other investigators (Kogan, 1965a; Tabenhous, 1953). The mechanism of action of these substances on the nature of scar formation was not discussed by these investigators. It is quite probable that in the presence of DOCA or ACTH the active proliferation of fibroblasts may not result in failure of regeneration, but their later maturation and transformation into scar forming collagen fibers may not be inhibited, as occurs in the presence of Piromen. The mechanisms of action of ACTH, DOCA, and Piromen are similar: They all activate the hypophyseal-adrenal system and thus cause the proliferation of cellular elements. During the administration of pyrogens, new enzymatic processes may appear, particularly the liberation of hyaluronidase which depolymerizes the mucopolysaccharides, which tend to form the ground substance of the connective tissue.

The use of cortisone and hydrocortisone as the inhibitors of the scarring process failed to give uniform results. Markovich, Voinesku, and Markovich, (1958), using cortisone in the cerebral injuries in dogs, demonstrated that a fine network of collagen fibers with a small number of fibroblasts and a slight proliferation of glial tissues develops after a period of two months. The penetration of collagen fibers from the scar to neighboring brain tissue was not seen in a single animal. The American workers (Clemente, 1955; Windle & Clemente et al., 1952) using cortisone, on the other hand, obtained negative results which they attributed to a reduction in the proliferation of mesodermal elements (Clemente, 1958). The administration of hydrocortisone to cats after the hemisection of the spinal cord resulted in delayed wound healing and the reduced formation of the mesodermal scar (Ortiz-Galvan, 1955, 1956). In Kogan's experiments (1965a), the use of cortisone as well as ACTH led to the restoration of function in rats after a complete transection of the spinal cord. However, the percentage of animals with functional restoration was less than with the use of Pyrogenal. Experiments using cultured cerebellar tissue to inhibit the collagenous scar following transection have been reported by Kao, Shimizu, Perkins, and Freeman (1970).

Experimental Studies of Pyrogenal and Trypsin in the Regeneration of Intraspinal Axons

For these experiments, we transected the spinal cord in 52 mature young dogs at the level of Th_6-Th_{11} (Brazovskaya, Iordanskaya, & Nesmeyanova, 1959; Nesmeyanova, Brazovskaya, & Iordanskaya, 1960a, 1960b, 1961; Brazovskaya et al., 1960, 1962; Nesmeyanova, Brazovskaya, & Arnautova, 1964). In view of the fact that trophic changes of the tissues in the transected area of the spinal cord may be affected as a result of circulatory damage which could affect the experimental results, the anterior spinal artery on the ventral surface of cord was preserved during operation in some experimental animals (animals of the second and third group). In others, the artery was transected along with the soft spinal membrane (animals of the first group). Dogs of the *first* group received Pyrogenal while those of the *second* group received rhythmic stimulation as well as Pyrogenal: a total of 26 dogs belonged to these two groups. The *third* group of 10 dogs received trypsin, and the *fourth* group of 16 dogs served as controls. The Pyrogenal was administered at doses varying from 5-10 μg/kg and its effect was verified by noting the leukocytic response.

Pyrogenal was given intravenously in three dogs and intramuscularly in the rest. The only difference in the reaction was that leukocytic responses appeared somewhat later in the second case. Pyrogenal injections were given 5-6 times a week in the first month, on alternate days in the second month, and starting with the third month, 3 times a week followed by a rest for 7 days. In the experiments lasting for a longer period, Pyrogenal was administered for a period of nine months after operation. The daily administration of Pyrogenal in the first month was done to ensure an uninterrupted effect on the scar. Furthermore, when we started the work no data was available on the duration of action after a single administration. It was particularly important to obtain an uninterrupted effect in the first weeks after the operation when scar formation was taking place. Administration of the preparation on alternate days after the second post-operative month was considered essential as it was necessary only to retard the development of collagenous tissue during this period. Later in the experiments longer intervals were employed in order to prevent adaptation. Clemente et al. (1951) reported that an interval of up to two weeks caused an invasion of collagenous tissue in the area of section. Accordingly, we used seven-day intervals. The above program for the administration of Pyrogenal was not changed during the experiments in order to avoid complications when analyzing the results obtained from individual animals.

A daily dose of 0.15 mg/kg double recrystallized trypsin* was given to the dogs intramuscularly, following the day of operation, for 10-12 days. The usual post-operative care was given to all the animals, which were kept in wooden cages whose floor was covered with fresh sawdust. The dogs were examined on the 3d, 6th, 14th, and 30th day and in 3, 6, 12, and 26 months after the operation.

The morphological investigation consisted of longitudinal sections of the region of the lesion and in the parts of the spinal cord close to it. Sections were stained with hematoxylineosin or hematoxylin-picrofuchsin with fixation according to Cajal and Shtern-Beltskii's methods, while the argyrophillic fibers of the scar were treated according to Voight's method. Serial sections of the cord were also impregnated with silver according to Bielschowsky.

Tests for the Restoration of Function. Objective evaluation of the degree of functional restoration resulting from regeneration of conducting fibers in the spinal cord during chronic experimental conditions was rather difficult since there was no reliable test available. The usual method followed by American investigators was the electrophysiological study of conduction of excitation through the region of the lesion during acute experiments (Scott & Clemente, 1951, 1952a). We also tried this method in control animals and found that after an acute experiment the spinal cord had suffered to such an extent that further morphological examination was extremely difficult.

*Purchased from the "Nutritional Biochemical Corporation" with an activity of 124 units.

In the Soviet Union, various tests were adopted for use in chronic experiments (Barsegyan & Krivitskaya, 1967; Kogan, 1965a; Matinyan & Andreasyan, 1961; Musalov, 1965). Although subjective evaluation was not excluded in all these tests, they were unable to show signs of regeneration in a majority of cases. An interesting experiment by Matinyan, Andreasyan, and Epremyan (1965) recorded the evoked potentials in the sensorimotor area of the cortex, in response to a single electrical stimulus of the sciatic nerve in rats having a complete transection of the spinal cord. Such evoked potentials were observed in the experimental animals, despite the fact that the presence of a single fiber or a small fascicle of growing fibers may not always result in the appearance of evoked cortical potentials even when they make contact with neurons in the other part of the cord.

After a long search for dependable tests of functional restoration as a result of regeneration, we were left with only three tests which satisfied most of our requirements.

Test #1. The scratch reflex from the chest area, i.e., the area innervated by the proximal part of the spinal cord.

This reflex was consistently observed in normal intact dogs. Its receptive field was that part of the chest innervated by the supraclavicular nerve entering the spinal cord at the level of C_4. The afferent volleys are carried through the tract of Flechsig and Gowers to the cerebellum, and parts of the extra-pyramidal system in the medulla oblongata from where the impulses are carried back to the ventral root of the lumbosacral segments of the spinal cord along the rubrospinal and reticulospinal tracts. The reflex appears in the form of a rhythmic scratching movement by an extremity limited to the side which is scratched.

In dogs with transection of the spinal cord at the thoracic level, the receptive field of the scratch reflex is considerably expanded, covering the animal's back and sides (Kozak & Westerman, 1966; Krid et al., 1935; Sherrington, 1906), but the scratch reflex never appeared in response to scratching the skin innervated by the proximal segment of the spinal cord (see above). Even the appearance of a minimal scratch reflex, in the form of weak movements of the hind leg evoked by scratching the chest, might be an indication of restoration of impulse conduction along the path of this reflex. In order to facilitate the evoked response, the toe skin of the ipsilateral hind limb was subjected to weak, rhythmic stimulation once every 2 sec by an electric current. The weak flexor contractions evoked by electrical stimulation also influenced descending excitatory impulses to the neurons which produced the flexor reflex and, thus, could change the amplitude and even the character of the response.

Test #2. Restoration of the sensory response of the skin and the muscles of the posterior extremities, the sides and the sacrum was tested by noting the response of the dog to strong pressure and pin pricks.

In patients with spinal trauma, the recovery of sensation begins with a feeling of deep pressure in the muscles of the proximal joints, then with touch and, last of all, with the return of pain (Khurina, 1956). According to Razdol'skii (1952), the continued feeling of deep pressure in an extremity is a sign of the absence of anatomical transection of the spinal cord. Hence, in conditions of complete transection of the spinal cord, deep pressure sensation could be considered as a sign of returning propagation of excitation along the spinal axons. This test, involving the sense of deep pressure on the gluteal muscles and on the muscles of the thigh, was a principal method of determining the restoration of sensation.

Test #3. The stability of weight-bearing by the posterior extremities.

In spinal dogs, as already reported, the tone of extensor muscles was never constant. Increased activity of muscle receptors during pressure on the sacrum of a standing dog produces complete relaxation of the muscles. This is explained by the fact that overstimulation by pressure produces activation of the tendon receptors which neutralizes the activity of the muscle receptors. Only the restoration of supraspinal control will produce stable activity in these systems during standing.

In our first experiments, the weight-bearing stability of the animal was determined visually. In subsequent experiments, electromyograms of the gastrocnemius muscle were taken during the application of pressure on the sacrum of a standing dog. In intact animals, the electromyograms did not alter when pressure was applied, but in spinal animals, there was a gross change. Cortical activity might disappear completely or reappear at the time of applying pressure. The stability of the electromyographic pattern during the application of pressure on the sacrum of an experimental dog, served as an indication of the restoration of connections between the two segments of the spinal cord.

Formation of the Spinal Scar

In all the cases under investigation, a significant difference was observed between formation of the scar in experimental and control animals. This difference was seen within three days after operation. By this time, fine bands of differentiating cells of a fibroblastic nature were seen in the region of spinal section in the control animals (Fig. 23B). In contrast, organization of the spinal scar was not observed in the experimental animals during this period (Fig. 23A).

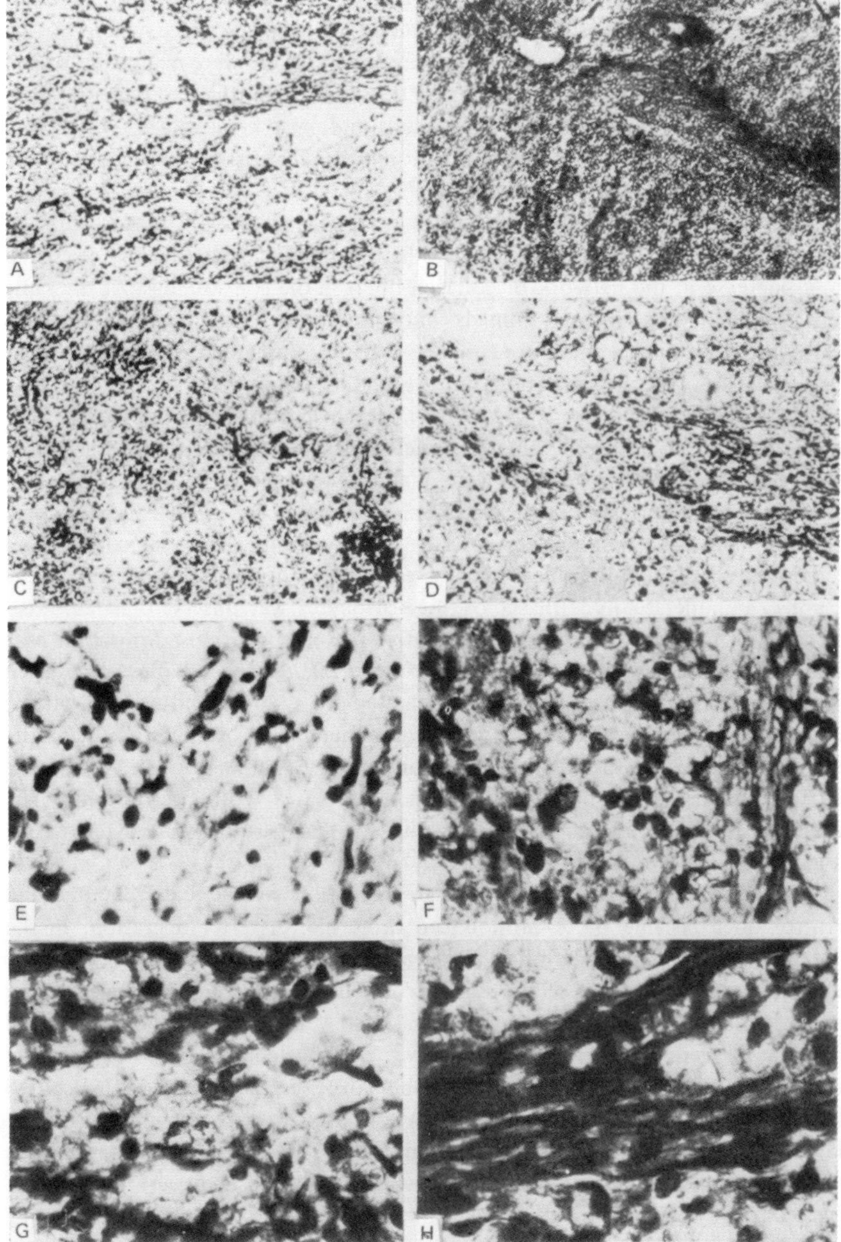

FIG. 23. Spinal scar of the experimental (left) and control (right) dogs in different periods after the operation.

A, B—after 3 days; C, D—after 6 days; E, F—after 14 days; G, H—after 30 days; Staining—hematoxylin-picrofuschin. Magnification: eye piece 10, objective 7 (rows 1 and 2 on the top); eye piece 10, objective 7 (rows 3 and 4 on the bottom).

After six days, the scar of the control animals showed a wide layer of connective tissue cells surrounding a blood clot in the place where a fine network of collagen fibers had already developed. There were many thin-walled blood vessels in the scar (Fig. 23D). At this same time, the experimental dogs only showed isolated collagen fibers surrounding a hemorrhage, which was accompanied by narrow bands of fibroblasts. The tissue continued to be penetrated by thin-walled blood vessels (Fig. 23C).

After 14 days, the progressive changes in the character of the scar in both the control and the experimental dogs were hardly significant and mainly consisted in an increase in the network of collagen fibers in the control dogs. At the same time, in all the experimental animals, only fine isolated bundles of these fibers were observed lying in the loose connective tissue. Numerous blood vessels were seen in the scar of the dogs of all groups (Fig. 23E, 23F).

A month after operation, there was little change in the nature of the scar in all experimental dogs so that the structural characteristics of the scar which were noticed after two weeks were mainly preserved (Fig. 23G). The fine bundles of collagen fibers were separated by a wide layer of cells containing a large number of macrophage cells as previously found. The scar contained a dense network of thin-walled blood vessels. In the peripheral part of the stumps, a moderate hyperplasia of the astrocytes was observed. In contrast, the control dogs in this same post-operative period showed the formation of a scar which had progressed significantly further. Thus, the bundles of collagen fibers had become denser and were separated by a corresponding thin narrow layer of loose connective tissue. In the peripheral part of the stumps, at the border of the scar tissue, there was a pronounced hyperplasia of the astrocytes and an astrocytic cell barrier was formed at places with interruptions. The number of blood vessels observed in the scar had already started decreasing (Fig. 23H).

The difference in the rate of scar formation in the experimental and control dogs became more pronounced three months after operation. In the experimental animals, a definite delay was observed in the development of the morphologic organization of the spinal scar. Though the number and thickness of the collagen fibers increased somewhat, the voids between them were still wide and were filled with connective tissue elements, including many macrophage cells. A considerable number of thin- and thick-walled blood vessels were seen in the scar (Fig. 24A). In the dogs receiving trypsin, the nature of the scar was more or less similar to that described above but the collagen bundles in it were, as a rule, wider and more compact. The scar of the control dogs contained thick spiral bundles of irregularly branching collagen fibers. Unlike the scar of the experimental dogs where the collagen fibers were stained pinkish red with picrofuschin, here they were stained bright red. Occasionally, a narrow layer of loose connective tissue was seen in

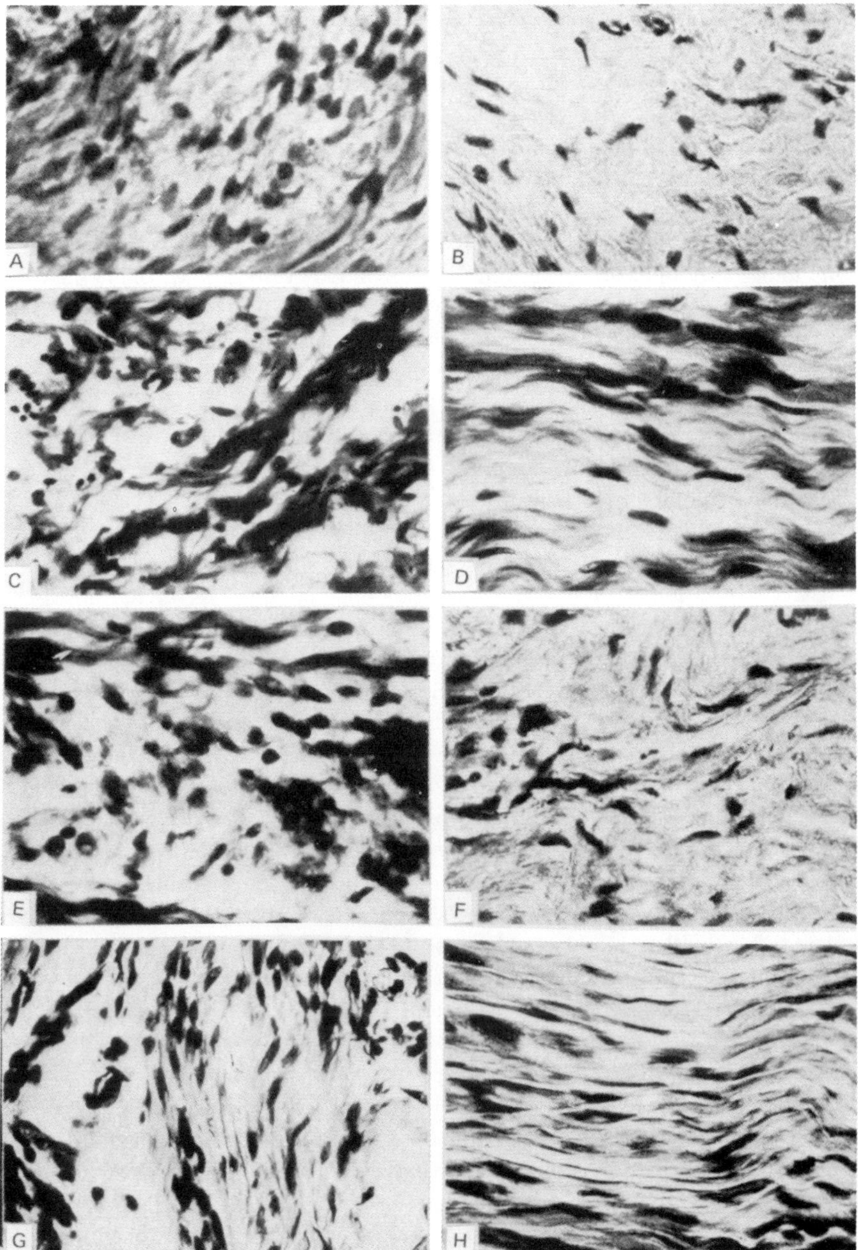

FIG. 24. Spinal scar of the experimental (left) and control (right) dogs in different periods after the operation.

A, B–after 3 months; C, D–after 6 months; E, F–after 13 months; G, H–after 26 months. Staining–hematoxylin-picrofuschin. Magnification–eye piece 10, objective 40.

which macrophages were absent. Only a small number of blood vessels were seen in the scar (Fig. 24B).

The delay in the rate of organization of the scar in the dogs receiving Pyrogenal appeared more clearly at a later date, e.g., 6, 12, or 26 months after operation. Six months after operation, the changes in the scar of the experimental dogs of the first and the second groups were insignificant, when compared with a three-month old scar. Even wider gaps in the networks of the bundles of collagen fibers were filled with connective tissue elements containing macrophages. The number of blood vessels was only slightly reduced (Fig. 24C). The scars of the experimental dogs of the third group still contained a small amount of loose connective tissue situated in the gap between the wide and compact bundles of collagen fibers.

In the region of spinal section in the control animals, the central and the peripheral zones of the scar were clearly identified by collagen fibers running in a parallel direction. The fibroblasts were situated between these groups of fibers. The blood vessels were absent in the scar tissue. There was a pronounced hyperplasia of the astrocytes in the peripheral part of the stumps (Fig. 24D). Twelve months after operation, only slight progress was observed in the organization of the scar of an experimental dog. As in the previous case, the relatively wide layer of loose connective tissue containing fibroblasts in the different stages of maturity was differentiated into histiocytes and a small number of macrophage cells. Thin- and thick-walled blood vessels were seen traversing the loose layers between bundles of collagen fibers and along the same bundles in the central part of the scar (Fig. 24F). In the control animals, the scar was further deprived of cellular elements during this period. The intervening gap between the loose connective tissues disappeared, the bundles of collagen fibers were oriented transverse to the axis of the spinal cord, where they were intertwined, and the nuclei of the fibroblast cells were markedly flattened. The vessels in the scar, generally, disappeared, leaving only isolated thick-walled blood vessels close to the spinal membranes (Fig. 24F).

A similar picture of slower scar formation with the use of Pyrogenal was seen as late as 26 months after operation. The direction of the collagen fibers in the central part of the scar was longitudinal to the axis of the spinal cord, which we never observed in the scar of control animals. This orientation certainly favors the growth of nerve fibers (Fig. 24G). The region of spinal section was replaced by a gelatineous scar in a control dog in this post-operative period, where the direction of collagen fibers was exclusively transverse (Fig. 24A).

It is well known that spinal scars following transection are formed mainly by proliferation of the cells of spinal membranes which penetrate the region of the lesion and form a layer in a direction transverse to the axis of the spinal cord. The proliferation of astrocytes is also of great importance and is responsible for the formation of a glial barrier separating the spinal stump from the region of the lesion. According to Clemente and Windle (1954), the glio-mesodermal membrane which has already been formed in the peripheral part of the scar by the 3rd day after transection of the spinal cord, consists of glial and connective tissue fibroblasts cells in various stages of differentiation which form a compact barrier by the 30th day. This membrane is absent in animals treated with Piromen and the formation of a coarse collagenous scar originating from the tough internal layer of the spinal membrane is considerably inhibited by this means.

From these observations, it appears that Pyrogenal significantly slows the rate of organization of the scar. Collagen fibers were still arranged in isolated bundles and loose connective tissue in the scars of dogs receiving Pyrogenal 13 and 26 months post-operatively and fibroblasts were found between them at different stages of maturation. The blood vessels in the form of capillaries were preserved during these periods.

However, when comparing our data with the results obtained by the American investigators who used Piromen (Clemente & Windle, 1954), a substantial difference was observed. In our experimental dogs, the proliferation of fibroblasts (connective tissue cells) continued, but their differentiation was delayed for a considerable period under the action of Pyrogenal. Similarly, the astrocytic reaction was very pronounced in the control animals but was delayed considerably by Pyrogenal and in all cases was less marked than that reported by Clemente and Windle.

The cause of delay in the astrocytic hyperplasia might have been due to better circulation in the region of the lesion in experimental dogs due to the formation of a capillary network. Snesarev (1946) has reported that hypoxia stimulates astrocytic hyperplasia which is always observed in a developing scar. The delay in the differentiation of fibroblasts and proliferation of astrocytes results in the scar being formed more slowly, and becoming more friable. This is in contrast to the results from the control dogs, where the collagen fibers in connective tissue were often arranged in a direction transverse to the axis of a spinal cord.

The positive influence of Pyrogenal on the formation of a spinal scar has also been observed in experiments on rats. In these experiments, the effectiveness of Pyrogenal was compared with a number of substances, especially with several pyrimidine derivatives (Kogan, 1965a, 1967). The appearance of the scar tissue and the functional restoration in experimental animals at different post-operative periods were improved with Pyrogenal. In addition to formation of a more friable scar, the collagen fibers were directed either irregularly or longitudinal to the axis of the spinal cord during the administration of Pyrogenal, and this favored the growth of nerve fibers along them. Pyrimidine derivatives cannot act as an inhibitor of scar formation, since they are responsible for the stimulation of RNA synthesis and favor the proliferation of fibroblasts and astrocytes and in this way hasten the condensation of scar tissue. Similar results have been reported by Kogan (1967).

In our experiments, trypsin, which was expected to inhibit the formation of a scar, was found to be similar in action to Pyrogenal, but only in its initial phases. After longer post-operative intervals, the action of trypsin ceased and the scar formed at the usual rate (Nesmeyanova, Brazovskaya, & Arnautova, 1964a).

Comparing the action of Pyrogenal and trypsin as inhibitors of the scarring process, Matinyan and his associates found a greater effectiveness for trypsin, particularly when compared to preparations containing hyaluronidase (Matinyan & Andreasyan, 1961; Matinyan, Andreasyan, & Epremyan, 1965). In the experiments of these investigators, crystalline trypsin was injected intramuscularly in the later post-operative stages after the rats had been treated with lidase. One and one half months, post-operatively, complete restoration of motor function was reported in the majority of animals (Matinyan, 1964, 1965). Histochemical investigation of the region of transection demonstrated a considerable decrease in the concentration of acid mucopolysaccharides in the ground substance of the connective tissue, 8–10 months after operation (Matinyan & Sarkisyan, 1965).*

Taking into consideration the specific action of trypsin, particularly its ability to split only the nonvital neural tissues, it is difficult to conceive that the use of trypsin could be particularly effective during the later stages post-operatively. In our own experiments, we found it to be inactive one month after operation, as we expected. It is possible that in Matinyan's experiments the success of the treatment was mainly due to lidase, which might have influenced scar formation. In fact, in the work of Oganisyan and Matinyan (1964) it was reported that the use of lidase with Pyrogenal in clinical practice, when administered by the subdural or subarachnoid route, gave the expected results. This suggests that the inadequate effect of trypsin in our experiments might have been due to its mode of administration. In the experiments of Freeman and his colleagues, much better results were obtained by subdural administration of this product (Turbes & Freeman, 1953). However, the same authors, comparing the action of both inhibitors of the scarring process, came to the conclusion that Piromen is more effective than trypsin (Gokay & Freeman, 1952).

From material which has been presented, it can be concluded that Pyrogenal has a number of advantages over other inhibitors of scar formation. It retards the formation of spinal scars in the early post-operative periods, as demonstrated by several clinical studies; it is also highly effective in eliminating the after-effects of the scarring process in the spinal cord and

*Martinian and Andreasyan (1976), *Enzyme Therapy in Organic Lesions of the Spinal Cord.* (English trans.)

other tissues at a late stage (Batkin, Petrov, & Frolov, 1965; Bogdanovich & Palamarchuk, 1965; Kogan, 1961, 1965a; Koptsiovskaya, 1965; Lubenskii, 1965; Patskikh, 1961, 1965; Selezneva, 1965; Selezneva & Drize, 1965; Vysheslavtseva, 1965; and others). The administration of Pyrogenal after an abdominal operation retards the development of peritoneal adhesions (Galkin, 1966; Galkin & Sorokin, 1966). The capillary networks are preserved for a considerably longer period in the region of the lesion by use of Pyrogenal in comparison to control cases in which the tropism in the stumps of a transected spinal cord was intensified.

It has been suggested that the presence of more capillaries in regenerating tissue increases the degree of tissue oxidation, and produces an acceleration in differentiation of cellular elements in the connective tissue which causes the scar to become condensed (Leites, 1945). This process is changed with a pyrogen, since the differentiation of the cellular elements is delayed considerably even in the presence of capillaries.

Thus, Pyrogenal initiates a chain of complex tissue reactions which are maintained by intracellular processes through the liberation of endogenous pyrogens. Tissue permeability is increased when the formation of mucopolysaccharides, the maturation of fibroblasts, and the proliferation of astrocytes are delayed, and thus help in the formation of a more friable spinal scar. The capillaries developed in the scar and lying in the area close to it provide a nice trophic stimulus to the growing nerve fibers, instead of hampering them.

Significance of the Blood Supply in the Reorganization of the Damaged Area

The formation of a gap in the region of a spinal section creates a serious obstacle in the path of growing axons. Preservation of the anterior spinal artery at the time of operation had a beneficial effect on the amount of necrosis and appearance of the gap between the stumps.* As a rule, the gap was smaller, and this produced conditions more favorable for the growth of axons through the lesion (Nesmeyanova, Brazovskaya, & Iordanskaya, 1963).

By comparing the character of the necrotic zone in dogs which had been subjected to different procedures (the first and second groups), it was observed that this zone was mainly composed of granules with markedly vacuolated bodies which displaced the oval nuclei into the periphery in animals of both the groups. In the dogs of the second group (Pyrogenal plus stimulation), the size of the necrotic zone was 1-2 mm in the cranio-caudal direction. This dimension may be as great as 6 mm in the animals of the first group.

*Study of the chemical characteristics of local schema after spinal cord trauma has shown the effect of steroids on potassium depletion (Lewin, Hansebout, & Pappius, 1974).

Fourteen days post-operatively, small gaps were formed in the necrotic zone and partially filled with an accumulation of round granules. The difference in gap size among animals of different groups was still negligible.

One month after operation, the difference in gap sizes and in the character of their formation could be clearly seen in dogs of different groups. While there was little change in dogs of the second group, the animals of the first group (unstimulated) already showed gaps with smooth walls which practically separated the stumps from the spinal scar (groups described p. 95).

Three months after the operation performed on dogs of the first group, the size of the gaps often reached 5-7 mm in the cranio-caudal direction and were very extensive. In the spinal cord of dogs of the second group (stimulated plus Pyrogenal), the gaps were also completely formed, but they never reached more than 3 mm in size. After 12 months, the gaps had only changed a little in this latter group but at the same time they had increased to 7-8 mm in the animals of the first group.

Several investigators have suggested that the cause of the formation of gaps in the necrotic zone is due to an impairment of the trophic response of tissue (Aleksandrovskaya, 1955; Bakulev, 1935; Stepanyan-Tarakanova, 1959; Yakovelev, 1956) and this is in agreement with our data. Even in an intact spinal cord, occlusion of the abdominal aorta leads to its degeneration (Turren, 1936). The size of the future gaps will be related to the size of the necrotic zone six days after transection when the arteries are severed.

The Growth of Nerve Fibers and Restoration of Function

Regeneration of axons and restoration of function were not observed in our experiments without the use of Pyrogenal. This supported the conclusion of a number of investigators that regeneration of axons in the untreated mammalian central nervous system was only abortive (Brown & McCouch, 1947; Cajal, 1928; Gorodinskaya & Minut-Sorokhtine, 1948; Rossi & Castaldi, 1935; Samarin, 1926; Windle & Chambers, 1950).

Histologic investigation of growing nerve fibers two weeks after operation demonstrated that the character and the rate of growth were similar in the experimental dogs of all groups. Growing nerve fibers were seen in an area adjacent to the injured zone of the stumps. They grew up to the scar in small numbers with irregular shapes filled with protoplasm, bulging here and there (Fig. 25). After a month, a small number of nerve fibers in the terminal parts of the stumps reached up to the scar in the control dogs, whereas they penetrated the scar in all experimental groups (Fig. 26). There was no restoration of functions in the experimental animals during a period of two months post-operatively.

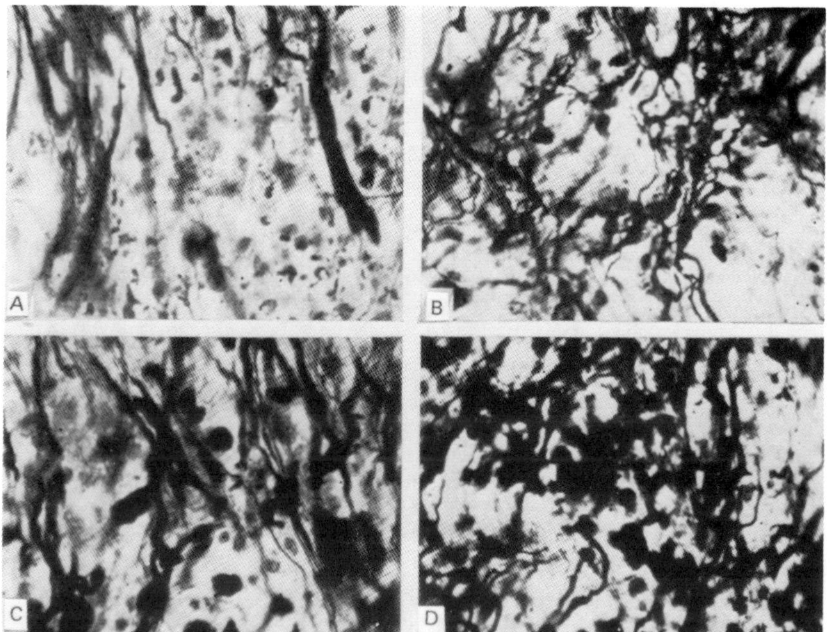

FIG. 25. Character of growing nerve fibers in dogs of different groups two weeks after operation.

A–Pyrogenal treated (first group); B–trypsin treated (third group); C–Pyrogenal treated plus rhythmic stimulation (second group); D–untreated control (fourth group). Silver impregnation. Magnification: eye piece–10, objective–20.

Examination 2 and 2½ months after operation showed that restoration of a weak scratch reflex took place in only one experimental dog of the second group after 2½ months, but response to the test of sensation did not appear in even a single animal. A weak scratch reflex appeared in 5 out of 11 experimental dogs after 3 months and a poor sensitivity to pain was noticed in 2 of them. The scratch reflex was absent in all control animals (Fig. 27).

Of the four dogs receiving trypsin, the scratch reflex and response to sensation returned in only one animal.

Histological investigation of the spinal cord of eight experimental and control dogs three months after operation demonstrated growth of nerve fibers in the scar of the experimental animals, as reported above. In two dogs of the second group, isolated nerve fibers penetrated through the scar to the opposite stump. In four experimental dogs and in all the controls, nerve growth was not observed through the scar.

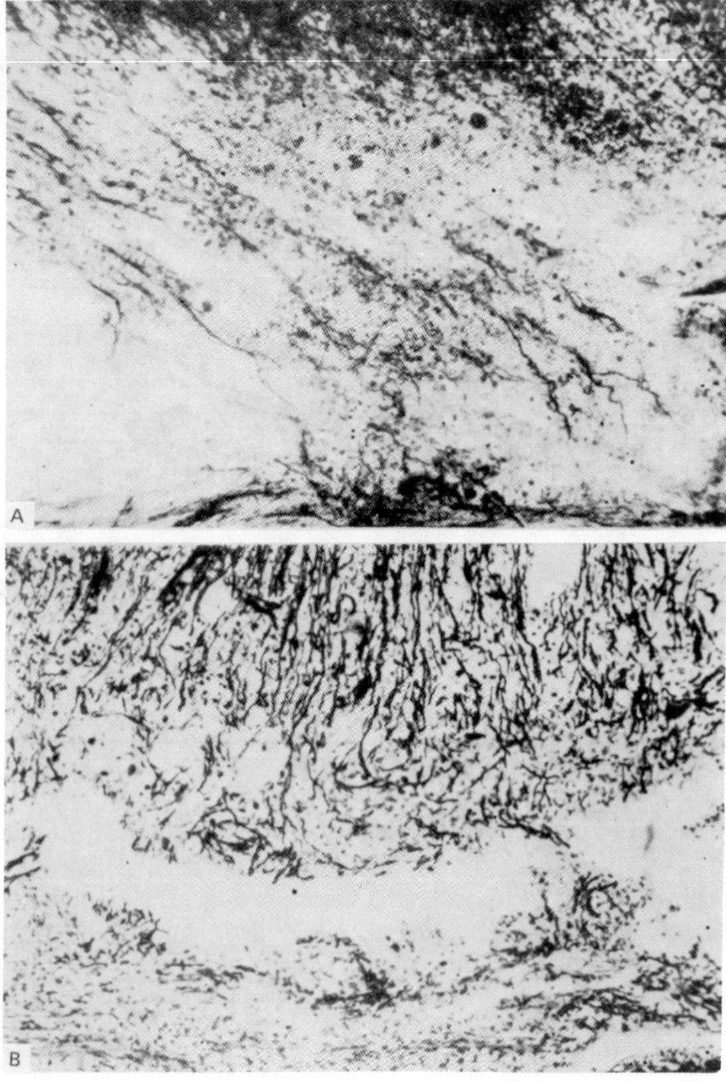

FIG. 26. Growth of nerve fibers toward the scar one month after the operation.

A–in dogs of the second group (Pyrogenal treated plus stimulation); B–in dogs of the fourth group (control). Silver impregnation. Magnification: eye piece–6, objective–9.

Five to six months after operation, the scratch reflex became better developed in the majority of the dogs receiving Pyrogenal and often appeared without the application of rhythmic stimulation (Fig. 28). In one animal, this

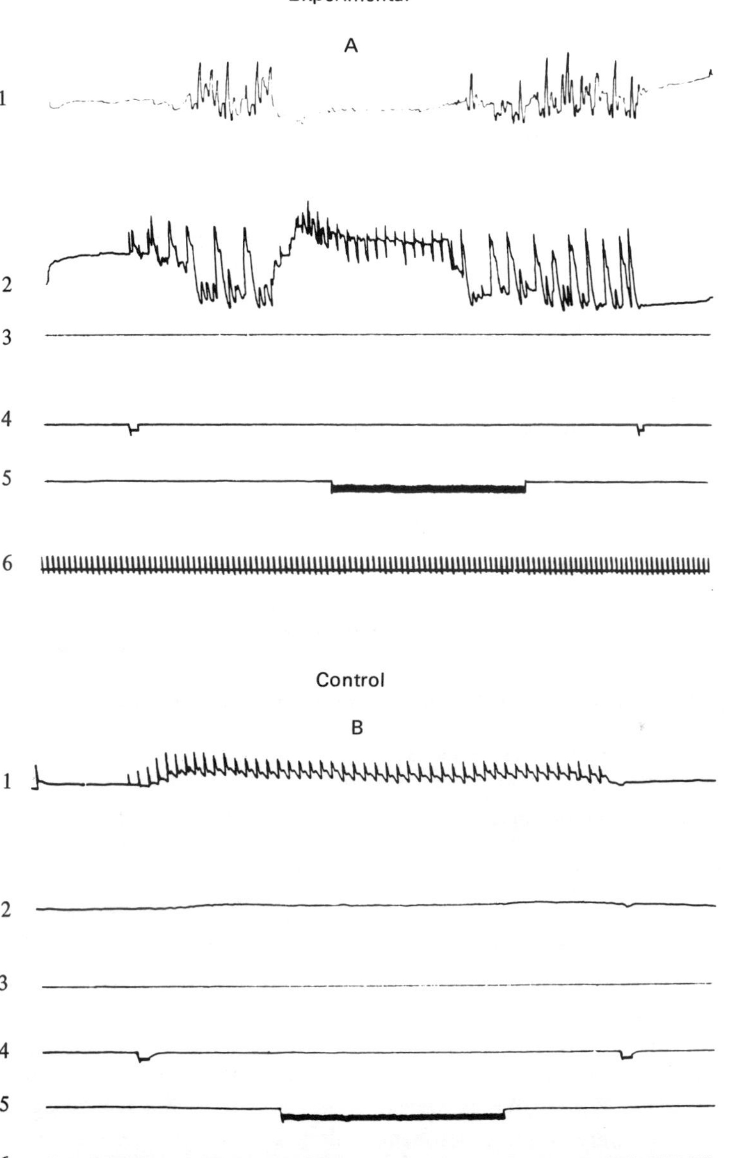

FIG. 27. Scratch reflex in experimental (A) and control (B) dogs in presence of a rhythmic stimulation of paw, 3½ months after operation.

1–movement of the ipsilateral (B) and the cotnralateral (A) extremities; 2–movement of the contralateral (B) and the ipsilateral (A) extremities; 3–movement of the tail; 4–mark of electric stimulations; 5–mark of scratching; 6–time, 1 sec.

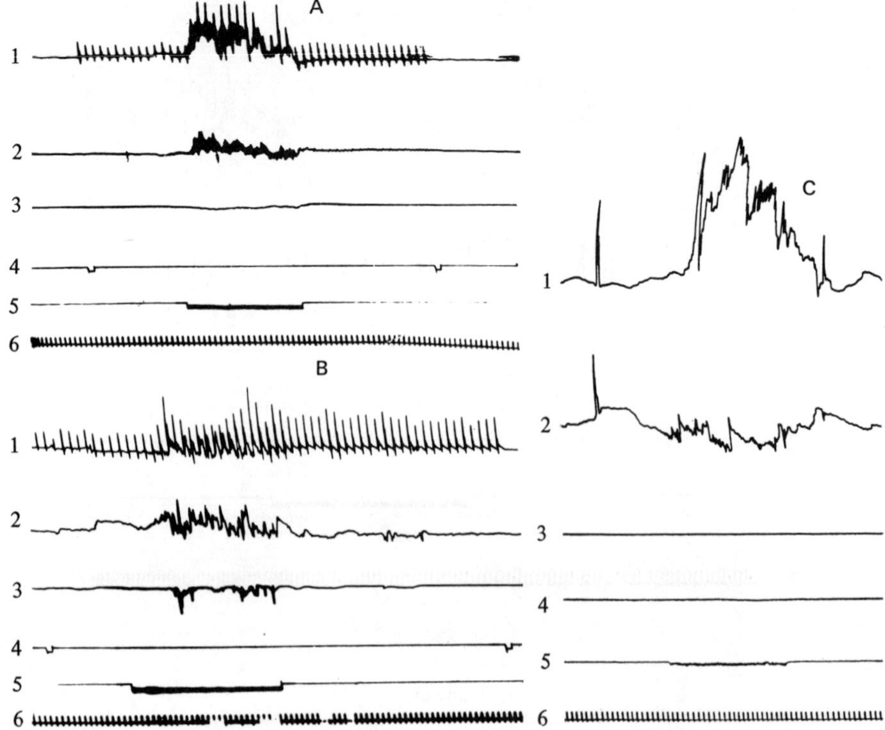

FIG. 28. Scratch reflex in experimental dogs in the presence of a rhythmic stimulation of the paw (A, B) and in the absence (C) six months after operation.

1–movement of the ipsilateral (B) and the contralateral (A) extremities; 2–movement of the contralateral (B) and the ipsilateral (A) extremities; 3–movement of the tail; 4–mark of electric stimulations; 5–mark of scratching; 6–time, 1 sec.

reflex barely emerged during this period, but the sensory response to pressure in some experimental animals was very prominent (Fig. 29A, 29B). The scratch reflex and sensory perception did not appear in a single case among animals of the control group.

The dogs receiving Pyrogenal and subjected to treatment, as a rule, possessed well developed muscles of the extremities and often were able to activate them (Fig. 30A). However, comparatively stable weight-bearing was observed in only one experimental dog during this period (Fig. 30B). Dystrophic changes of muscle were not pronounced in the absence of treatment in the dogs receiving Pyrogenal (Fig. 30C), but this was a characteristic feature of all control animals (Fig. 30D, 30E).

The penetration of isolated nerve fibers across a lesion to the opposite stump was demonstrated histologically, in dogs which had shown functional

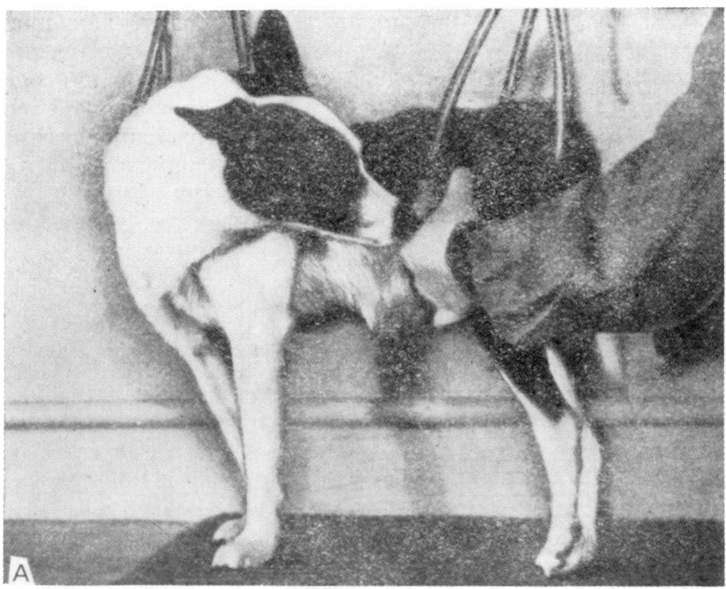

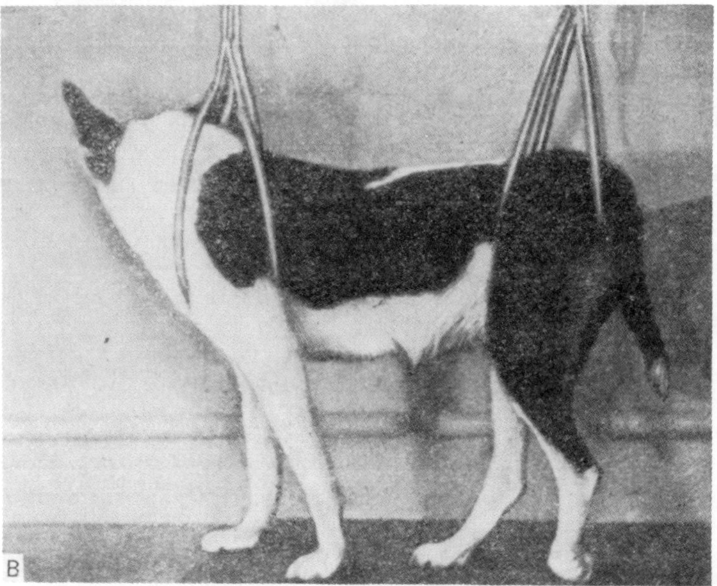

FIG. 29. Reaction of the experimental dogs to pressing of the muscle of the thigh. A–in the left hind paw; B–in the right hind paw.

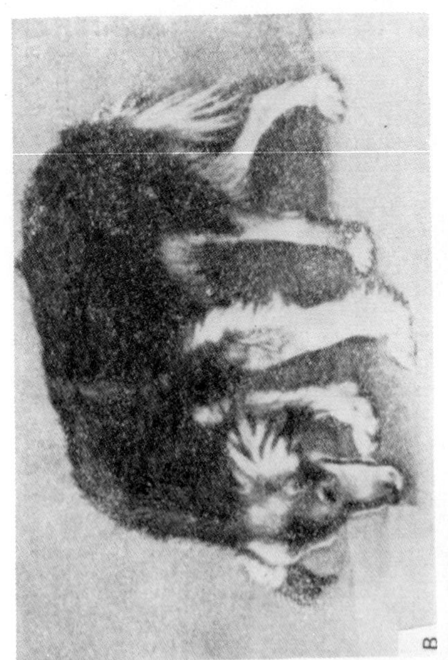
B

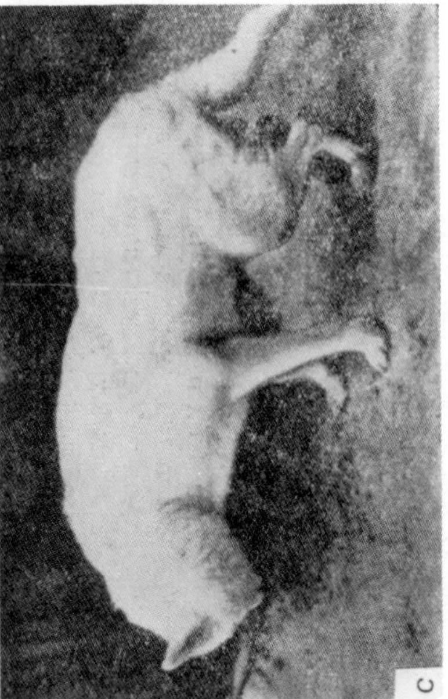
C

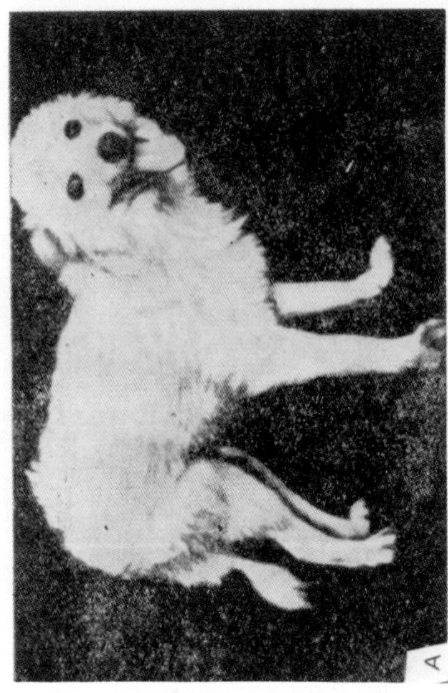
A

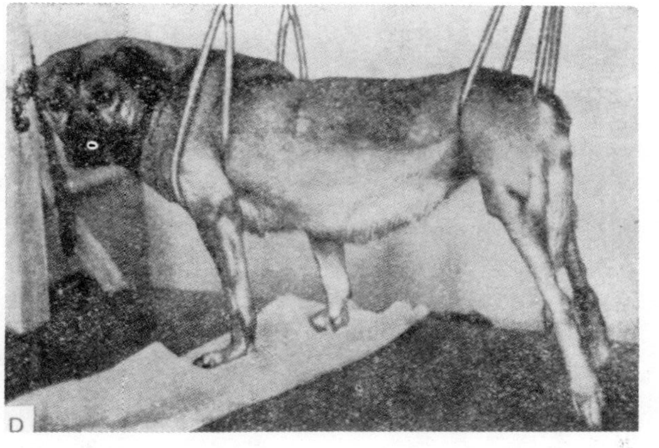

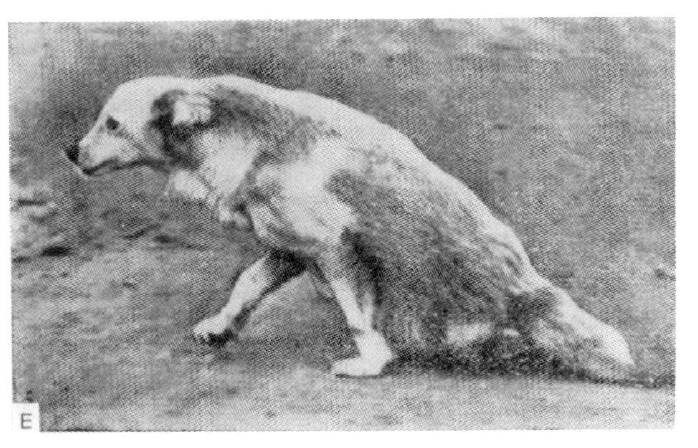

FIG. 30. Treated (A, B) and untreated (C) experimental dogs, as compared with treated control dogs (D, E).

recovery six months after cord transection. This occurred only in those places where the collagen fibers penetrated the friable connective tissue in a direction parallel to the axis of the spinal cord. As the collagen fibers were primarily arranged in a transverse direction, the growing nerve fibers seldom reached the opposite stump (Fig. 31). As a result, regeneration of nerve fibers through the scar was not observed in those animals where function was not restored.

More or less similar results were obtained during examination of dogs 12 months after operation. Functional restoration, which had been observed 3 to 6 months after operation, remained during this period.

Histologic examination demonstrated the presence of isolated nerve fibers growing through the region of section in dogs of the first group and also small groups of fibers in the dogs of the second group. The growing nerve fibers, as a rule, were closely associated with the blood vessels or with the collagen fibers of the friable connective tissue (Fig. 32A). When large gaps occurred in the lesion area of the spinal cord in dogs of the first group, this often obstructed the growth of fibers through the area.

Nine months after the first operation, a second spinal transection was made in two experimental dogs and one control dog one segment below the previous site. The functions which had been restored after the initial transection in the experimental dogs were lost, but in the control animal the increased tone of the extensor muscles was quickly restored, even after the second transection, and consequently, this could not have depended on the conduction of impulses along regenerated nerve fibers. This control experiment to a certain extent validated the tests selected for determining the restoration of function as a result of regeneration. In an experimental dog with considerable restoration of function which survived for 2½ years post-operatively, retrograde changes started after 15 months and a typical paralysis developed within 2 years. Histologic examination of this dog did not show growing nerve fibers; instead there were signs of degeneration of newly grown axons (Nesmeyanova et al., 1960a). American investigators have similarly observed the reversal of restored function in Piromen treated dogs, 12 to 18 months after operation. They believed that the cause of this fiber degeneration was due to pressure exerted by the associated scar (Littrell, 1955; Windle, 1956). It is possible that along with the pressure exerted by the scar, impairment of the trophic response of tissue was an important factor in the development of degeneration. This response might later hamper the myelination of axons and make them more sensitive to an unfavorable environment.

The delay in formation of a dense scar in the region of a spinal section under the influence of Pyrogenal was very important. This, in fact, decided the intraspinal growth of the axons, since the growth of nerve fibers in our

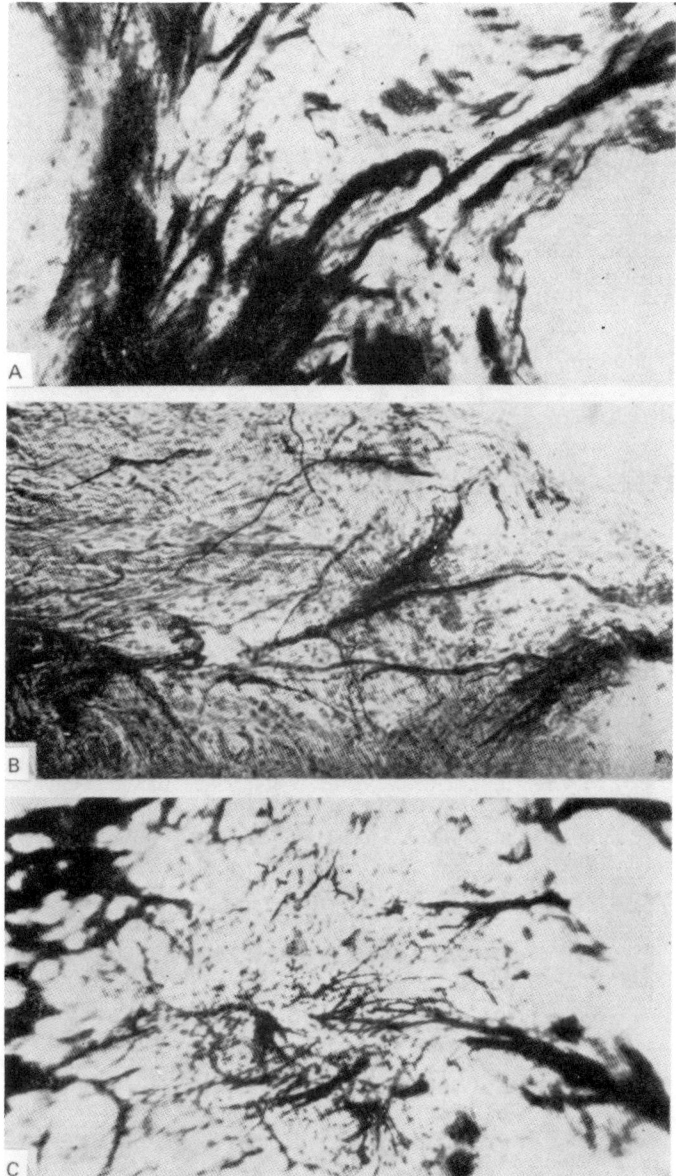

FIG. 31. The growth of nerve fibers in the area of cord section in dogs six months after operation.

A–first group (Pyrogenal); B–second group (Pyrogenal plus stimulation); C–third group (trypsin). Silver impregnation. Magnification–A (eye piece 40, objective 7), B, C (eye piece 20, objective 7).

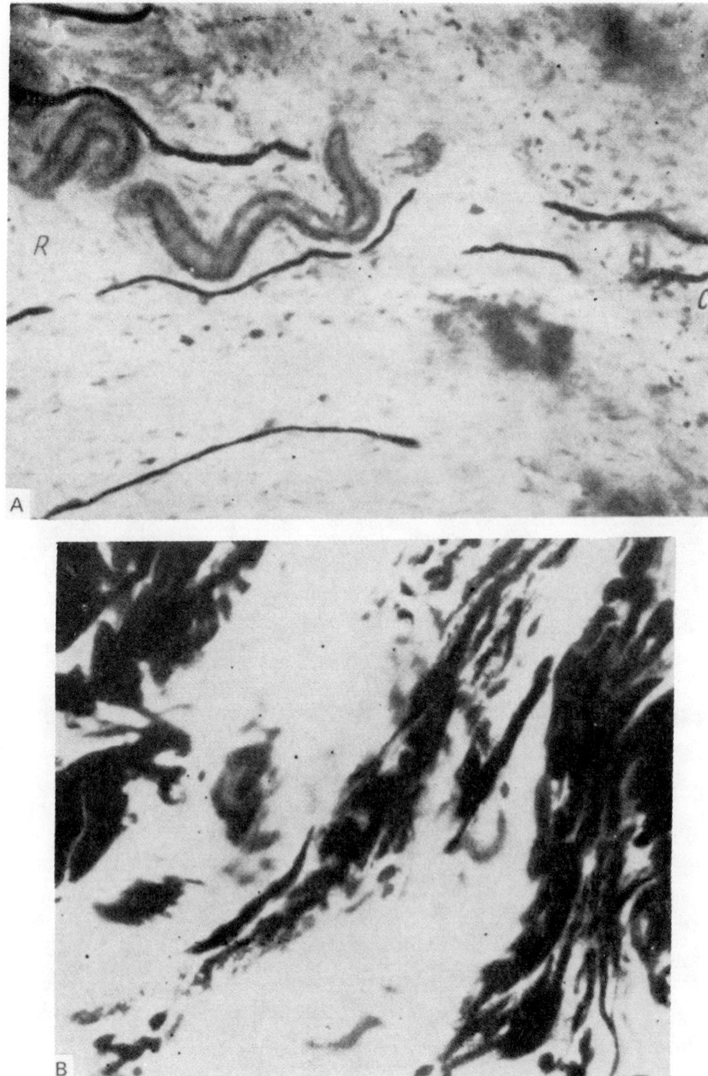

FIG. 32. The growth of nerve fibers along blood vessels and collagen bundles in dogs treated with Pyrogenal.

A–after 13 months; B–26 months after operations. Silver impregnation. Magnification: A–(eye piece 20, objective 10); B–(eye piece 40, objective 10).

experiments started only a week after operation, when the formation of a scar had already been established. This opinion is also supported by the result of Yakovleva (1956).

Our experiments on the appearance of the sensory and motor function (scratch reflex) as well as weight-bearing by the hind legs indicate that the growth of fibers takes place both from rostral as well as caudal stumps of the spinal cord: Thus, the fibers belonging to the descending and ascending systems of the spinal cord may both be restored. We failed to show the selective growth of the fibers in either of these systems as reported by Yakovleva (1956).

Restoration of function was not observed in the experiments of Windle and Chambers (1950, 1951) when spinal cats were given Piromen. In later work, restoration of muscle tone, reflex activity, and sometimes even coordination in movement of the extremities were present in the experimental animals. Restoration of sensation was not recorded in a single case (Littrell, Bunnell, Agnew, Smart, & Windle, 1953). Our experiments demonstrated that the motor reflexes, the muscle tone, and even the ability to move the hind limbs unsteadily in forward movement often depended on effective treatment of the animals by electrostimulation and therefore, never served as a dependable sign of regeneration. This was established more convincingly by Scott and Clemente (1951, 1952a) who recorded the conduction of impulses through the region of section.

The difference between experimental and control animals in the development of motor functions largely disappeared 12 to 18 months after operation (Littrell, 1955; Windle, 1956), which is in agreement with our findings. These authors reported that the development of a dense fibrous scar led to degeneration of the nerve fibers which had previously regenerated, and, as a result, the motor functions which had initially recovered, subsequently disappeared. We observed reversal of these functions and the degeneration of the nerve fibers in the scar of an experimental dog, 18-24 months after operation. It is possible that administration of Pyrogenal at less frequent intervals than we adopted would have been more effective than the method used by the American investigators. Our evidence indicates that Pyrogenal was more effective than Piromen. In an experimental dog which was kept under observation over a long period of 26 months, the histologic picture of the scar was similar to that of control dogs, 13 months after operation. It is possible that an inadequate trophic response might have hampered myelination of axons and been a further important factor in development of the degenerative process in growing axons, in addition to the mechanical pressure exerted by the scar. These factors might have made the axons more sensitive to an unfavorable environment.

Even the slight recovery of function obtained with Pyrogenal in dogs having a spinal transection demonstrated the possible viability of the newly grown axons.

There are major differences in the mechanism of functional recovery based primarily on either neural regeneration, or on the effect of compensatory treatment of spinal animals. When regeneration was present, normal function returned to a slight extent, based on conduction of excitation along the spinal cord through the damaged area.

It is interesting to investigate the possibility of formation of synaptic contacts by regenerating nerve fibers and to follow their development.

The Formation of Synaptic Connections by Regenerating Nerve Fibers in the Spinal Cord

The following studies investigated the restoration of conducted excitation along a spinal reflex arc after transection and subsequent regeneration of a dorsal root, the purpose being to examine the dynamic changes involved in the formation of new synaptic terminals (Bernstein & Bernstein, 1973; Illis, 1973a).

Several investigators have shown how these may be formed by the regenerated terminals of the preganglionic sympathetic fibers. Regeneration of synaptic knobs was observed after transecting preganglionic fibers of the cervical sympathetic ganglion and subsequent restoration of conduction 44 days post-operatively in cats (Gibson, 1940). In this case the contacts formed by the regenerating fibers were selective; the fibers in S_1 connected only with the cells of S_1, etc. The rate of conduction was decreased although the synaptic delay was only increased to 4 msec as compared to 3 msec observed in control animals.

The possibility of formation of heterogenous synapses was investigated by Baron (1935) who conducted the following experiment: Dorsal roots were transected in the sacral region of the rat spinal cord and their central stumps were sutured to the central stump of a transected sciatic nerve. After two to three months, stimulation of the central segment of the sciatic nerve produced movement of the tail. Histologically, the presence of immature synapses among the neurons of the ventral horn of the spinal cord was observed. Thus, the central end of a peripheral nerve was found capable of growing inside the spinal cord and of forming synaptic connections with its neurons. It was established by Lavrent'ev and his associates (Fedorov, 1934; Lavrent'ev, 1934a, 1934b) that during heterogenous regeneration the character of a synapse is determined by the recipient neuron, i.e., the formation of synapses depends on the functional characteristics of the innervated cells. Even the mechanical contiguity of the growing axons with a nerve ganglion, partially fixed in alcohol, causes the appearance of synapses which later die due to inactivity Fedorov (1935a). The live neurons attract substances closely related to enzymes which are liberated by growing axons and stimulate their growth. The possible ramification of neurons inside a ganglion was reported by Fedorov (1935b) in the same manner as the ramification of a peripheral neural sprout and was shown to contain several neurons.

These results suggest that regenerating central axons when approaching a neuron form synaptic vesicles. Indirect evidence concerning the formation of synapses was provided by electrophysiological investigations of Thulin (1960) who recorded by inserting an electrode in the ganglion and showed that the latent period of the response after stimulation depends primarily on the synaptic delay. The partial restoration of motor function that was demonstrated also proved that synaptic contact was made by regenerating fibers.

Histologists have tried to follow the growth of fibers and the formation of synapses after the transection of a dorsal root and noticed that the pia-glial barrier obstructed the penetration of fibers into the spinal cord (Moyer & Kimmel, 1948; Moyer, Kimmel, & Winborne, 1953). However, it was found that the regenerating fibers which were able to overcome this barrier and penetrated inside the spinal cord continued to grow in the substance of the central nervous system (Illis, 1973b). From this it may be concluded that the environment inside the spinal cord was favorable for the growth of axons (Kimmel, 1955).

To overcome this scar-like barrier, the central stump of a transected dorsal root was transplanted within the spinal cord. For this purpose, a small longitudinal incision was made in the dural membrane and the root fibers were inserted under the membrane in the area of the ventral horn. As a result of this procedure, it was found possible to elicit muscle contraction in response to stimulation of the transected dorsal root after 1 to 1½ years. Histologically, synapse-like structures could be seen with special stains but structures on the neurons of the corresponding area from control animals only took the usual stains. Without this artificial transplantation, the restoration of motor function was not possible (Turbes & Freeman, 1961).

Investigation of the recovery of conduction in a spinal reflex arc following transection and subsequent regeneration of a dorsal root was conducted on rats weighing 150–170 gm and comprised two series of experiments (Arnautova & Nesmeyanova, 1964, 1966). In the first series (Ia) of experiments, the dorsal root fibers in L_5 or L_6 were transected 3 mm proximal to the ganglion in one group of animals. In the remainder of the animals (Ib), the same fibers were sectioned just before entering the spinal cord. In both cases, the cut ends were joined together and were wrapped with a fibrinous membrane which was fixed with a drop of liquid adhesive (BF-8) or sutured with thread. Fixation of the transected ends gave hope that the growing fibers from the root might follow the old framework of Schwann cells.

In our second series (II) of experiments, the dorsal root was not transected but crushed with fine forceps in order to preserve the membrane. Whether the pressure was complete or not was determined by noting the transparency of the membrane. These experimental procedures were such that the preparation of the roots for subsequent acute experiment was considerably easier. All the operated rats received injections of Pyrogenal at a dose of 10 μg/kg daily during the first month, then on alternate days, and later 3 times a week, followed by a rest for 7 days.

In the first series (Ia and Ib), 17 rats were operated for chronic study and in the second series (II) 40 animals were selected for an acute experiment following a period from 3 days to 8 months after initial operation. To prevent the movement of the lumbosacral region of the spine, during the preparation and operation the rats were fixed in a special stand with the help of two rods running through the chest and lumbar regions. After laminectomy, the dorsal and the ventral roots of L_5 and L_6 were exposed. The exposed roots were sectioned near the ganglion excepting those previously transected which were sectioned lateral to the previous transection.

Method

In order to investigate the condition of a damaged reflex arc, the following acute experiment was performed. The dorsal roots of L_5 or L_6 were stimulated by rectangular impulses through bipolar electrodes. The electrical response was monophasic in the L_6 ventral root but rarely in L_5 which was recorded with bipolar electrodes having a distance of 6 mm between them. The response from the neighboring reflex arc (usually DL_5-VL_5) served as a control where the dorsal roots were left intact. The potentials were photographed from the screen of a cathode ray oscillograph during a single trace. An alternating current amplifier UBP 1-01 was used to record the potentials from the surface of the spinal cord using a circular electrode at the place of entry of the dorsal root.

Results

The results of these experiments indicated that during an early phase (from the first to the third days of our investigation) monosynaptic responses were not recorded from the ventral root during stimulation of the dorsal root transected between the ganglion and the spinal cord; however, polysynaptic responses of small amplitude with a greater latent period than in the control were observed. Later, beginning with the fourth day and up to 2½ months after operation, no responses appeared in the ventral roots by dorsal root stimulation (Fig. 33). This observation is in agreement with the reports available in the literature showing the development of degenerative changes in a reflex arc (Kostyuk & Savos'kina, 1959; Vera & Luco, 1958). This

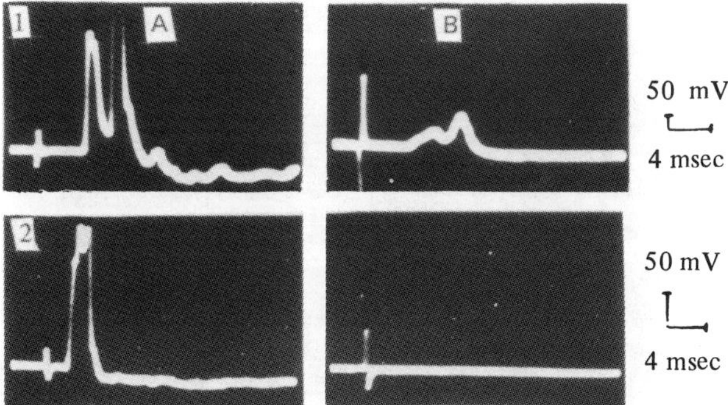

FIG. 33. Ventral root potentials evoked in response to stimulation of the dorsal root after its transection.

A–control side; B–transected side. (1) second day and (2) fourth day after operation.

degenerative process first affects the more delicate structures–axon terminals (De Robertis, 1959; Wedell & Zander, 1951) but within 48 hours after operation, the synapses became swollen and within 72 hours were transformed into an irregular mass (Gibson, 1940; Pchelina, 1951). According to Illis (1963, 1964), this degeneration is noticed not only in the synapses of the transected fibers but also in the neighboring intact ones. The absence of impulse propagation in a damaged reflex arc from the third day up to a period of three months, demonstrates that, in fact, there is no restoration of synapses by the irreversibly, damaged fibers. The presence of regenerating fibers was essential for synapse formation.

Recovery of impulse conduction in a damaged reflex arc was observed from the third month after operation. When this first appeared, the potentials were ansynchronous and their amplitude was smaller than the control. As a rule, they consisted of individual peaks having different latent periods and only in isolated cases did these potentials resemble a typical polysynaptic response (Fig. 34). The latent period of the response was considerably increased in a damaged reflex arc. In normal circumstances, the latent period during stimulation of an intact dorsal root varied from 1.2–2 msec, but during stimulation of the regenerating fibers and recording from the ventral root of that particular segment, it was increased to 4–12 msec.

At a later stage of investigation (5½ to 8 months after operation), the recorded potentials were more synchronous with greater amplitude than those recorded in the early stages. However, the latent period was still considerably longer and, on the average, was 6.5 msec. In the experiments where only monosynaptic peaks were recorded, the latent period varied from 2–3 msec or, in other words, it was very close to those recorded in normal cases (Fig. 35).

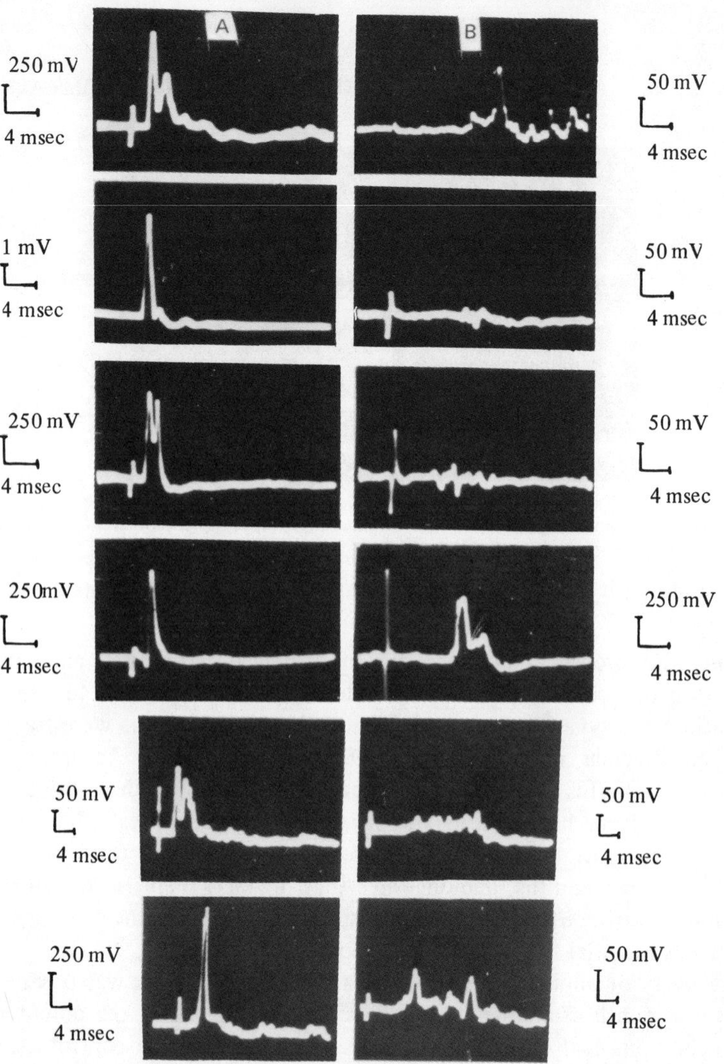

FIG. 34. Comparison of the character of the electrical activity recorded in the ventral roots in respose to stimulation of (A) an intact and (B) a post-operated dorsal root.

Latencies and thresholds of the evoked potential of the responses at different time intervals after surgery (3–5 months post-operation).

No. row	Time interval after surgery (months)	Latencies/msec		Thresholds/v	
		Column A	Column B	Column A	Column B
1	3.0	1.3	7.7	0.5	2.0
2	3.5	1.2	8.8	0.5	0.5
3	3.5	2.0	4.0	–	0.5
4	3.5	1.6	6.0	0.5	1.5
5	4.5	2.0	4.5	0.5	1.0
6	5.0	2.0	12.0	0.5	1.5

Stimuli applied to A and B in a given experiment were always equal.

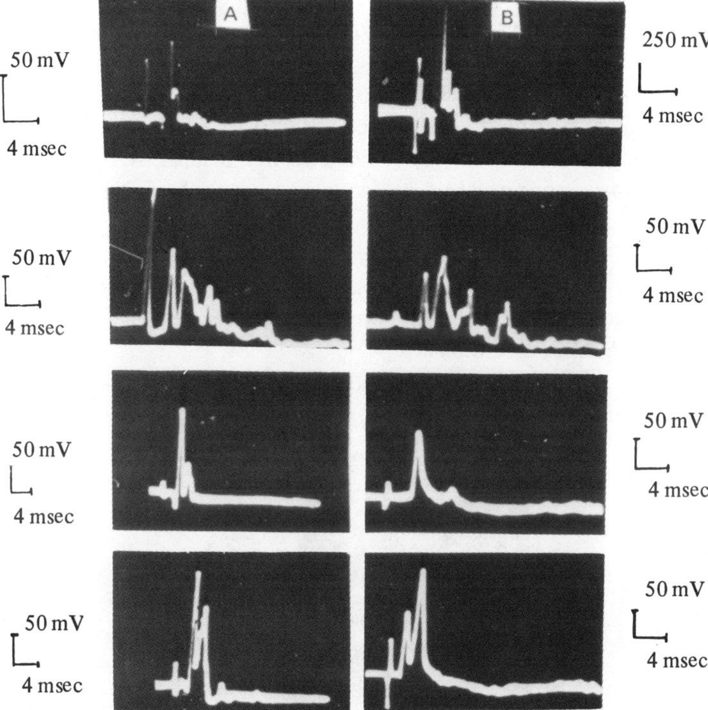

FIG. 35. Comparison of the character of electrical activity recorded in the ventral roots in response to the stimulation of an intact dorsal root (A) and a dorsal root, 5½ to 8 months after operation (B).

Latencies and thresholds of the evoked potential of the responses at different time intervals after surgery (5–8 months post-operation).

No. row	Time interval after surgery (months)	Latencies/msec		Thresholds/v	
		Column A	Column B	Column A	Column B
1	5.5	2.1	2.1	0.5	6.0
2	5.5	2.0	6.5	0.8	1.5
3	5.5	2.0	6.4	0.6	4.5
4	7.0	2.0	2.0	0.5	4.8

Stimuli applied to A and B in a given experiment were always equal.

The mean arithmetic difference between them was 1.7 ± 0.93, msec where $P > 0.05$, i.e., the difference not being statistically significant.

When the latent period of the different parts of the reflex arc was determined by stimulating the dorsal root and recording from the ventral root, it was found to vary from 4–12 msec. By comparison, the latency of the potentials recorded from the surface of the spinal cord in response to dorsal root stimulation varied hardly 0.1 msec (Fig. 36).

If the dorsal root in a rat was crushed severly instead of transected, it was possible to record monosynaptic peaks within a period of 3½–5 months after operation (Fig. 37). The duration of the latent period was 3.6 msec (varied from 2.4 to 9.0 msec, on the average, i.e., it was considerably shorter than in the rats having a transected dorsal root during the same period). Statistical evaluation demonstrated that this was significant when compared with the control ($x = 3 \pm 0.99$; $P < 0.05$).

In the damaged reflex arc, threshold of stimulation was 2–3 times that of the control. The electrical activity recorded during the recovery of conduction

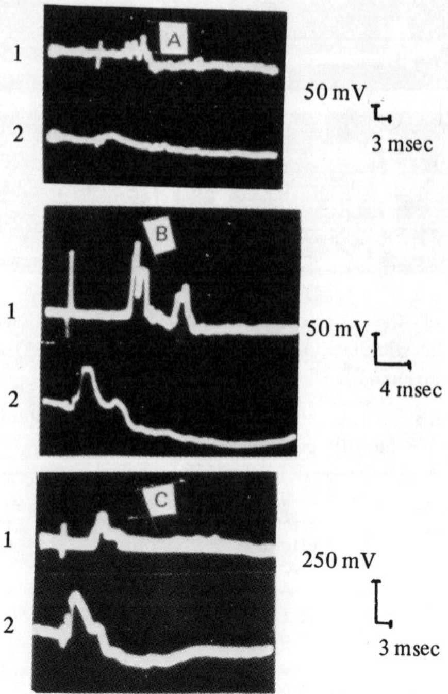

FIG. 36. Comparison of the latent period of a response recorded from a ventral root (1) and from a dorsal surface of the spinal cord (2) when evoked by dorsal root stimulation.

A–4 months; B–5½ months after transecting the root; C–3½ months after crushing the root.

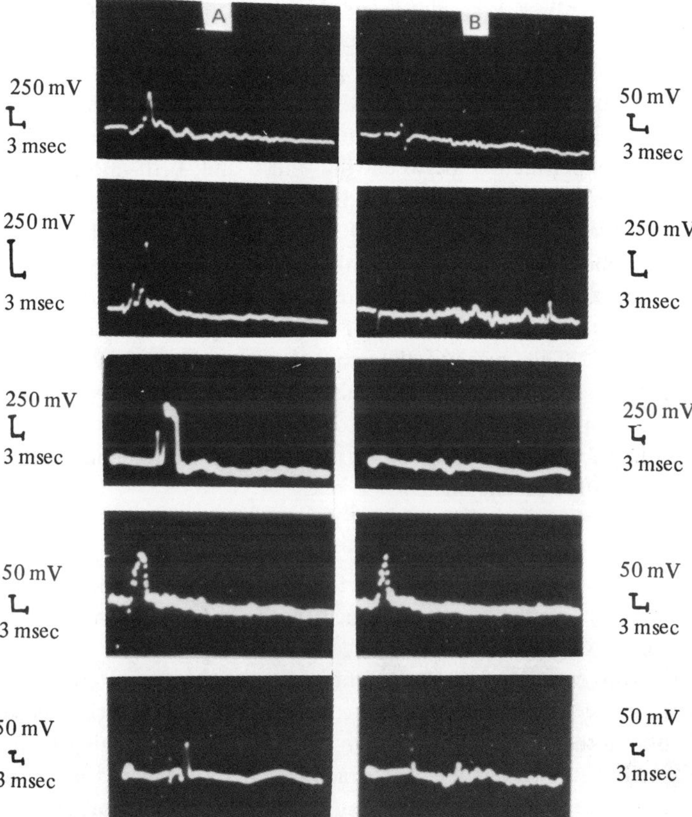

FIG. 37. Electrical activity recorded from a ventral root in response to dorsal root stimulation (3 to 5 months after crushing the dorsal root).

A–control side; B–crushed side.

Latencies and thresholds of the evoked potential of the responses at different time intervals after surgery.

No. row	Time interval after surgery (months)	Latencies/msec		Thresholds/v	
		Column A	Column B	Column A	Column B
1	3.5	2.4	3.0	–	–
2	3.5	1.5	9.0	–	1.6
3	3.5	1.1	6.6	1.1	16.5
4	4.0	2.0	2.4	0.62	1.0
5	5.0	1.8	4.4	1.6	3.1

Stimuli applied to A and B in a given experiment were always equal.

was characterized by a very short latent period in the afferent part of the reflex arc, i.e., it was exclusively related to the time involved in synaptic transmission. This fact, along with the polysynaptic character of the response, indicates that the synaptic contact of the growing fibers in this particular case probably took place through interneurons. The characteristic feature is that, in a number of experiments, between the third and fifth month, the polysynaptic response appeared with individual spikes having different time intervals, possible due to an absence of synchronization in synaptic activity or to the involvement of a smaller number of synapses. After a longer postoperative interval, the nature of the response and the duration of its latent period were, as a rule, changed and gradually resembled that recorded from an intact reflex arc. This suggests the gradual restoration of synaptic endings, possibly due to an increase in the number of new synapses or to a rapid liberation of a large quantity of mediator through the membrane forming new synaptic endings. The possibility of formation of a spontaneous contact with motoneurons cannot be excluded.

The high percentage of recovery and the earlier appearance of a response in the experiments where the roots were crushed indicate that this method of damage was more favorable than the transection, for the regeneration of a dorsal root. These results are in agreement with other investigators (Gutmann, 1942; Gutmann & Sanders, 1943; Falin, 1962).

Results from experiments where the roots were transected at different intervals from the ganglion lead to the conclusion that transection close to the point of entry into the spinal cord is considerably more damaging than section near the ganglion. However, less retrograde degeneration would be expected in the first case since more axoplasm is left in the transected root, and this is an important factor for preventing the development of degeneration, according to the results of Liu (1955). The severity of trauma caused by the lesion is indicated not only by an absence in restoration of impulse transmission in a damaged reflex arc, but also there was a reduction in the reflex conduction of neighboring segments in a large number of cases. It is possible that the failure of other investigators to obtain regeneration of a transected root was principally due to severe trauma, the causes of which are not clear.

We have observed an area of scar in which the growth of protoplasmic threads were oriented in the direction of an intact root and entered the spinal cord along with it, but we are uncertain about their origin. It is possible that they originated from Schwann cells, growing with the nerve fibers and later making contact with the cell bodies. It seems probable that they were coming from intact root fibers, as a compensation for tissue damage similar to that noted by a number of investigators in the case of dorsal roots (Kostyuk, 1962; Liu & Chambers, 1955) and spinal axons (McCouch, Austin, Liu, & Liu, 1958) which is known as "sprouting" (Bernstein & Bernstein, 1973). There is another possibility: The transected root may cause the growth of nerve fibers from its own ganglion which do not grow along the old framework of Schwann sheaths but rather in a new one formed by the protoplasmic threads growing in the direction of the intact roots.

In one of the experimental rats the spinal ganglion of a transected dorsal root was removed. After three months, no branching of the fibers in the root was noticed (Arnautova & Nesmeyanova, 1966). This led to the conclusion that branching occurred from the transected root and not from the neighboring ones, i.e., there was regeneration of the damaged root fibers rather than sprouting. It follows from these results that in spite of the abortive nature of the growth of intraspinal axons in mammals, the use of Pyrogenal produces regeneration, however insignificant it may be, by inhibiting the rapid formation of a spinal scar. The neural circuit is completed by making synaptic contact with individual regenerating nerve fibers. However, the rate of the growth of the intraspinal fibers was so slow that even a delay in the scar formation was not great enough to complete the growth of a large number of axons. It was therefore, necessary to find methods for stimulating the growth of intraspinal axons in order to increase the effectiveness of these procedures.

CHAPTER IV

STIMULATION OF THE GROWTH OF INTRASPINAL AXONS

Degeneration in the Central and Peripheral Fibers of the Nervous System and its Significance for Regeneration

It is known that motor nerve cells react by increasing their protein synthesis in response to transection of their peripheral axons (Brattgard, Edström, & Hydén, 1957; Fischer, Lodin, & Kolonsek, 1958; Gutman, Jakoubek, Hajek, Rohlicek, & Skaloud, 1962; Lajthe, 1964). Even the neurons of the hypoglossal nucleus, which are related to a central axon, react by increasing their protein synthesis in response to transection of the hypoglossal nerve (Haddad, Jucif, & Cruz, 1969). However, it has been reported in the previous chapter that the growth of central axons occurs more slowly than the growth of a transected peripheral fiber.

On the basis of evidence reported by Nasonov, Polezhaev, and other investigators, who studied the effect of degenerative products on the regeneration of organs and tissues in different types of animals, we may ask whether the absence of regeneration in intraspinal axons is due to the lack of an active process of degeneration in the area of the lesion. There is evidence that intense proteolysis and subsequent protein synthesis are carried out in those places where the corresponding enzymes and the materials for such synthesis are available. Perhaps the factors regulating regeneration are the same for all tissues and organs, irrespective of the animal species and the degree of differentiation of tissue. If this assumption is correct, the process of degeneration appearing in transected nerve should have a different character in a nicely regenerating peripheral nerve from that of slow growing fibers of the CNS. It is possible that degeneration inside a nerve is a process preparatory for subsequent regeneration, as has been observed during the regeneration of the organs in lower vertebrates (Urbani, 1965). However, immediately after the transection of a peripheral nerve one observes an abrupt activation of the Schwann cells, whose number increases 15 times within 14 days after the transection (Abercrombie & Johnson, 1942), although disintegration of the axons and myelin sheaths of the neuron becomes clearly evident within 72 hours, when excitability in the nerve fiber is lost (Falin, 1954; Gutmann & Holubar, 1950).

The activity of proteolytic enzymes increases soon after the transection of a peripheral nerve (particularly the acid proteinase taking part in the hydrolysis of the cellular protein and the dipeptidases connected with the synthesis of protein) (Urbani, 1965). That author considered this to be due to an increase in the number of Schwann cells (Fig. 38). Similar degeneration in the optic nerve, which is related to the central nervous system, starts at the end of the first week and continues for several months (Van Crevel, 1958). McCaman and Robins (1959a) reported a temporary marked difference in the activity of a number of enzymes during the degeneration of the central and peripheral fibers. In particular, a maximum rise of peptidase activity was noticed within 14 days in the tibial nerve but only after 100 days in the optic nerve. The number of satellite cells was increased within 14-15 days in the tibial nerve, but only after 200 days in the optic nerve (McCaman & Robins, 1959b).

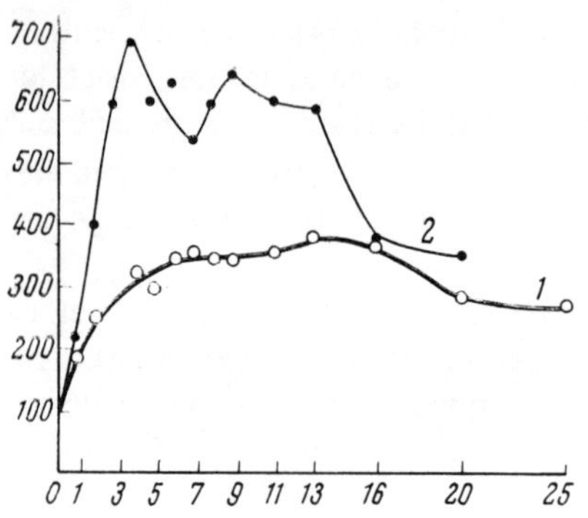

FIG. 38. The activity of proteinase (1) and acid dipeptidase (2) in the process of degeneration of a peripheral nerve (adopted from *Urbani,* 1965).

On the abscissa–days of investigation; on the ordinate–the activity of the enzymes (in units).

Evidently, there is a difference in both the rate and character of the degenerative process in the central and peripheral nervous systems. It may be that the slow growth of the CNS fibers as compared to peripheral axons can be explained by this. To examine this hypothesis, it was necessary to follow the course of degenerative processes by using several methods simultaneously in peripheral and CNS fibers.

Experimental Method

We conducted such experiments using both sciatic and optic nerves in rabbits and rats (Nesmeyanova, Gutmann, & Gaek, 1966). The optic nerve is typical of central neurons and is composed of fibers varying from 1 to 8.5 μ in diameter which are myelinated (Bishop, Jeremy, & Lance, 1953). Degeneration of the optic nerve was produced by unilateral enucleation and that of the sciatic nerve by transecting it in midthigh. The process of degeneration was studied from the morphologic, physiologic, and biochemical aspects.

For morphologic investigation, sections were impregnated according to Bielschowsky's and Fleming's methods. The number of glial cells in the cross sections of an optic nerve was determined in 5 μ-thick sections stained with hematoxylin-eosin. From each nerve, 10 sections were also taken for counting the nuclei. Morphologic studies in rats were obtained at intervals of 3, 5, 7, 14, 20, and 30 days after the enucleation and the transection of the nerve; those in rabbits, after 7 and 18 days. Excitability of the optic nerve was studied by electrophysiological methods. Action potentials were evoked by stimulating it with rectangular pulses of 0.5 msec duration at a frequency of 35 per sec and an amplitude not exceeding 14 volts, and recorded on a cathode ray oscillograph. The excitability of the nerve was studied in rabbits 4, 5, 6, and 7 days after enucleation or transection.

The enzymatic activity of cathepsin was determined at *pH* 4.0. The isolation of hemoglobin was carried out after extracting the nerve in physiological saline by Anson's method (Anson, 1938-1939). The quantity of tyrosine degraded in both cases was measured colorimetrically by Folin's method. The activity of the enzyme was determined by calculating the nitrogen content of protein in a nerve extract by the micro Kjeldahl method. The proteolytic activity of the enzyme was investigated in rabbits 4, 7, and 18 days following the enucleation or the nerve transection.

The protein synthesis was studied by determining the incorporation of the ^{35}S-methionine. Intravenous injections of the latter were given rats at a dose of 100 μCi per 100 g of body weight. The optic and sciatic nerves were isolated one hour after injection and the specific activity of the protein precipitate was measured in a scintillation counter. Protein synthesis was studied in rats 4, 7, and 9 days after the enucleation or transection.

Results

While all the fibers in the peripheral nerve were found to be in a state of morphologic degeneration on the third day after transection, the fibers of the optic nerve were still completely intact (Fig. 39A). The degeneration only started in these neurons after the fourth day (Fig. 39B) and complete degeneration of the nerve was not observed until 14 days after the enucleation (Fig. 39C). However, some widely separated thin unmyelinated fibers were not subject to degeneration. Perhaps they were the resistant central fibers responsible for carrying rapid impulses. It was also found that the resorption of degeneration products was carried out more slowly in the optic nerve than in sciatic. The proliferation of glial cells only doubled their number within 14 days of enucleation, although the number of Schwann cells increased 15 times within this period.

The excitability of the optic nerve was maintained for a longer period than the excitability of the peripheral nerve. In the latter, it disappeared within 72 hours, while in the optic nerve it was maintained for 6 days and disappeared only on the seventh day. The latent period of the evoked potentials in the degenerating nerve was somewhat longer than in the control; this may be explained by a slower degeneration of the fine fibers and slower propagation of impulses.

The proteolytic activity of cathepsin was found to differ sharply in these two cases. The comparative enzyme activity is shown in Fig. 40 as a percentage of control values. It can be seen that the cathepsin activity in the peripheral nerve rose quickly to a marked degree, reaching nearly 549% of the control by the 18th day, while, at the same time, there was no change in the enzyme activity of the CNS fibers.

Investigation of protein synthesis of an enucleated optic nerve showed that the incorporation of ^{35}S-methionine did not increase in a single case both *in vivo* and *in vitro* experiments, when compared with an intact nerve, at different experimental intervals. In comparison, the protein synthesis in a transected sciatic nerve increased sharply, reaching 205% of control by the fourth day and 311% by the seventh day (Fig. 41).

Thus the simultaneous investigation using several techniques for the study of peripheral and central axons revealed considerable differences in the rate and character of their degenerative changes. These processes began immediately after a transection in the peripheral nerve and progressed rapidly, while in the CNS fibers, they appeared at a considerably later stage and progressed slowly. The degenerative process might be considered a phenomenon which is not progressive from the beginning. In actual practice, the rapid disintegration of the axons and the myelin sheaths as well as the activation of the Schwann cells were observed immediately after the

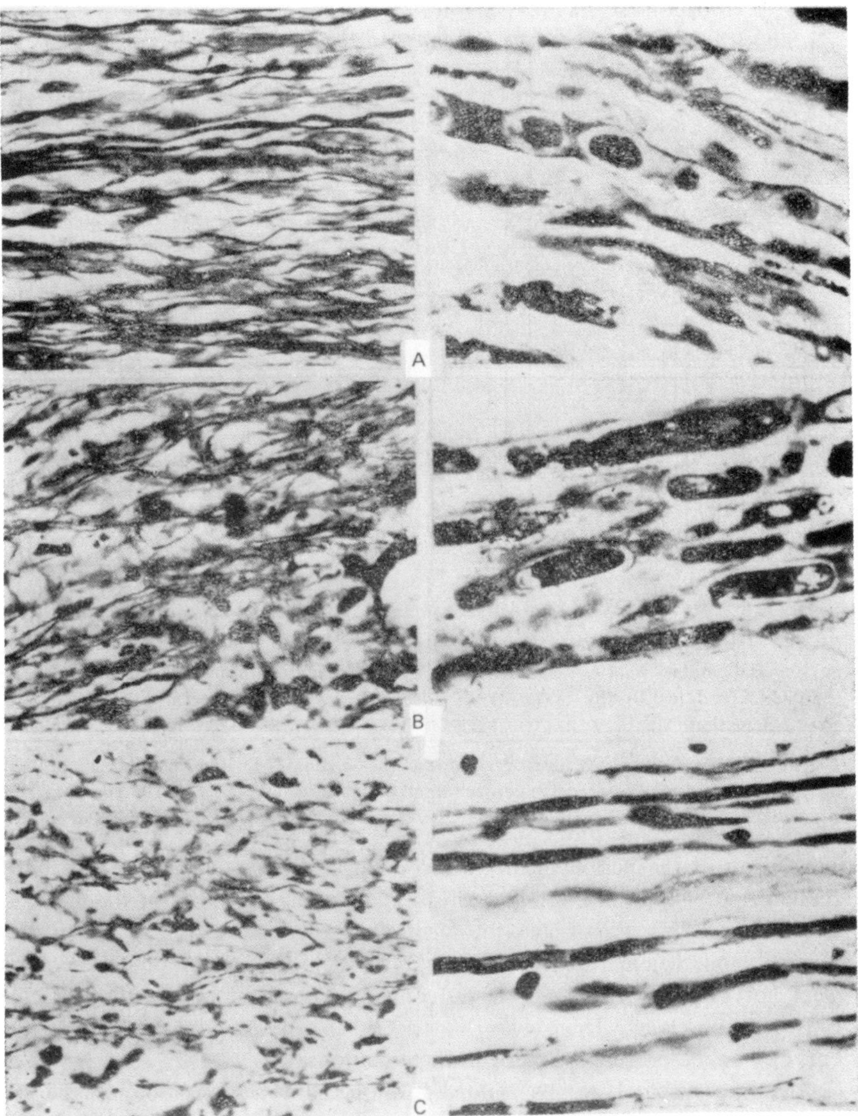

FIG. 39. The degeneration of axons in the optic (left) and sciatic (right) nerves.

A–after 3 days; B–after 4 days; C–14 days after enucleation or transection. Silver impregnation. Magnification 1 : 1000.

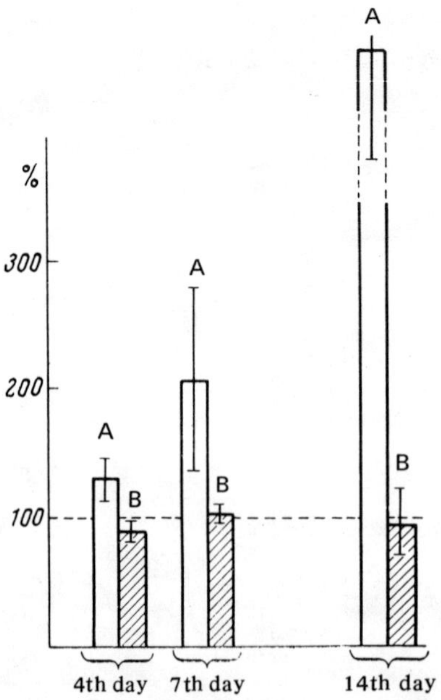

FIG. 40. Comparative catepsin activity in (A) the rabbit sciatic nerve after transection and in (B) the optic nerve after enucleation.

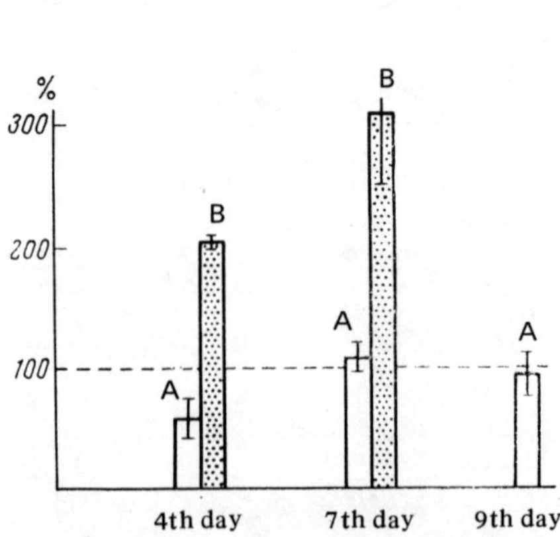

FIG. 41. Protein synthesis in (A) the rat optic nerve after enucleation and in (B) the sciatic nerve after transection.

On the abscissa–days of investigation; on the ordinate–relative change in protein synthesis. The degree of protein synthesis in an intact nerve was taken as 100 percent.

transection of the peripheral nerve accompanied by a rapid rise in activity of the enzymes responsible for proteolysis and protein synthesis in the neurons, i.e., the processes responsible for successful growth of the nerve fibers. In a central axon, where regeneration is slow, the initial phases of degeneration were not especially pronounced and only a very slight proliferation of glial cells was observed. There was no rise in the proteolytic activity of the enzymes or the protein synthesis in these neurons.

The experimental results obtained during this investigation of the degenerative process correspond with the theoretical expectations of biologists, namely, that an increase in the products of tissue disintegration in a growing area is mainly responsible for the successful regeneration of these tissues and organs (Fedotov, 1943; Nasonov, 1941; Polezhaev, 1933a, 1933b; Zelinskii, 1946). The success in regeneration of peripheral nerve was also linked to a rise in the quantity of the disintegration products in the damaged area (Borovskii, 1958a, 1958b).

In the light of the present investigation, it is possible to discuss the phenomenon of neurotrophism, first reported by Tello (1911), in which it was proposed that the direction of growth of a nerve was determined by the chemical environment of the surrounding media. The existence and the nature of this phenomenon has been questioned for the last 50 years.

Ramon y Cajal considered that neurotrophism had an influence in the growth of nerve fibers and suggested that the liberation of substances resembling an enzyme could help the assimilation and growth processes. Similar trophic properties are manifested by Schwann cells after the transection of a nerve. It was reported by Yakovleva (1954) that intraspinal and root fibers will grow along the strands of Schwann cells, as has been found in transplants.

Great attention has been paid by investigators to the trophic effect of different degenerating tissues. In the experiments of Tello (1923), the implantation of transected peripheral nerve into the white matter of brain led to the growth of axons in it. Even the implantation of pieces of elder soaked in a brain extract showed the growth of axons in this piece of wood. Sugar and Gerard (1940) filled the gap of a transected spinal cord with a piece of a muscle or fetal brain or with an isolated sciatic nerve. Substantial regeneration with restoration of functions was subsequently observed, particularly in the last case.

Later, it was demonstrated that a degenerated muscle, when inserted into the body close to a transected nerve, accelerates its regeneration (Harreveld, 1947). The homogenate from denervated nerves and muscles, when administered intramuscularly to a rat, caused the growth of fine ultraterminal fibrils from the nerve endings within 48 hours (Hoffman, 1951, 1952, 1955; Hoffman & Springell, 1951). They suggested that the growth stimulating factor was “neurocletin” containing several fatty acids which could easily penetrate through a cell membrane and thus decrease the viscosity of the protoplasm.

Acceleration in the growth of regenerating nerve fibers under the action of degenerated tissues has been observed in the undamaged tracts of spinal cord lying close to those which had been transected. The latter were subjected to degeneration and the growth of axons took place from the intact nerve cells (sprouting) (McCouch et al., 1955, 1958). Detailed studies to localize the accelerated growth of axons demonstrated that this was restricted to a narrow area adjoining the degenerated tissue and depended on the degree of degeneration of the implant (Liu & Chambers, 1958). They thought that the disintegration products of myelin, i.e., the protein, were the active growth-stimulating factors in degenerated tissue. Another observation which showed the importance of metabolites for successful regeneration was made on the cat spinal cord after transection where the majority of the regenerating nerve fibers were observed near blood vessels in which metabolites were concentrated (Liu & Scott, 1958).

In spite of a large number of observations supporting the trophic effect of degenerating tissues or the effect of metabolites directing the growth of axons, a number of investigators denied the existence of neurotrophism on the basis of negative results obtained from similar types of experiments (Barnard & Carpenter, 1950; Clark, 1942, 1943). In the experiments of Brown and McCouch (1947), smearing the transected ends of the spinal cord with an emulsion prepared from a degenerated nerve or the administration of the latter in the spinal gap in cats and dogs failed to stimulate the growth of nerve fibers through a scar. On the contrary, these transplants produced an abundant growth of collagen fibers and favored the formation of a dense scar. Weiss and his group, mainly using tissue culture methods, showed that the direction of growth of nerve fibers was determined exclusively by the presence of ultrastructures represented by the filaments of growing axons and was not influenced by the trophic action of degenerating tissue (Weiss, 1934, 1950, 1955; Weiss & Hoag, 1946; Weiss & Taylor, 1944). However, these authors do not deny the nutritive effect of degenerating tissue which is essential for the growth of axons. The absence of neurotrophic action directing the growth of axons (neurotaxis) was similarly reported by a number of other investigators (Bernstein & Guth, 1961; Guth, 1962, 1963; Young, Holmes, & Sanders, 1940).

Negative results obtained by Brown and McCouch (1947) are explained by the fact that even the improvement of trophism could not favor the growth of the axons through a scar tissue, which was rapidly formed by the action of the disintegration products.

It may be presumed that neurotrophism also has a nutritive effect on the growth processes and undoubtedly plays a positive role. The question of neurotaxis remains unsettled. However, it is beyond dispute that there are differences in the chemotaxis of the nerve fibers of different tracts and their selective contact is based on this specificity, i.e., the presence of chemotaxis (Attardi & Sperry, 1963; Hooker, 1930; Sperry, 1960).

Use of Resorptive Transplants as Stimulators for the Process of Regeneration*

From the data presented above, the possibility arises that activation of the disintegration processes, i.e., degeneration, will enhance the regenerative

*Editor's note: The author's use of the phrase "resorptive transplants" calls for the following clarification: She stated, "From experiments on neurotrophism it has been suggested that degenerating tissue may have a nutritive effect essential for the growth of

processes in an injured region of the spinal cord. This idea suggested experiments in which resorptive transplants were used for the activation of the disintegration process (Nesmeyanova, Brazovskaya, & Arnautova, 1964a, 1964b).

We used resorptive transplants from spinal tissue or from nerves on the assumption that after disintegration they might have accumulated fragments of protein molecules which would be essential for the synthesis of axoplasm. The regenerative process could also be intensified by the possibility of attracting a large number of macrophages having the capacity to synthesize nucleoproteins in a traumatized area. It was also expected that since the structure of the transplants was similar to that of the spinal cord, they would give a better support to growing axons (Anokhina, 1953; Yakovleva, 1954). In some of the experiments transplants were made from pieces of spinal cord preserved in formalin. This particular fixative preserves some of the biological properties of tissue (Anokhin, 1944; Anokhina, 1953; Voino-Yasenetskii, 1961), so that its proteins retain the capacity for hydrolysis, although this process is considerably delayed (Nasonov & Aleksandrov, 1944). Therefore, the disintegration of tissues in such transplants is continued for a prolonged period, and this might be useful for the success of regeneration if the slow growth of the axons is taken into consideration. Transplants from a degenerated nerve were used because of their trophic action.

Experimental Procedures

The spinal cord was completely transected at the level of Th_{10}-Th_{12} on 30 young dogs while the anterior spinal artery was carefully preserved. These dogs were divided into four groups.

In these procedures, the first group of 18 animals received a formalin treated spinal transplant which had the form of a cone, with a thickness of 1 mm at the dorsal and 0.5 mm at the ventral surface, which was introduced transversely, filling the dorsal half of the lesion site. This piece of transplant was taken from the spinal cord of another dog and preserved in 10% formalin for a week. It was then thoroughly washed in physiological saline a day before

axons. It might be presumed that activation of the disintegrative processes, i.e., degeneration, will promote the acceleration of the regenerative process in an injured region of the spinal cord. Resorptive transplants were used for the activation of the disintegration process. We used transplants of spinal tissue or nerve on the assumption that after disintegration they might have left (accumulated) fragments of protein molecules which would be essential for the formation of axoplasm." It appears that the resorptive transplant would first promote protein denaturation within itself, forming a stored pool of fragments which could then be used when placed in the experimental lesion to promote and accelerate the formation of new proteins at the site of the lesion into which the transplant was placed. (The concept is described in Polezhaev, 1972.)

the operation. The animals of this group were observed at periods of 2 weeks, 1 month, 3 months, and 6 months after operation.

The second group included five dogs who received the same size of transplant as the first group, but the transplant was taken from the freshly removed spinal cord of a dog, which was refrigerated at 4°C for about an hour. It also filled the whole dorsal half of the experimental lesion. The animals of the second group were observed for periods of two weeks and one month post-operatively.

The third group included five dogs. They received a freshly dissected transverse section of dog sciatic nerve which had been removed from the donor two weeks earlier. It was of approximately the same size as the transplants used in the animals of other groups and also filled the whole dorsal half of the lesion. These animals were observed for a period of two weeks and some of them for three months.

The fourth, control group, included two dogs. Here a piece of wax of approximately the same form and size as the other transplants was introduced. It occupied the whole dorsal half of the lesion. These animals were observed for a period of two weeks after operation. Pyrogenal was administered to the animals of all the groups, according to the schedule described earlier.

Histologic studies consisted of a series of longitudinal sections stained with hematoxylineosin, hematoxylin-picrofuchsin, and impregnated with silver according to the method of Bielschowsky and Gross.

The post-operative period in all the dogs with transplants passed without any complication.

Results: Two Weeks Post-operative

Histologic investigation of the spinal cord which received the transplant prepared from a formalin-treated spinal cord showed that this was not favorable for directing the growing axons. They grew around the transplant and penetrated the scar only in its ventral part—the region opposite to the implant. However, the transplant was of importance due to its own slow resorption in the delayed formation of a collagenous scar.

The use of various transplants influenced the rate of growth of the nerve fibers but not to a uniform extent. Study of the silver impregnated preparations showed that two weeks after operation there was a significant difference in the quantity and condition of the nerve fibers growing toward the scar in the animals with resorptive tissue transplants (first, second, and third groups) as compared to the control, nonresorptive transplants (fourth group). In the latter, the growth of fibers toward the scar was rather insignificant, and the peripheral part of the stumps were thick with divided fibers filled with protoplasm (Fig. 42A), as had been observed in animals without any transplants (Fig. 42B). In the experimental dogs of the first three

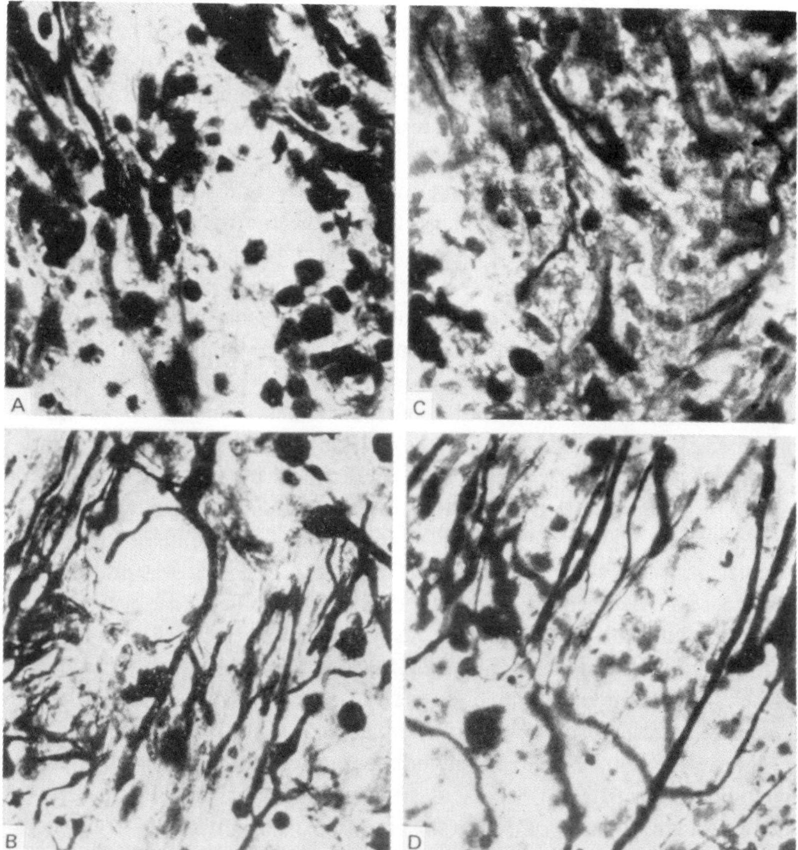

FIG. 42. Condition of the growing nerve fibers two weeks after operation.

A–in the case of a transplant made of wax (fourth group); B–without any transplant; C–in the case of a formalin-treated transplant (first group); D–in the case of a transplant prepared from a degenerated nerve (third group). Silver impregnation. Magnification : eye piece 7, objective 40.

groups, the number of growing fibers was considerably higher, and they were clearly impregnated with silver. In these animals the phenomena of abnormal swelling and irregular division of fibers were absent. It was possible to observe some characteristics of a nerve fiber from their contours (Fig. 42C, D).

Results: One Month Post-operative

One month after operation, the difference in the character of growth of the nerve fibers in the animals of the first, second, and third groups became evident, particularly in the animals in the first group. In all these three groups, an abundant growth of nerve fibers was noticed at this time; however, in dogs of the first group, the fibers were observed to be growing in columns and fasciculi, which was not the case in the animals of the other groups. The growth of nerve fibers through the area of scar ventral to a transplant was observed in 25% of the dogs with resorptive transplants one month following operation (Fig. 43).

Later observations, three to six months after operation, showed that an abundant growth of nerve fibers surrounding the transplant occurred in all the experimental dogs of the first, second, and third groups (Fig. 44A). Growth of nerve fibers through the scar was noticed in 70 percent of the animals in these groups. At this time, also, a greater response was seen in the dogs of the first group with the formalin-treated transplant. In three animals of this group, the growth of nerve fibers was very pronounced and it was possible to follow their course. In one case, bundles of nerve fibers penetrated the scar in its ventromedial part (Fig. 44B). On the basis of the observations in a series of longitudinal sections, it appears that these fibers belong to a long ascending system. In another case, the growth of axons through the scar was observed in the central part of the right lateral column involving the descending fibers of the corticospinal and rubrospinal tracts. Growth of axons was also noticed on both sides of the ventral parts of the lateral column, i.e., in the ventral spinocerebellar and possibly in the spinothalamic tracts (Fig. 44C). In the third case, bundles of nerve fibers of the right lateral column connected both of the spinal stumps. Probably, these fibers were related to the lateral tectospinal, vestibulospinal, spinothalamic, and spinotectal tracts and also to the intersegmental fibers, i.e., including both the descending and ascending fibers. For comparison, we present photomicrographs showing the growth of axons through the site of lesion in the animals receiving no transplant and only Pyrogenal (Fig. 45). It can be seen that the growth toward the scar and through it was considerably less pronounced than in the cases with resorptive transplants. It was not possible here to follow the course of the growing fibers in the tract.

Restoration of impaired function was observed in 70 percent of the animals in the first three groups and this correlated with the histologic picture of the growth of nerve fibers. As a rule, it appeared in these animals earlier than in those using Pyrogenal alone. Thus, in five out of eight dogs of the first group, the scratch reflex appeared, in a mild degree, within 2-2½ months after operation (Fig. 46A) at which time sensitivity to pressure on the thigh was noticed in four dogs.

In the three cases reported above, where a marked response followed receipt of the transplant, there was abundant growth of nerve fibers in certain tracts and restoration of function was particularly pronounced. In one dog, which was kept under observation for three months, the growth of ascending fibers with the restoration of sensation was noticed. In the second case, the

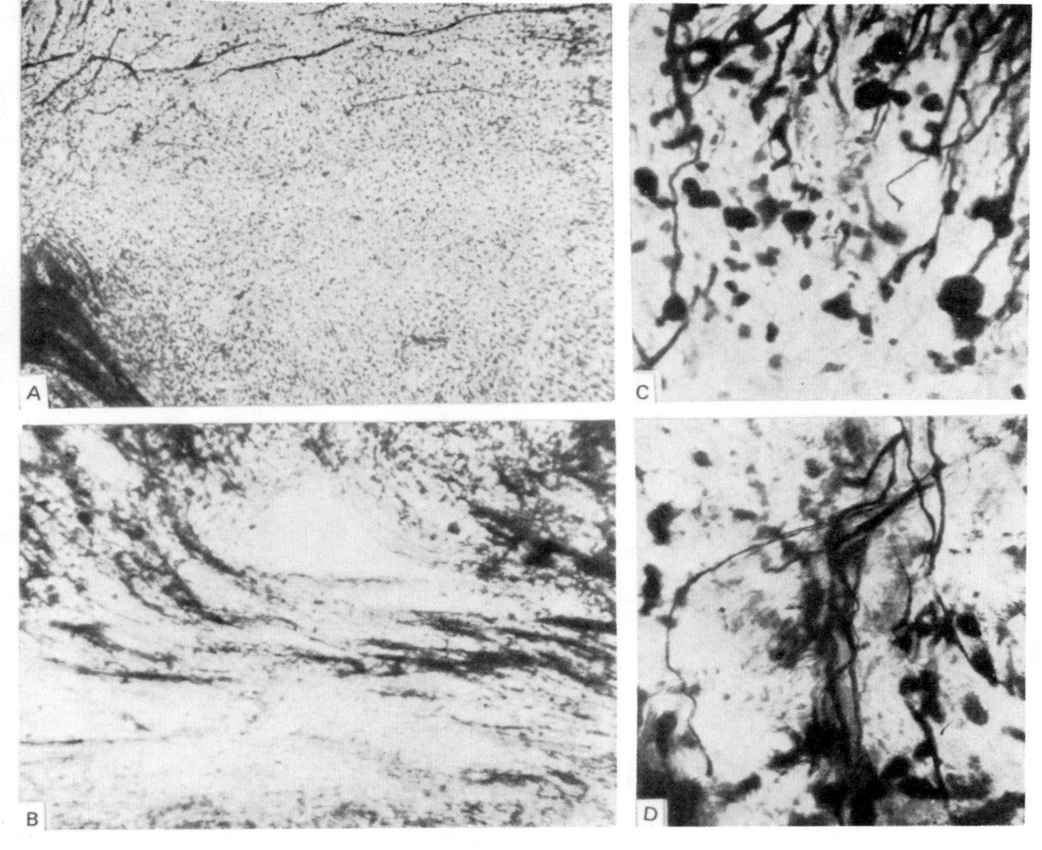

FIG. 43. Growth of the nerve fibers (A, B) toward a transplant and (C, D) through the area of section, in the presence of resorptive transplants.

A, C—two weeks after operation, B, D—one month after operation. Silver impregnation. Magnification—A, B—eye piece 6, objective 9; C, D—eye piece 6, objective 90.

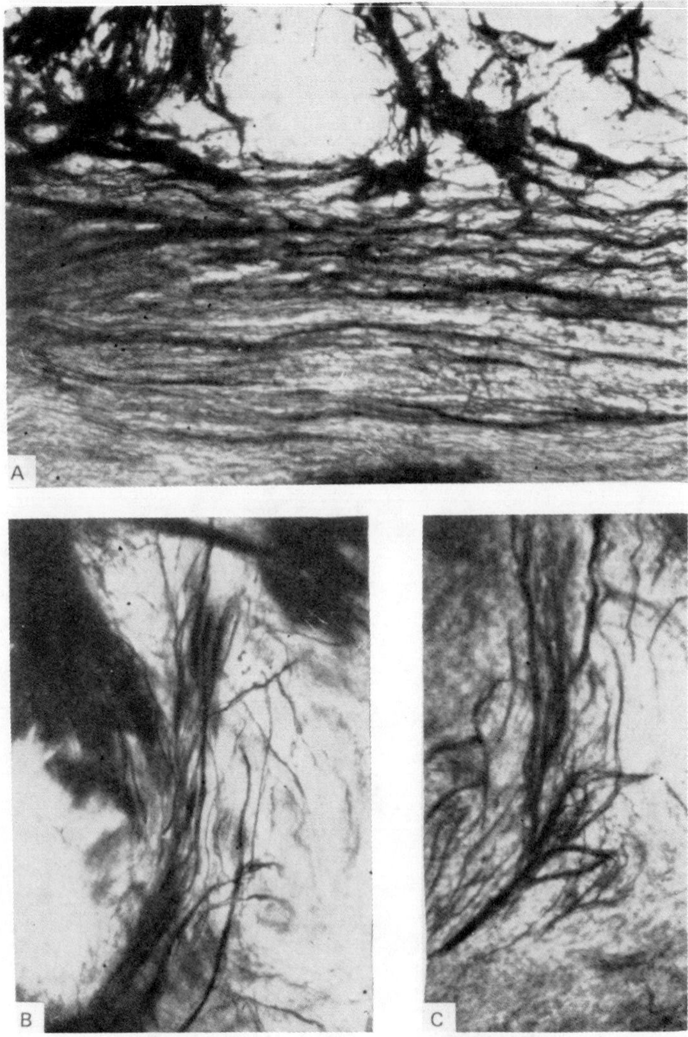

FIG. 44. Growth of the nerve fibers toward (A) a transplant (as in first, second, & third groups) and (B, C) through the site of the lesion in the presence of resorptive transplants (first group) three months after operation.

Silver impregnation. Magnification—eye piece 6, objective 20 (A), eye piece 6, objective 90 (B, C).

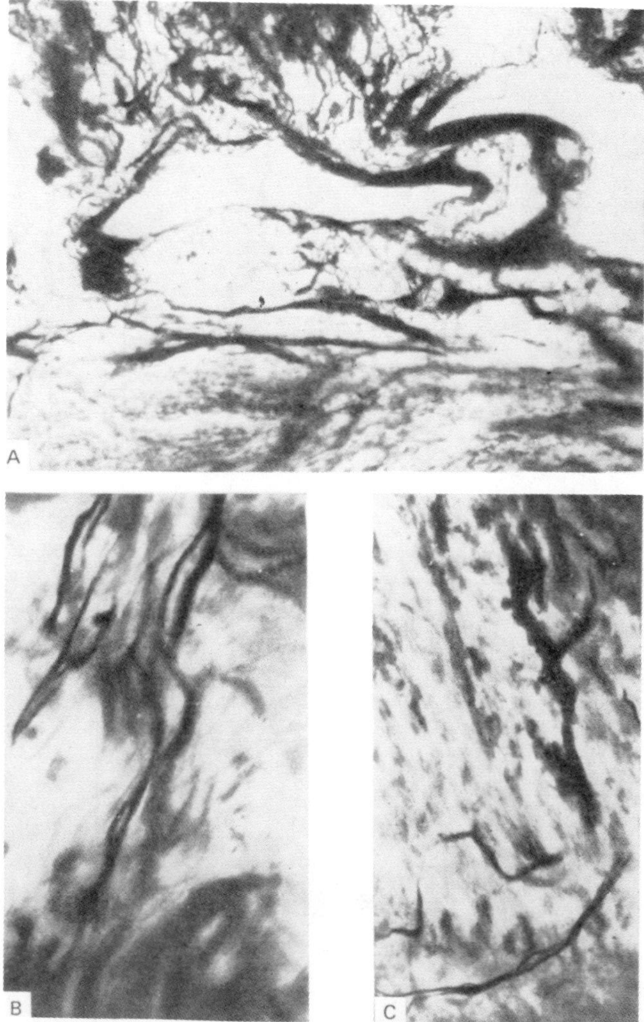

FIG. 45. Growth of nerve fibers (A) toward the scar and (B, C) in the site of section, in dogs receiving only Pyrogenal, three months after operation.

Silver impregnation. Magnification—eye piece 6, objectives 20 (A) eye piece 6, objectives 90 (B, C).

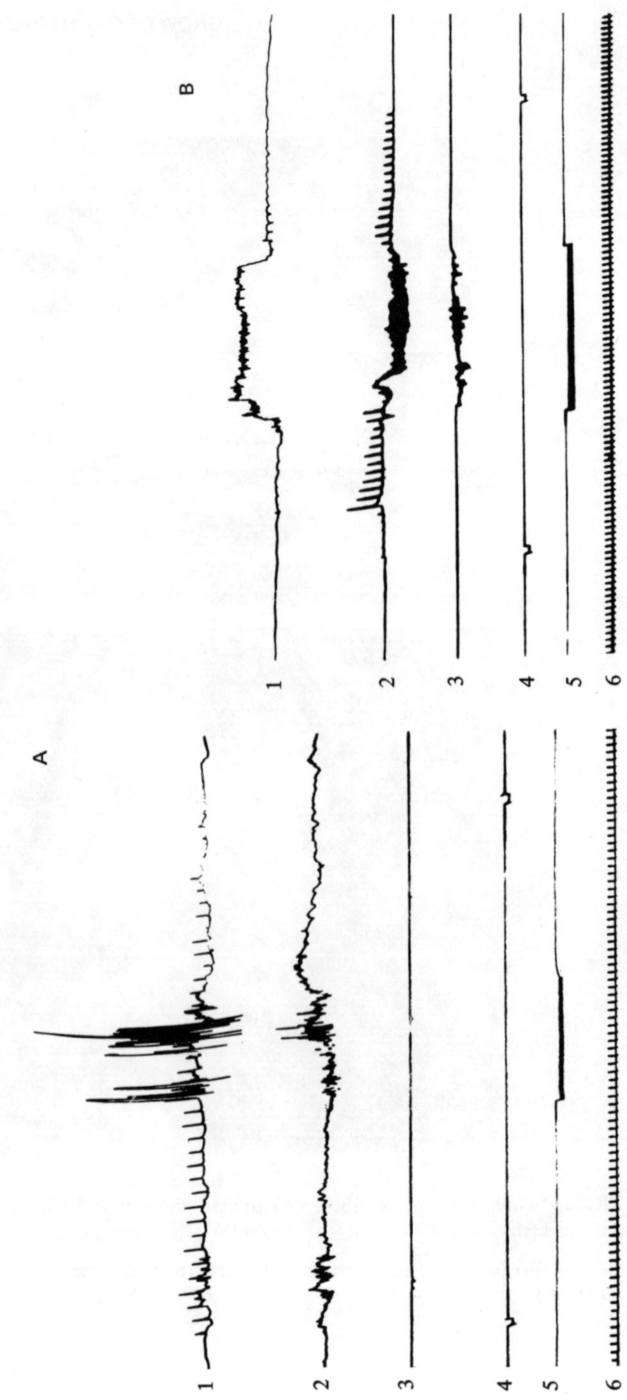
A
1
2
3
4
5
6
B
1
2
3
4
5
6

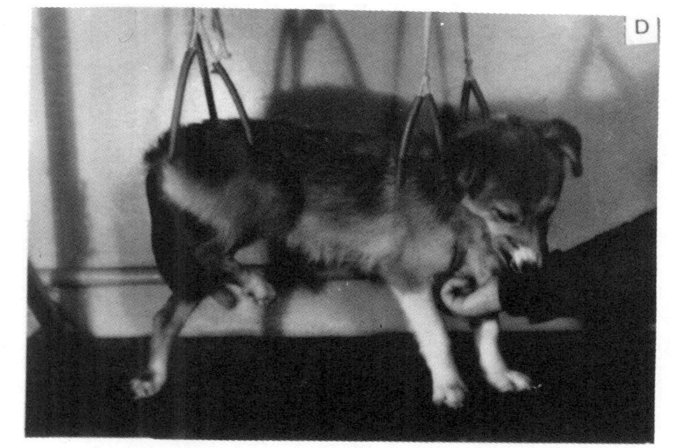

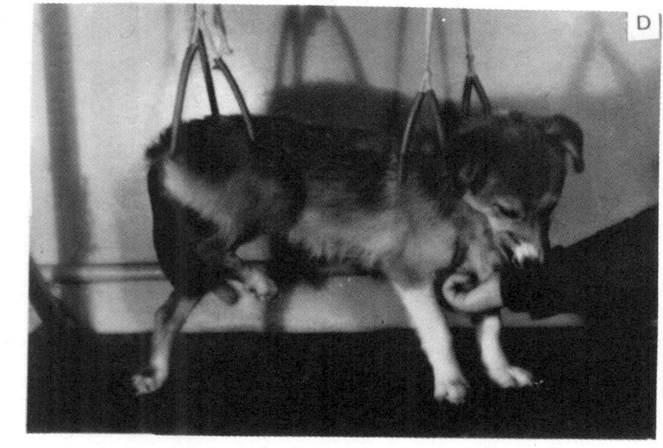

FIG. 46. Scratch reflex in experimental dogs (first group) (A) and (B, C) three months post-operative; (D)—picture of dog at the moment of scratching.

1—movement of ipsilateral extremity; 2—movement of contralateral extremity; 3—movement of tail; 4—mark showing the beginning and end of electrostimulation; 5—mark of scratching; 6—time, 1 sec.

scratch reflex was very pronounced (Fig. 46B) but sensation was not restored. In the third case, the dog was kept under observation for six months, and showed a scratch reflex (Fig. 46) and return of sensation, both of which were pronounced. The latter appeared not only in response to pressure over the thigh but also on pricking the skin of the sacrum and thigh (Fig. 46D). It was found that this dog was capable of voluntarily moving its right hind limb when called upon to do so. Morphologic examination showed that the spinal cord in this particular dog had been transected completely at the initial operation. Thus, the use of transplants prepared from spinal tissue subjected to resorption, as well as the predegenerated nerve, stimulated the growth of intraspinal axons, while the control transplants prepared from nonresorptive tissue did not show such an effect. Mechanical stimulation failed to affect the growth of the intraspinal axons as well as peripheral nerve, according to the observations of Fuks (1959).

It may be thought that the main factor accelerating the regenerative growth of axons was the more intensive and, possibly, more prolonged disintegration of tissues in the lesion as compared to the experimental transection without any transplants. The experimental results showed that the formalin-treated transplants, in which resorption was carried out for a long period, were the most effective. Probably prolongation of the processes providing trophic response was essential for the slow-growing intraspinal axons. It was clearly shown that the spinal scar formed in dogs of the first group was more friable than in the dogs of any other group. This provided an opportunity for regeneration of intraspinal axons in the ventral part of the cord which was not in contact with the transplant. The duration of growth and the time in making synaptic contact were both reduced. Restoration of function took place two to three weeks earlier in these dogs than in the experiments using Pyrogenal alone and their functions were relatively more developed.

Morphologic studies of nerve fiber growth in experimental animals conclusively showed that this occurred equally from the rostral and the caudal stumps. We failed to show any preferential growth of the nerve fibers from any particular group of spinal cells. The observed restoration of function in the experimental animals was judged to involve both efferent and afferent fibers. In the experiments of Clemente and Windle (1954), growth of fibers was primarily observed in the efferent tracts of the lateral and ventral columns. Yakovleva (1956) investigated the regenerative potential of axons in the early phase after transection and came to the conclusion that more intensive growth was observed in the afferent systems, mainly in the posterior columns of the caudal stump. It is possible that these contradictions are due to the difference in the periods of observation, the use of different animal species, or, most importantly, to the absence of stimulating agents intensifying the growth of the axons. Thus, in cases where only Pyrogenal was used, it was not possible to discriminate the structures in which the principal growth of the axons took place.

The positive results in the experiments with transplants which intensified the degree and duration of the disintegration process in an area of a spinal trauma support the hypothesis that degeneration (tissue disintegration) is a progressive phenomenon and preparatory for a subsequent regenerative process. The loss of this property in the highly differentiated brain tissue likewise led to a loss of regenerative capacity.

On the basis of experimental results presented above, it seems likely that the restoration of regenerating capacity is guided by the same general rule which is true for other mammalian tissues as well as the organs of the lower vertebrates (Polezhaev, 1956, 1959b), and the only difference is that disintegration in the central nervous system does not produce, on its own, the dedifferentiation of the nerve cells. This process is not necessary for the growth of the transected axon. The essential factor for effective growth is the increased resynthesis of the axon proteins and their transport to the periphery, i.e., to the site of the lesion.

In other cases, when investigators have tried to increase multiplication of nerve cells in the cerebral cortex with the help of suitable agents, dedifferentiation of some neurons and formation of new neuron-like cells from undifferentiated cambian cells of the ependymal layer were observed (Polezhaev & Karnaukhova, 1963; Polezhaev & Reznikov, 1966; Renznikov, 1965). Consequently, physiological regeneration of nerve cells, even in the central nervous system, was possible before their dedifferentiation.

The positive results of experiments using slow resorptive transplants as stimulators of regeneration (which intensified the disintegration of tissues in an injured area and prolonged its duration) led to the idea that stimulation of protein synthesis in the cell body and in the periphery is mainly responsible for enhanced axonal growth. The intensification of protein synthesis can be encouraged by the presence of raw materials such as fragments of protein molecules and an increased number of macrophages which convert these into round granules. The latter supply the products of protein disintegration to the cells in a form which can be used in subsequent synthesis (Kedrovskii, 1945).

Stimulation of nerve regeneration with the use of "resorptive transplants," placed in the experimental lesion of the spinal cord, and the effect of the degenerative processes on the growth of the axons led us to reconsider the trophic connection of a nerve cell body with a growing axon, although they are situated at a great distance from each other. This question has not been studied adequately. As previously noted, the neuron reacts to the transection of its axon by stimulating protein synthesis in response. Growth may start within three days of transection of a peripheral nerve (Gutmann & Holubar, 1950). Thus the axon is capable of sending signals to the cell body of a neuron immediately after transection. In the opinion of Gutmann (1964), the trophic connection between the axon and the cell body is established by some means without involving an impulse. However, it is difficult to say, at the present moment, how this is accomplished. The connection between a neuronal cell body and a growing axon can be maintained actively by axoplasmatic flow involving all the substances necessary for the construction of tissue and maintenance of vital neuronal function. These include the nucleoprotein particles, enzymes, and mediators. The movement of axoplasm is possible in two directions, from the body of a cell to the periphery and vice versa, as shown by Zelena and Lyubinska (1962) using a cholinesterase stain. However, it is difficult to conceive that the promotion of axon growth during the onset of regeneration is exclusively due to intensification of protein synthesis in the cell body and the flow of substances to the tip of an axon. A trophic function has been shown for Büngners bands which are formed from Schwann cells both during the process of degeneration and also the process of regeneration in a peripheral nerve. To some extent, they can help the formation of axoplasm in the periphery. The role of neuroglia is not clear during stimulation of the trophic processes which promote regeneration of the central axons. Therefore, we started investigating this problem.

The Role of Neuroglia in the Central Nervous System: Particularly in Relation to Regeneration of Central Neurons

In spite of the absence of sophisticated methods and high resolution optical instruments, it was shown in the early years of this century that neuroglia played an active role in carrying out the vital functions of nerve tissue (Cajal, 1906; Penfield, 1924). The trophic function of neuroglia was reported by Friede (1953) both from his own observations and after reviewing the literature. Snesarev (1946) and Alekandrovskaya (1950) concluded that neuroglia, particularly the astrocytes, constitute an intervening nutritive system situated between the blood vessels and the nerve cells.

Electron microscopic observations have confirmed that neuroglia are involved in trophic function and have shown that they are closely related to the neurons by metabolic processes. It was shown that neuroglia are involved in transporting the end products of neuronal activity to the blood vessels (Polak, 1965), thus maintaining the constant internal ionic composition of a neuron (Friede, 1965). According to modern concepts, neuroglial cells form part of a functional system with neurons (Hydén, 1960). The distribution of oligodendrocytes in the central nervous system of a rabbit is such that it provides a close connection between the neurons and the small blood vessels (Jao Yhu Shu, 1964). As a result, the oligodendrocytes are capable of active participation in the metabolic processes of nerve tissue. They have a considerably higher sensitivity to hypoxia than the astrocytes, i.e., there is a higher rate of oxidative processes (Pope, 1958). The higher DNA concentration in the nuclei of oligodendrocytes as compared to astrocytes (Pia, 1963) shows their more active participation in protein synthesis.

The oligodendrocytes also have a significant role in the myelination of the nerve fibers. Small vesicles can be seen in the cytoplasm closely surrounding an axon from which concentric layers are organized to form the typical structure of the myelin membrane, i.e., the myelination in the central nervous system is characterized by the process of myelin synthesis inside the cytoplasm of the oligodendrocytes (De Robertis, 1964). Hydén (1963a) observed that whereas only the Schwann cells are necessary for myelination of peripheral nerve, a considerable number of oligodendrocytes connected by protoplasmic threads with an axon are essential for myelination of central neurons.

Since neuroglial cells are satellites of neurons, they react by proliferating when neurons are damaged, in addition to their active participation in the metabolic processes. They will encircle a dying cell and finally resorb the products of its disintegration; likewise they will actively engulf the products of myelin disintegration by converting them into round granules (Avtsyn & Il'ina 1961; Horrocks, Toews, Yashon, & Locke, 1973). This capacity to resorb the disintegration products may subsequently lead to an increase of protein synthesis. Kedrovskii (1945) has reported that the round granules split up the protein molecules into amino acids, i.e., transform them into a form suitable for future protein synthesis, and in this way the neuroglial cells may participate in the metabolism of a neuron.

The functions of neuroglia are not restricted to metabolism, although a discussion of other aspects is beyond our purview. A review of the work on the physiology and morphology of the glia in the last five years has been presented by Mats (1968).

Recent experimental methods have provided data relating to the connection between the glial cells and neurons. The metabolic processes of the individual components of the nervous system in different functional states and phases of growth was investigated by Hydén (1960) who reported that neuroglial cells, especially the oligodendrocytes, normally supply high-energy substances to the neurons, whereas during increased functional stress the most easily available energy is derived from its intrinsic protein synthesis.

Adenosine triphosphatase, which is essential for the liberation of energy from ATP, is contained primarily in the glial cells while the ATP is found in the nerve cells (Hydén, 1964; Hydén & Egyhazi; 1964). It was their opinion that ATP-ase liberates energy for the transport of nutrients from the capillaries to the neuron surface.

Experiments using the application of a vestibular stimulus showed that the quantitative relation is changed between the high-energy compounds and other substances connected with protein synthesis in the nerve cell and the glia. Thus, in a nerve cell the concentration of RNA and respiratory enzymes increases and the protein synthesis is accelerated during stimulation, while these processes decrease in the glial cells, and there is increased anerobic glycolysis in the glial cells (Hydén, 1959, 1963b). This emphasizes that glial cells and neurons belong to a single system of interconnected metabolic processes.

As a result, there is no doubt about the active participation of neuroglia in carrying out many of the vital functional processes of nerve tissue. Naturally, it may be expected that glial cells should participate actively in the process of regeneration of damaged nerve fibers. As demonstrated above, the spontaneously proliferating Schwann cells invariably participate in the regeneration of a nerve.

There are reports showing the participation of neuroglial cells in the metabolic processes during regeneration of a hypoglossal nerve (Sjöstrand, 1966). It has been shown that as soon as two to four days after the compression of a hypoglossal nerve, there is proliferation of glial cells in the hypoglossal nuclei which reaches its maximum on the sixth day. At this time, hypertrophy of the glial cell body and activation of the number of enzymes are observed. The author concludes that during regeneration of a nerve cell, neuroglia play a significant role in the transport of substances between the capillary system and the perikaryon.

It is suggested that stimulating regeneration of conducting axons in the central nervous system causes neuroglia to proliferate and thus to play an active role in regeneration.

Counting the glial cells (Nesmeyanova & Vorob'eva, 1967) in a growing area of the spinal cord, both after application of resorptive transplants and in the controls, should provide an answer to this question.

Investigations were performed on 30 μm thick longitudinal sections of a dog's spinal cord stained with hematoxylin-picrofuchsin. All types of glial cells, except microglia, were counted. Two areas from the segment proximal to the lesion of the spinal cord (each measuring about 4 mm^2) were selected for counting. The number of glial cells was analyzed statistically and the mean number of cells in individual groups of animals was compared with the help of the "student's criterion," including gray matter and a narrow stip of white matter.

The first area was situated 1-1.5 mm proximal to the boundary of the scar tissue (Fig. 47). It may be characterized as a zone with a maximum number of the growing nerve fibers and with degeneration of a large number of neurons. The second area was situated two to three segments proximal to the

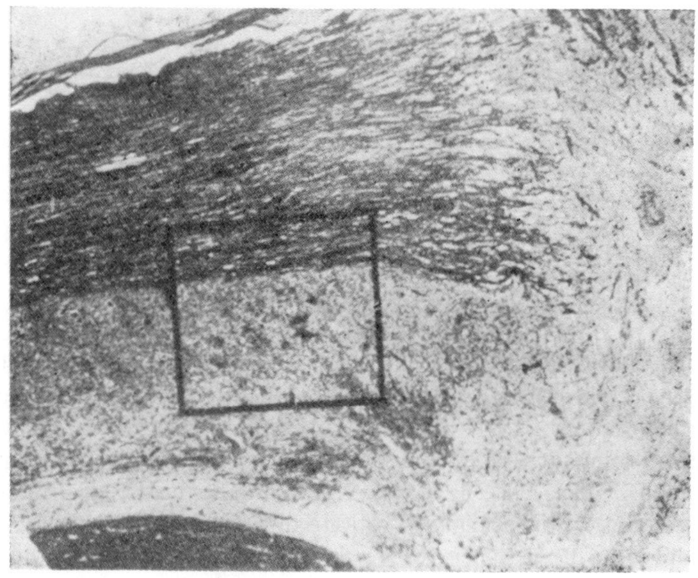

FIG. 47. An area selected for counting glial cells in a section of spinal cord. Silver impregnation. Magnification X 10.

first one. A large number of intact axons and neurons were seen as well as those undergoing degeneration. The spinal cord of these animals was examined 2, 4, and 12 weeks after transection. Animals with resorptive transplants were included in the experimental group. Some control animals received only Pyrogenal while others did not. Animals of the two control groups were combined into one on the basis of glial cell counts. The control group also included animals in which wax transplants were introduced as well as Pyrogenal

Two weeks after operation, comparison of the number of glial cells in the two selected areas revealed that there was no statistically significant difference between them and hence, in the later experiments, only cells in the first area were counted.

The results of counting the glial cells in gray matter and some peripheral white matter in an area of growth are shown in Fig. 48. Two to four weeks after operation, the number of glial cells was greater in the dogs with resorptive transplants than in the controls, and the difference was statistically significant. After 12 weeks, the number of glial cells in both groups increased further but the difference between the number in the experimental and control animals decreased and was not statistically significant.

The difference observed in the increased number of neuroglia is in agreement with the data on growth of nerve fibers in the experimental

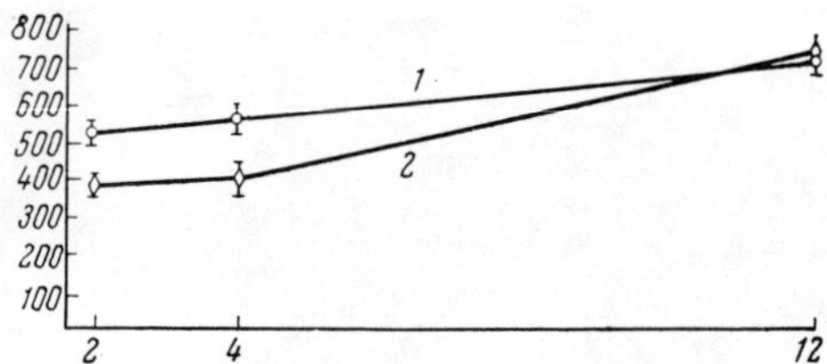

FIG. 48. Comparison of the number of glial cells between (1) experimental and (2) control dogs at different periods of investigation.

On the abscissa–time (in weeks); on the ordinate–number of cells in 0.01 mm^3.

animals. In "growing" areas of the cord, where a large number of glial cells was observed, there was greater growth of nerve fibers and they appeared more nearly normal; there were less degenerative changes and more fibers growing in columns. These observations, once again, support the possible participation of the glial cells in carrying out trophic functions in the nervous system, and suggest their ability to activate the metabolic processes, simulating the condition in the periphery where the Schwann cells proliferate during the nerve damage and thus provide support for a growing fiber and supply of its building material.

A similar increase in the number of glial cells was observed two weeks after operation, both in an area at some distance from the site of the lesion where the neurons were intact and also in a zone close to the area of disintegration where axon growth was more pronounced. This may indicate that there is a connection through the metabolic processes between glia and the neuronal cell body as well as with growing axons. In particular, it has been reported that the glial cells help in the movement of axoplasm along an axon (Pomerat, Altman et al., 1964).

Thus, enhancement of the disintegration process in a lesion site resulting from the use of resorptive transplants favors the proliferation of neuroglia and this may possibly facilitate protein synthesis carried out in the neuronal body and in the periphery of a growing axon as in the case of Schwann cells.

We were also interested to observe a uniform rise in the number of glial cells in the spinal cord of all the categories of dogs 12 weeks after operation, both in the control and experimental groups. Probably it was not connected with growth processes, but with an increase in the motor activity of the front legs of the dogs, which might have affected the number and condition of neuroglia in the proximal segments of the spinal cord responsible for this motor activity.

A similar phenomenon was observed in the experiments on rats maintained in "enriched" and "impoverished" conditions. The number of glial cells in the cerebral cortex of rats in the first group increased by 14 percent more than that in the rats of the second group (Diamond, Law, Rhodes, Lindner, Rosenzweig, & Krech, 1966).

Stimulation of the Regenerative Process in Intraspinal Axons by Promoting the Synthesis of Nucleoproteins

Role of RNA in the Regeneration of Organs and Tissues

The results described above show the importance of the disintegration process which provides the substrates for protein synthesis to a neuron and for the proliferation of neuroglia promoting protein synthesis. This confirms the assumption that the main factor involved in the regeneration of the central axons is the stimulation of protein synthesis in those neurons whose axons have been transected.

Nucleic acids are the essential constituents of protein synthesis inside a cell. Consideration of the relation between protein synthesis and the participation of RNA in this process, as well as the dependence of the synthesis of RNA from the genetic apparatus, led Brachet to conclude that "DNA produces RNA, and RNA produces protein." Or, in other words, DNA connected with genes is essential for the synthesis of nuclear RNA which is then transferred to the cytoplasm. The energy necessary for the synthesis of protein is supplied to the mitochondria inside a cell by high-energy compounds (i.e., compounds rich in phosphorous), while the building materials are amino acids. RNA is an essential component of this process. Addition of the enzyme ribonuclease which inactivates RNA leads to a complete inhibition of protein synthesis inside a cell (Brachet, 1960).

If RNA synthesis is stopped when there is a rise in the level of protein synthesis, during functional stress, the dry weight of the ganglion cells, like the grandular cells, decreases, indicating an inhibition of intracellular protein synthesis (Brodskii, Aref'eva, & Kuznetsova, 1966; Brodskii & Nechaeva, 1966). On the other hand, during administration of dinitrylmalonic acid, the amount of RNA is increased in Deiters' nucleus in rabbits (Egyhazi & Hydén, 1961). The change of RNA during such an enhancement of protein synthesis is not limited to a quantitative increase but there is also a qualitative change as well: It is converted into a more active state (Brattgard et al., 1957).

In accordance with the hypothesis put forward by Jacob and Monad (1961), the activity of metabolic processes in an organism is regulated by stimulation or inhibition of the synthesis of enzymes connected with the activity of cellular genetic apparatus. Based on these ideas, Meerson (1963, 1967) developed and experimentally substantiated the theory of plastic functions by an organism: i.e., the synthesis of nucleoproteins leading to formation of new compounds, instead of destruction during a vital process, is regulated directly and indirectly by a complex mechanism. Any process of activity vital to an organism (its growth or the activity of individual systems) requires the synthesis of nucleoproteins, i.e., it is dependent on the genetic apparatus of the cell. It has been shown that memory (ability to consolidate the developed conditioned reflexes and even the development of new ones) was connected with the capacity to synthesize DNA, RNA, and proteins (Meerson & Kruglikov, 1966; Meerson, Kruglikov, & Kolomeitseva, 1965). Inherent pathological processes as well as aging of an organism depend on the alteration of its plastic functions (Gutmann et al., 1962; Meerson, 1967).

Naturally, it has been thought that regeneration is controlled by some factor which accelerates the interdependent processes of the synthesis of nucleic acids and protein. In fact, investigation of the concentration of RNA in the regenerating limbs and tails of lower vertebrates showed that the quantity of RNA was increased, but in a mammalian amputated stump RNA remained unchanged (Barakina, 1951a, 1951b, 1952). The rise in concentration of RNA in regenerated tissue was maximum during differentiation (Teplits, 1964a), i.e., during the formation of specific cells in each tissue.

Sectioning of an axon to sever it form its mammalian nerve cell is similarly associated with sharp changes in the Nissl bodies which are connected with an acceleration of the synthesis of nucleoproteins (Bodian, 1947). The incorporation of ^{14}C-oratic acid is increased by 100 percent above the control, on the eighth day after compression of the axon when there is chromatolysis (Brattgard et al., 1958). Synthesis of RNA in the neurons of the hypoglossal nucleus started increasing 12 hours after the transection of their axons and reached a maximum between the 7th and 14th day as determined by noting the incorporation of hydrogen labeled uridine (Haddad et al., 1969). Brodskii (1966) has reported that a considerable change in the amount of RNA was necessary during the active phase of a cell. He suggested that replacement of specific RNA may be due to the utilization of the disintegrated products of RNA, mainly the fragments of the "functional" RNA which have participated in the biosynthesis of protein. In his opinion, RNA has several different forms of participation in the synthesis of cellular protein, apart from acting as a messenger in the transmission of information from DNA to protein and acting as a carrier of amino acids for transcription. RNA must also play a role of some importance in the catabolic phase of protein metabolism. The intensity of the nucleic acid synthesis which facilitates favoring the synthesis of protein in a cell may be changed by the administration of different biogenic stimulators and chemicals (Hydén, 1947; Lazarev & Felistovich, 1954; Polezhaev, 1966a; Reznikov, 1967). It is possible that among the substances stimulating the synthesis of nucleic acids, some substances could be found which would actively stimulate the process of axon regeneration inside the central nervous system.

Hydrolyzates and Extracts as Stimulators of Regeneration

The effort to encourage the regenerative processes with the help of different agents appeared as soon as the principal mechanisms guiding protein synthesis were known. Administration of all types of products from disintegrated tissues was reported by investigators in an effort to control the regenerative processes at every stage.

Several Swiss investigators (Jent, Koechlin, Muralt, & Wagner-Jauregg, 1945) isolated two substances during the search for an active principle in the tissue extracts: one which accelerated and the other which retarded regeneration. The nerve-regenerating factor isolated by these workers, termed as NR, had certain specificity; it did not contain protein, was relatively stable to heat, and was destroyed during autolysis, i.e., it was not an autolytic product. Koechlin (1955) reported that the best source of NR was rabbit or calf brain, possibly the white matter, or else a degenerated or normal sciatic nerve. Extracts of spleen, liver, or embryo were found inactive. Luescher and Muralt (1947) thought that pyrimidine derivatives were the active ingredients of NR.

Frequent attempts to use hydrolyzates and extracts for various purposes have been reported in the Soviet Union.

Tushnov (1938) obtained lyzates by autolysis of individual organ tissues which showed a specific action after their administration in an organism by stimulating the function of that organ from which the lyzates had been prepared.

Filatov (1953) worked out a method for application of "biogenic stimulators" whose action was based on the rise of resistance of an organism as well as the activation of its growth processes. These gave nice results in a hospital for eye diseases. Rumyantsev (1951) employed preserved tissues as biogenic stimulators, in the belief that when administered in an organism, these would produce a stimulating effect favoring the formation of substances which would utilize the dying tissue.

Zelinskii (1946) suggested the role of hydrolyzates in the process of regeneration in the belief that hydrolyzates helped in the formation of new proteins based on the successful utilization of cartilage hydrolyzate for the regeneration of an additional limb in axolotl [in experiments conducted by Nasonov (1941)]. More or less similar explanations have been given by Polezhaev; he considered that the hydrolyzate acts as an activator of the nucleoprotein synthesis and this is possibly due to the presence of protein degradation products. He and his coworkers successfully used the hydrolyzates of corresponding tissues in different types of procedures involving regeneration of an amputated extremity in a rodent (Polezhaev & Ramenskaya, 1950) and also for healing myocardial damage in rats and dogs (Polezhaev et al., 1965). Restoration of regenerating capacity after radiation in an axolotl was achieved by the administration of muscle homogenates, acidic proteins, and with highly polymerized RNA (Polezhaev, 1959b, 1966b; Polezhaev, Tepkits, & Ernakova, 1961; Polezhaev, Teplits, & Tuchkova, 1962). The action of substances restoring the regenerative capacity was based on a rise in concentration of nucleic acids in the regenerating part of the tissue which was found to show an increase, with a maximum in the initial phases of tissue differentiation (Teplits, 1964a, 1964b).

Thus, the effect on the synthesis of nucleic acids which had favored the regeneration of organs and tissues was not capable of stimulating regenerative neural growth.

Nerve Growth Factor (NGF)

Very interesting work was conducted by a group of scientists in St. Louis, Missouri on the study of a new factor promoting the growth of axons, which had initially been isolated from rat sarcoma and later from snake venom and the salivary glands of rodents. The basis for utilizing tumor tissues was obtained from the experiments of Duncan and Belledie (1948). They found that a Walter rat sarcoma implanted in the gap between the stumps of a transected rat spinal cord was penetrated by the nerve fibers from the posterior columns and dorsal roots. Similarly, an intense growth of intraspinal fibers was noticed in a transplant during the extradural transplantation of rat sarcoma 319 (Duncan, 1955). The character of myelination and staining of the fibers were changed so that they resembled peripheral nerves.

Levi-Montalcini alone and in collaboration with Hamburger (Levi-Montalcini, 1951, 1952; Levi-Montalcini & Hamburger, 1953) similarly transplanted pieces of mouse sarcoma 180 and 37 in a chick embryo which was incubated *in vitro.* They reported that the cells of sensory and sympathetic ganglion invaded and filled the tumor with their sprouts. In an attempt to study the mechanism of action of the neoplastic factor, Levi-Montalcini, Mejer, and Hamburger (1954) used a suspended drop type of *in vitro* method and determined the rate of axonal growth in the spinal ganglion separated from the body of a chick embryo, in the presence and absence of a piece of sarcoma. The results demonstrated that when a piece of sarcoma was present in a suspended drop preparation, a complete halo of axons was seen to surround the ganglion within the first 24 hours, although this was not observed in the control. The authors concluded that the neoplastic factor acted directly on the nerve cells.

Subsequent efforts of these investigators were directed toward studying the chemical nature of this active factor (Cohen, Levi-Montalcini, & Hamburger, 1954; Levi-Montalcini, Cohen, & Hamburger, 1954). It was shown that the active principle of NGF was present in the microsomal fraction of the tumor homogenate and was a thermolabile substance, containing 66% protein, 27%

RNA, and 0.2% DNA. The same group investigated snake venom and its protein fraction to determine the exact nature of the growth factor (Cohen & Levi-Montalcini, 1956; Levi-Montalcini & Cohen, 1956). It was found that snake venom even in a crude form was an even more effective stimulator of the growth of afferent and sympathetic nerve fibers than the neoplastic factor. A nondialyzable, thermolabile substance isolated from venom was tested on the growth of axons *in vitro*; it was found to be 1000 times more active than a purified fraction obtained from a neoplasm (Fig. 49).

Cohen (1959) came to the following conclusion in the course of his attempts to investigate the nature and mode of action of this active substance. Though the snake venom was rich in enzymes, the active principle was not associated with them, as the activity of all the enzymes was found to be lower in the purified fraction of the venom than in the crude extract. The potential for growth effect in the ganglion was tested by the application of a number of growth hormones in tissue cultures; none of these produced any acceleration of growth. A question was then raised about the action of the growth-stimulating substance on the synthesis of protein and nucleic acids. The incorporation of labeled amino acids into nuclear RNA and DNA, both in the presence and absence of NGF, was studied. It was found that the incorporation of ^{14}C-lysine into nucleic acids was accelerated by 58–72 percent in the presence of NGF, while the rate of incorporation of ^{14}C-adenine in RNA was increased by 84–94 percent. In the study of incorporation of ^{14}C of adenine into RNA, an increase of 40–69 percent was noticed, while the incorporation in DNA in the presence of NGF was not increased. The increase in synthesis of RNA due to the action of NGF during *in vitro* experiments was also confirmed by other investigators (Angeletti, Toschi, Salvi, & Levi-Montalcini, 1960).

Thus, the growth factor isolated from a neoplasm, snake venom or, later, from the salivary glands of rodents distinctly increased the synthesis of cellular RNA but did not affect the synthesis of DNA. The energy source of this synthesis was investigated by Cohen (1959). The necessity of glucose for the growth of axons was determined by the fact that growth began in its absence but did not continue. The addition of ^{14}C-glucose to the tissue-culture medium intensified the oxidative processes during the action of the growth factor by 41–54 percent. Among the several amino acids studied, phenylalanine was found to be essential.

Considering the chemical properties, biological activity and other characteristics, growth factor may, in all probability, be related to a class of substances occupying a position between the enzymes and hormones (Levi-Montalcini & Angeletti, 1968).

These investigations gave valuable evidence on the factors enhancing the growth of afferent fibers in a chick embryo during an *in vitro* experiment. It

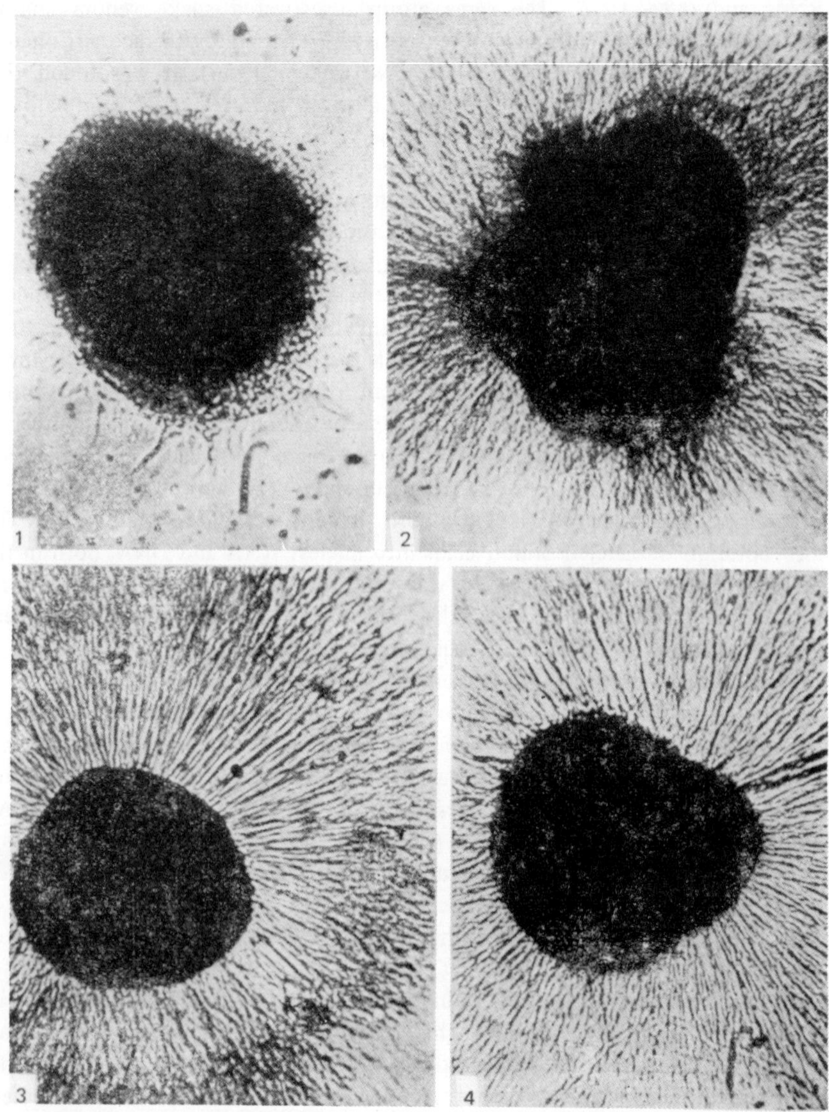

FIG. 49. Microphotographs of the sensory ganglion from a 7-day-old chick embryo after incubation at 37°C for 18 hours.

1–in a standard control medium; 2–in a medium containing crude snake venom at a concentration of 7 μg/ml; 3–in a medium containing the active fraction obtained from snake venom at a concentration of 0.3 μg/ml; 4–in a medium containing 250 μg/ml of "protein fraction" obtained from a sarcoma 180 (adopted from *Cohen and Levi-Montalcini,* 1956).

was found necessary to repeat the experiment on mammals (Bueker, Schenkein, & Bane, 1960; Levi-Montalcini & Booker, 1960). The action of an active fraction isolated from the salivary glands of mouse was tested in *in vitro* experiments on mammalian sympathetic ganglia, especially in a human embryo. The results were more or less similar to those obtained with a chick embryo. The administration of an active fraction to a newborn and an adult mouse produced a definite rise in the size of the sympathetic ganglion. Its size varied with the age of the animal, the amount and the frequency of administration of the extract.

The action of NGF on mammalian spinal neurons was reported by Scott and Liu (1963, 1964). A transection of the dorsal spinocerebeller tract was performed on a kitten weighing 700-800 g. The neuro-regenerating substance with a known unit of activity was administered subcutaneously to three kittens daily for a period of 14, 22, and 28 days, respectively, after operation. In the first case, 2200 units was given per day; in the second, 280 units; and in the third, 860 units. Piromen was given twice at a dose of 10 μg each. The best results were obtained by the administration of the maximum dose of NGF, and observed 50 days after operation. The axons, after growing through the area of transection, continued in a compact manner into the rostral stump up to a distance of 6.3 mm. The conducted nerve impulse was recorded at a distance of 8 mm rostral to the section. With smaller doses, the results were less striking. The authors concluded that NGF could promote the regeneration of afferent nerve fibers; later they supported the hypothesis that an underlying cause of the abortive regeneration of intraspinal axons is their inadequate potential for growth. The nature of the fibers subjected to stimulation is not clear from this particular work. In a discussion of this question, Glees (1964) suggested that they grew from the fibers of the dorsal root ganglion. This conclusion was based on the nature of the growing fibers, the growth potentiality of which was well known. Trevor (1964) similarly supported the view that the growing fibers had originated from a root.

In another experiment on rats, Scott, Gutmann, and Horsky, (1966) compressed the dorsal root of S_1 and then compared the degree of incorporation of ^{3}H-leucine in the spinal ganglion cells following an intraperitoneal administration of NGF. The other side of the cord served as the control. It was shown that incorporation of ^{3}H-leucine in the ganglion cells on the side of the crush was increased by 14 ± 4% as compared with the control. Without the administration of NGF, no increase in incorporation of leucine was observed.

Thus, the incorporation of labeled amino acids in the cells of spinal ganglion was considerably increased by the action of NGF, which indicates an accelerated intracellular synthesis of nucleoprotein. The above results confirm the correctness of our assumption that the stimulation of the regenerative process occurs by accelerating the synthesis of nucleoproteins in nerve cells having a transected axon, when substances activating the synthesis of nucleic acids are administrated.

Search for Substances Stimulating the Growth of Nerve Fibers

Repeated attempts have been made to stimulate regeneration of peripheral nerves by the administration of pharmacological compounds or by accelerating the function of the neuron. Hoffman (1952) tried to influence the regeneration of peripheral nerves by changing the "synthetic activity of a neuron." This was achieved by electrically stimulating the spinal cord or the roots and by administration of the dye, Pyronin. This work proceeded from the discovery by Hydén (1943) and by Barr and Bertram (1951) who showed that Nissl substance can be changed as a result of stimulation. The use of Pyronin was based on the fact that it causes an acceleration of growth in Drosophila by participating in the formation of constituent parts of nucleic acids. He, then, noticed that when Pyronin was administered to a rat orally for four successive days preceding nerve transection, about 80.8 percent innervation was observed on the seventh day after operation as compared to 24.7 percent in the control. Electrical stimulation of the roots of the sciatic plexus or the spinal cord also produced a significant increase in the growth of peripheral nerve. Gamble and Jha (1959) used Pyronin in rats after compression of the peripheral nerve and similarly obtained acceleration of growth and myelination of the regenerating nerve, but to a lesser degree. These authors suggested that Pyronin acts not directly by increasing the protein synthesis, but by changing the enzyme activity of the intracellular components.

Considering the above data cited from various sources and our own observations, an attempt was made to select a pharmacological compound which could stimulate the growth of intraspinal axons. The pyrimidine derivatives might be such agents as they are the constituents of nucleic acids. Lazarev and Felistovich (1954) isolated two of the less toxic water-soluble compounds, metacil and pentoxyl, by hydrolyzing nucleic acids. Both the substances, particularly pentoxyl, showed the following effects: (1) Successfully increased the number of leukocytes in the blood dyscrasias, (2) accelerated the healing of corneal and cutaneous wounds; (3) stimulated the mitosis of the endothelial, muscular and connective tissue cells; and (4) significantly accelerated the multiplication of yeast cells. Lazarev suggested that the action of pentoxyl and metacil was due to their interference with the metabolism of nucleic acids. It is possible that they inhibit the depolymerization of nucleic acids by affecting their enzymes. Thus, they may change the equilibrium by increasing the polymerization of nucleic acids and this leads to a rise of their concentration in cells and thus causes an acceleration of protein synthesis (Lazarev, 1960).

The effect of pentoxyl on the nucleic acid metabolism in rats was confirmed in a number of organs (Minkina, 1958). She also suggested that the principal action of pentoxyl was due to its inhibition of depolymerases. When testing the action of pentoxyl on the regeneration from experimental damage to the sciatic nerve in albino mice, it was found that it stimulated the above process (Kustov, 1959). Animals with experimental injuries received pentoxyl at a dose of 40 mg/kg body weight (Chumak, 1959, 1960). The main advantages of this preparation are that it can be given orally and its use for therapeutic pruposes is permitted by Farmakomitet (the Drug Control Authority). In all the experiments with muscular and cutaneous injuries as well as in gastric lesions, pentoxyl stimulated healing by promoting quick formation of scar tissue and by regenerating the cells of a particular tissue. It has also been reported that pentoxyl is very useful for the treatment of cerebral injuries (Lemus, 1960). Pentoxyl seemed to be a prospective stimulator for the regeneration of axons in the central nervous system.

The results of our experiments conducted on rats and dogs demonstrated that such an assumption was correct (Nesmeyanova, Arnautova, & Brazovskaya, 1965). Pentoxyl was administered intramuscularly to a rat at a dose of 15 mg/kg for a period of six days after transection of the spinal cord. Pyrogenal was given simultaneously and the growth of the nerve fibers near a scar was found to be more abundant within two weeks after operation as compared to the application of Pyrogenal alone (Fig. 50). The rate of growth of the nerve fibers inside a scar was observed and in all cases was uniform from the rostral and caudal stumps of the spinal cord; this might indicate an enhancement of growth of both the sensory and motor nerve fibers.

The dogs receiving pentoxyl orally for a month at a dose of 15 mg/kg on every fourth day along with Pyrogenal did not differ much in either time or degree of functional restoration from the dogs which had received resorptive transplants.

The morphological investigation of serial spinal sections, impregnated with silver three to six months after operation, showed the presence of bundles of nerve fibers near a scar and their growth into an area where there was no cyst formation. Growth of nerve fibers inside a scar was observed on both the rostral and caudal sides of the stumps. The majority of the growing fibers were thick, resembling nerves showing increased argentophilia (Fig. 51).

The spinal scar in all the experimental dogs was friable, and the collagen fibers were arranged obliquely transversely and in some places, longitudinally.

Thus, substances which affect RNA synthesis in an organism were found to stimulate neural regeneration to a certain extent. This led to a search for a more effective stimulating agent which would cause pronounced regeneration of intraspinal axons.

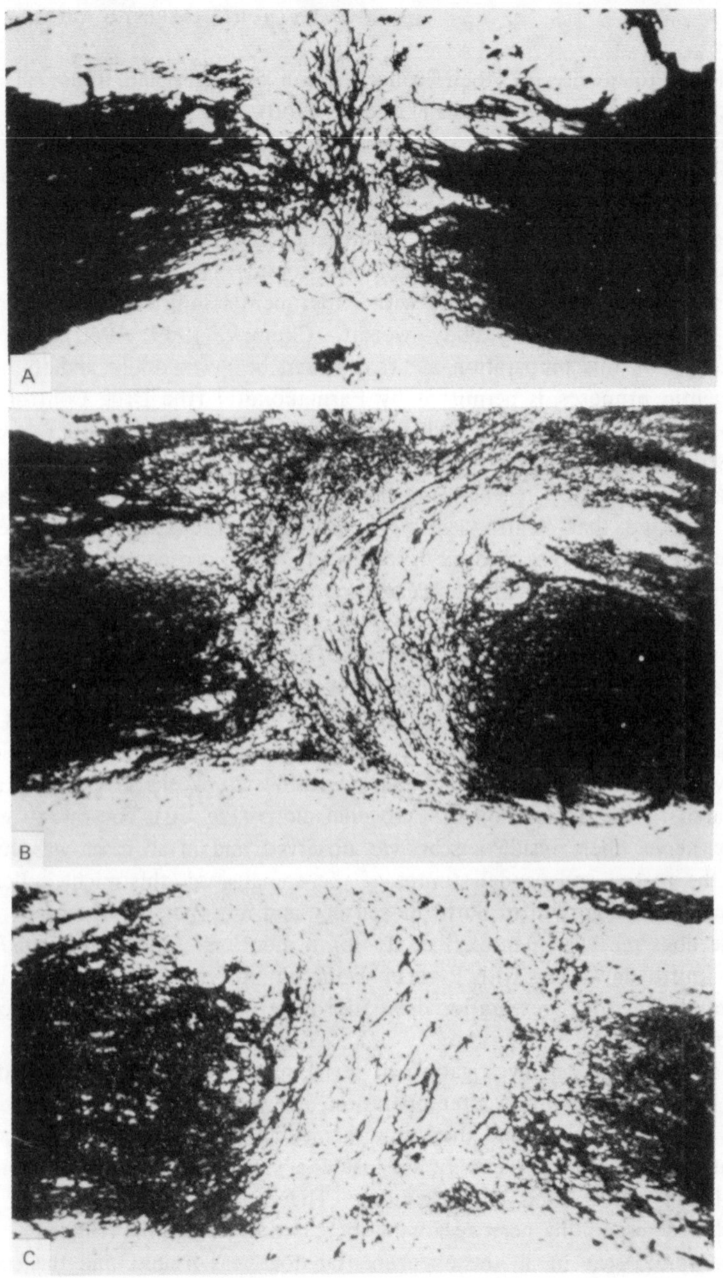

FIG. 50. Growth of nerve fibers through the area of section in experimental rats, two weeks after operation.

Rats receiving: A–dinitryl malonic acid + Pyrogenal; B–pentoxyl + Pyrogenal; C–Pyrogenal. Silver impregnation. Magnification, eye piece 3, 5 objective 7.

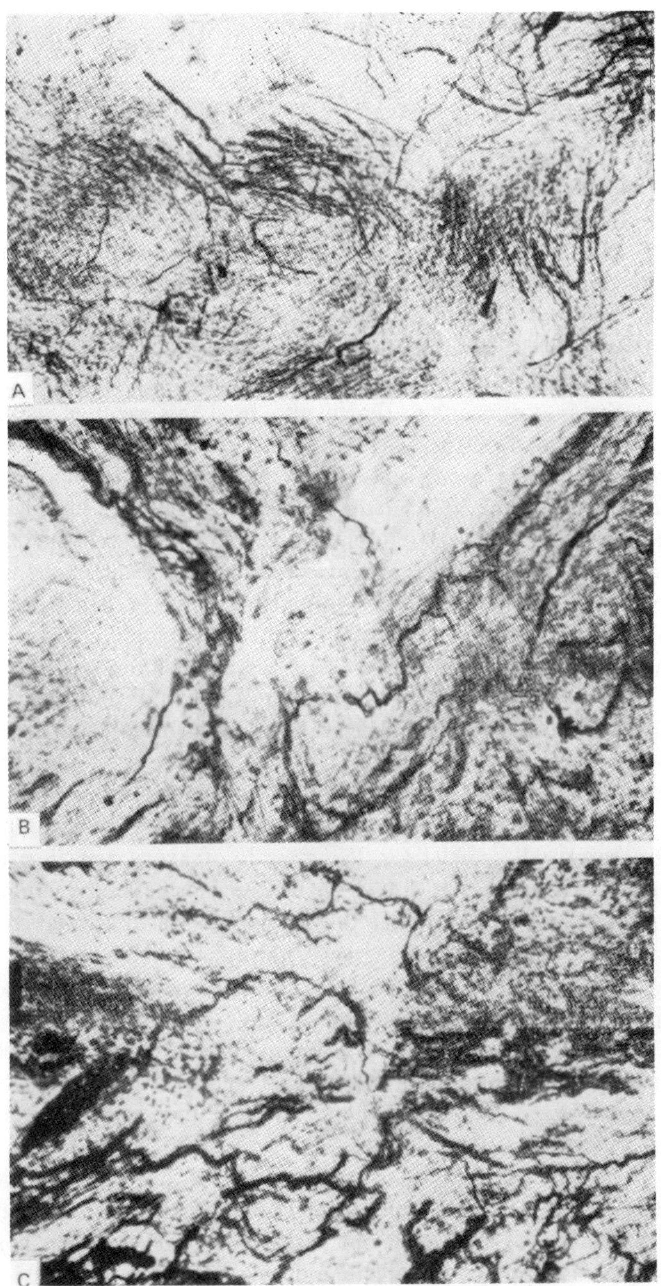

FIG. 51. Growth of the nerve fibers through the lesion site in dogs receiving pentoxyl.

A, B–three months after operation; C–six months after operation. Silver impregnation. Magnification–objective–7, eye piece–20.

Dinitrylmalonic Acid as a Stimulator of Intraspinal Axon Growth

Dinitrylmalonic acid (malononitrile)–CH_2 $(CN)_2$–might well be an effective stimulator of intraspinal axons regeneration. The administration of this compound to an animal produces a change in the cytochemical composition of its nerve cells (Hydén, 1947). Thus, intravenous administration at the rate of 4 mg/kg body-weight has been observed to produce a significant rise in the concentration of RNA, both inside the nucleoli and in the cytoplasm of a cell within an hour; subsequently, the concentration of protein was practically doubled in the motor neurons. Hydén also used this agent in schizophrenic patients due to the fact that mental diseases produce an alteration of the metabolism of RNA in nerve cells where the nucleolus is poorly developed and the concentration of RNA in the cytoplasm is low. He suggested that an acceleration of both RNA and protein synthesis in nerve cells increased their functional ability. Twenty-nine patients received this agent in a dose of 3-5 mg/kg for a total of 10 intravenous administrations. The beneficial effect of dinitrylmalonic acid on mental capabilities differed among individual patients. The effect appeared within 48 hours after administration and continued for 10 days. It was believed that the mechanism of action of dinitrylmalonic acid depended on a rise of RNA concentration in the neuron (Egyhazi & Hydén, 1961).

Experiments conducted by Nesmeyanova (1968a) confirmed the hypothesis that the use of dinitrylmalonic acid, the agent accelerating the synthesis of RNA in a nerve cell, accelerates the growth of axons and thus promotes regeneration. This agent was found to be the most effective stimulator of regeneration in our experiments. During its application for a total course of 4 injections at a dose level of 4 mg/kg every third day, the nerve fibers in all 10 rats grew abundantly. Within two weeks, numerous fibers were seen near the periphery of the spinal scar and a large number inside it, filling it completely in a loose and diffused manner. The fibers fully connected both the stumps, growing from both the caudal and the cranial direction. The growing nerves were smooth without any swelling and were intensively impregnated with silver (Fig. 50A).

For comparison, Fig. 50B shows the growth of fibers during the use of Pyrogenal alone. Interesting results were obtained related to formation of a scar during the use of dinitrylmalonic acid. The developed scar possessed a considerably more friable structure than during the use of Pyrogenal alone–as judged from a preparation impregnated with silver and counterstained with carmine.

A pronounced functional recovery was observed in a dog which survived for a long time and received dinitrylmalonic acid, in agreement with the data on the growth of nerve fibers in rats. Though sensation and scratch reflex in this dog were not restored, the locomotor functions and weight-bearing left no doubt about the restoration of conduction along the spinal cord. The dog began to rise and stand within 2½ months and weight-bearing became comparatively stable by 3½ months and remained unchanged for a period of 2½ years, i.e., for the rest of the life of the dog. The muscles of the hind legs atrophied in the initial period after operation, but were restored and became enlarged and resilient within four months. The same type of muscle tone as in an intact animal developed, which allowed stable support to the hind limbs. In Fig. 52A, the electromyogram from the gastrocnemius muscle was recorded during standing and on applying pressure over the sacrum. For comparison, the electromyograms obtained in control spinal dogs under the same conditions are presented simultaneously (Fig. 52B, C). It can be seen that while the character and degree of activity were changed in the latter, they remained unchanged in the experimental animals. Due to the presence of the well-developed stable tone of the extensor muscles, this particular dog used the hind legs effectivly which enabled it to run with comparative success (Fig. 53). The reversal of function which took place in dogs receiving only Pyrogenal was not observed here, even after a lapse of 2½ years following operation.

Morphologic study of the cord sections demonstrated that transection of the spinal cord in this dog was complete, and in the friable part of the scar,

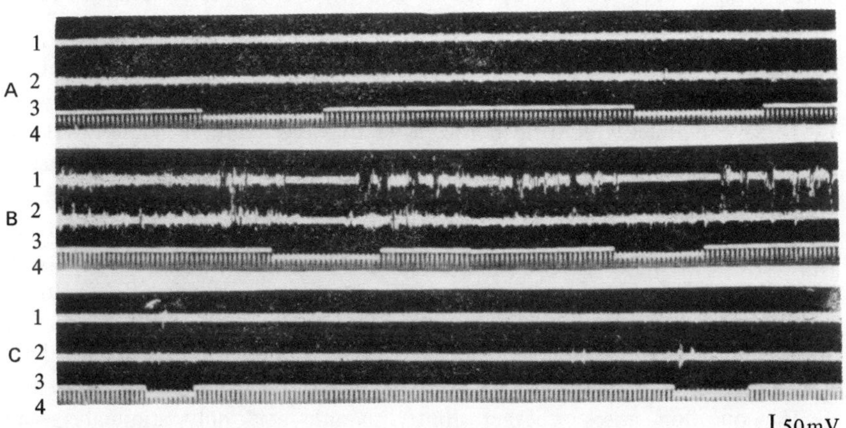

FIG. 52. The change of activity in the calf muscles of (A) a dog receiving dinitrylmalonic acid and (B, C) in control dogs without any treatment on pressing the sacrum at the time of standing.

1–m. gastrocnemius (right); 2–m. gastrocnemius (left); 3–mark of pressing the sacrum; 4–time, 20 msec.

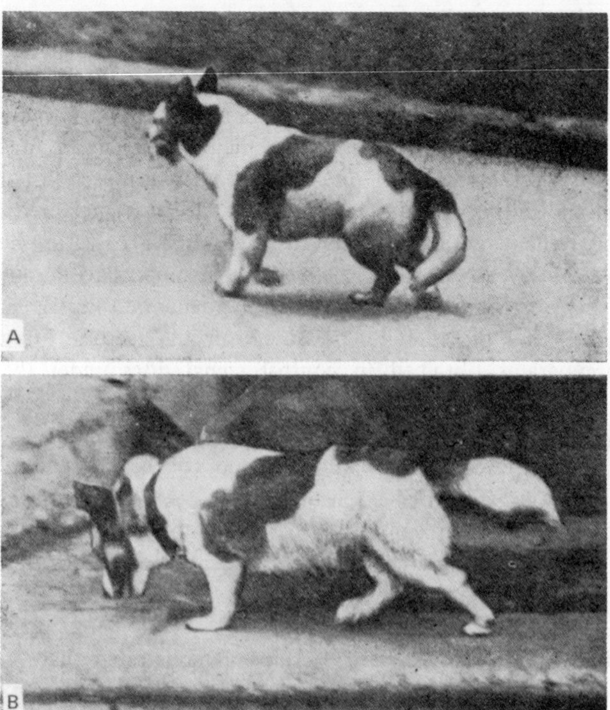

FIG. 53. Dog treated with dinitrylmalonic acid (A) one year after operation; (B) 2½ years after operation.

abundant growth of the intraspinal and root fibers from both the stumps of the cord was observed.

These experiments confirmed the belief that regeneration of the intraspinal axons in mammals can be stimulated with the administration of substances which accelerate RNA synthesis in the organism. The difference in the results obtained with pentoxyl and dinitrylmalonic acid could be due to the different effect of these preparations on this synthesis but the great disadvantage of dinitrylmalonic acid is its high toxicity, according to Hydén (1947). In our experiments, during its use in dogs, signs of poisoning were observed and there were cases where the animals died. According to Hydén, hyposulfite reduces the toxicity of this substance.

The question arises whether dinitrylmalonic acid only stimulates nerve regeneration or also activates functional recovery due to an increase in RNA synthesis in the neurons. In that case, compensatory processes will be developed to a greater extent than regenerative ones. In our experiments with dogs receiving dinitrylmalonic acid, growth of nerve fibers through the lesion site as well as restoration of motor function were observed; both effects tend to confirm the presence of functional regeneration. The restoration of motor functions by these dogs differed considerably both in character and degree, as was previously reported after compensatory restoration in a treated spinal dog. The possible effect of dinitrylmalonic acid on the development of compensatory processes cannot be excluded.

Another interesting fact is that dinitrylmalonic acid and pentoxyl activated the regeneration of both descending and ascending fibers while nerve growth factor (NGF), as reported by Levi-Montalcini and co-workers, only affected the growth of the afferent and sympathetic fibers. It is possible that these substances selectively affect the synthesis of nucleic acids in specific types of nerve cells, but there are reports that dinitrylmalonic acid and NGF are comparable between themselves in their mode of action (Houlihan & Da Vanzo, 1964). The observations of Liu (1951) about the absence of changes in the synthesis of nucleoproteins in a nerve cell with dinitrylmalonic acid are probably incorrect.

The success achieved with these preparations led to the search for a substance which was not so toxic as dinitrylmalonic acid but would considerably accelerate the synthesis of nucleic acids. The use of Pyronin by Musalov (1965) gave results similar to whose obtained with pentoxyl, based on the preliminary data.

The substances which need testing are the derivatives of dinitrylmalonic acid–tricyanoaminopropane (tricyan) and succinodinitryl (dinitrylsuccinic acid, SDN). Within an hour of the administration of 5 mg of tricyan, the amount of RNA inside a neuron is increased by 25 percent while that in a glial cell decreases by 40 percent (Hydén & Hartelius, 1948). Likewise, activity of cytochrome oxidase, calculated for a single nerve cell, is found to increase to 300 percent. When they received tricyan for a period of three days, mice did not respond with convulsive shock to normally effective electric stimulation (Essman, 1966). Brain tissue showed a considerable difference in RNA concentration when the experimental and control animals were compared.

Partial motor asymmetry was produced in a pigeon by unilateral destruction of the cerebellum. Subsequent transection of the spinal cord, in this case, did not abolish this asymmetry, if the operation was done more than 45 min after destruction of the cerebellum. The use of a malonic acid derivative reduced the time necessary for producing irreversible asymmetry to 30 min (Gerard, Chamberlain, & Rothschild, 1963). These authors considered that the more rapid effect was due to a change of the form of RNA as a result of the tricyanoamino propane.

The second substance–succinodinitryl–was studied by Swiss scientists. They found that changes in the coefficient of absorption of the nucleoproteins in ultraviolet light showed that there was considerable rise in the concentration of these substances in the nucleoli and cytoplasm after treating rabbits with succinodinitryl. The quantity of Nissl substance was, likewise, increased and possibly showed a structural change (Bammer & von Muralt, 1955). They concluded that succinodinitryl interferes with the nucleoprotein metabolism of nerve cells affecting the synthesis of nucleic acids. While dinitrylmalonic acid possesses a strong toxic action, succinodinitryl is relatively nontoxic (König, 1953). When succinodinitryl was administered to a rabbit at a dose of 25 mg/kg, it was found to be toxic, but a dose of 15 mg/kg given for 3 consecutive days or at an interval of 1 to 2 days for 11-26 days was not toxic (Bammer & von Maralt, 1953). The toxicity of a high dose of succinodinitryl was probably related to suppression of the oxidative phosphorylation in the tissue (Houlihan & Da Vanzo, 1964).

These data indicate that the factor deciding the success in the growth of intraspinal axons is an acceleration of the synthesis of nucleoproteins in the neurons whose axons have been transected. Thus, the regeneration of central axons requires the same process which is responsible for the growth and development of different types of tissues and organs after their destruction in various types of animals. The regenerative capacity of neurons, which has been lost as a result of the unusual and pronounced differentiation of the nervous system during the process of phylogenesis, may be restored by influencing the synthesis of nucleic acids in nerve cells whose axons have been damaged. This process may be carried out with the help of various pharmacologic preparations.

CHAPTER V

RESTORATION OF MOTOR FUNCTION IN THE LOWER EXTREMITIES OF PATIENTS WITH COMPLETE OR PARTIAL LOSS OF CONDUCTION IN SPINAL NEURONS

Possible Means of Developing Motor Function

Analysis of the functional peculiarities of a transected spinal cord (such as the capacity to organize new motor reflexes, the stability of developed reactions, and the maintenance of neuronal apparatus in a normal state by treatment), which have been demonstrated in previous chapters, allows us to evaluate the significance of these factors relating to the restoration of function in patients with complete or partial loss of conduction in spinal neurons (Roaf, 1972).

Restoration of function following spinal trauma may take place in several ways. The following are the most important:

1. Regeneration of neurons in the spinal cord.

2. Functional recovery, i.e., the restoration of impulse propagation along an uninjured axon of the spinal cord. This may appear immediately after trauma or at some later stage of the restorative treatment if these fibers fail to

function initially, due to the development of dystrophic processes in the spinal cord.

3. Compensatory development of alternate motor functions which may substitute for those previously injured, namely: (a) compensation by involvement of muscles usually not participating in a given movement; (b) development of activity in muscles innervated from a distal spinal segment; (c) compensation by the utilization of fibers in the sympathetic nervous system.

Let us examine what is known about this problem and the information available concerning restoration of lost functions as a result of spinal trauma.

Regeneration of Intrinsic Fibers in the Spinal Cord

Brown-Sequard (1892) first reported the possibility of regeneration in conducting paths of the human spinal cord. In a review dealing with this problem, Druckman (1955) cited a number of cases from the literature in which growing nerve fibers were found near the damaged area of the spinal cord. Mair and Druckman (1953) noted similar nerve fibers in the spinal cord of patients with a prolapse of the intervertebral disc. In another review, a number of cases were reported to show the presence of regenerating nerve fibers inside the spinal cord (Lockhart, 1955). These growing fibers may belong to dorsal roots having a high potential for growth, as suggested by Lhermitte (1919). However, following the experimental compression of the spinal cord in kittens, it was observed that the central fibers began to resemble the peripheral ones and neuroglia turned into neurolemma (Duncan, 1954, 1955; Duncan & Bellegie, 1948) and from this Druckman (1955) concluded that the growing fibers observed by these investigators were intraspinal.

The restoration of function due to regeneration following damage to the spinal cord has been reported by several investigators (Fickler, 1905; Zemlyanskaya, 1940). Enhancement of tone in the antigravity muscles of patients with a complete transection of the spinal cord, as observed by Foerster (1936) and Riddoch (1937), can probably be explained by restoration of the connections between spinal segments, since the tone of these muscles is determined by the presence of supraspinal control over the gamma-motoneurons.

A case involving complete transection of the spinal cord (caused by a bullet injury at the level of Th_{10} with subsequent suturing of the stumps) was reported by Lockhart (1955) and Windle (1959). The restoration of several motor functions, such as weight-bearing and protopathic sensation, was reported in this patient, indicating the regeneration of spinal axons. Windle suggested that infection of the urinary bladder, causing liberation of pyrogens, might have favored the growth of the nerve fibers. This patient survived more than 20 years following the injury but lost the restored functions within a few years. A dense collagenous scar in the injured area was found upon examining the cord in histologic sections.

The possibility of axon regeneration in a damaged spinal cord and of the restoration of corresponding altered functions in man can be considered by presenting a few facts.

Recovery of Function

Recovery may take place in cases of partial or almost complete loss of conduction in the fibers of the spinal cord (e.g., during its release from compression). An essential condition for recovery is to keep the neuronal apparatus of the spinal cord in good condition which can be attained through its increased activity by use of physiotherapy methods. A summary of experimental treatment applied after spinal cord injury in the monkey has been reported by Black, Markowitz, Cianei, and Dunn (1974).

Methods for the treatment of patients having spinal trauma have been worked out in the Soviet Union and other countries (Rogan, 1975; Nakamura, 1973; Steinberg, 1975). Great importance has been attached to physiotherapy, such as massage, electrotherapy, and other similar methods. This type of treatment improves the blood supply to the organs and favors the conduction of excitation along the spinal cord (Gorinevskaya, 1933, 1938; Heinmanovich, 1943; Khoroshko, 1941; Mokreeva, 1950; Moshkov, Freidin, & Ratova, 1944; Prikhod'ko, 1940; Sozon-Yaroshevich, 1934; Uarova-Yakobson, 1940). Physiotherapy differs from other methods of treatment in that the patient participates actively. This is particularly important for the return to normal of both somatic as well as psychic function (Moshkov, 1944, 1963).

The treatment of patients with spinal injuries has been well organized in England. The Stoke Mandeville Hospital, a rehabilitation center for the last 25 years, has been directed by Prof. L. Guttmann, who, together with his medical and paramedical colleagues, has achieved considerable success in saving the life of spinal patients and sending them back to work (Guttmann, 1942, 1946, 1957, 1959, 1973a, 1973b). The first-aid care and nursing of patients has been developed and has been used successfully. Here, the patients' posture is taken into consideration when caring for them as it affects the future development of the extensor muscle tone (Guttmann, 1953). Proper care is taken of the pelvic organs (Guttmann & Frankel, 1966). Great attention is paid to physiotherapy as applied in the form of passive movements of the extremities, and, later, intensive treatment is started in which the long muscles of the trunk and shoulder girdle are included. The patients with partial transection of the spinal cord begin to stand up and learn to walk. Direct stimulation of the muscles, particularly of the extensor muscles of the extremities, has been recommended to prevent the development of atrophy

(Guttmann, 1953). A review of physiological problems in paraplegia has been published by Eccles (1972).

In other countries, as, for example, in the USA, the treatment of patients with spinal injuries is based more or less on the same principles as described here. Great importance is given to physiotherapy for the maintenance of normal function of an organism and in training the motor systems innervated by the proximal segment of the spinal cord. Both of these help in the restoration of normal activity after partial cord transection (Dinken, 1943; Freeman, 1949a, 1949b; Joster & Boche, 1941; Lorme, 1946; Rusk, 1958).

In Czechoslovakia, patients with a partial transection of the spinal cord are usually treated in such a way as to provide the maximum possible restoration of function (Benes, 1958).

Prof. Ugryumov and his colleagues achieved considerable progress in the treatment of spinal patients (Ugryumov, 1956a, 1956b, 1960, 1961; Ugryumov, Kruglyi, & Vinarskaya, 1964). Application of physiotherapy methods, which were worked out individually by them for patients with an incomplete transection of the spinal cord, led to partial restoration of normal motor function. Kruglyi (1956, 1958) attached greater importance to early lifting of the patient to a vertical position on special crutches with suitable splints and applying the methods of physiotherapy. This promoted the development of motor activity in patients and helped to develop the muscles, joints, and bones. These measures also prevented the development of dystrophic processes (Skotnikov, 1956) and considerably improved the condition of the peripheral nerve-muscle apparatus (Kruglyi, 1960).

The therapeutic treatment of patients with trauma of the spinal cord—involving recovery of function of the pelvic organs, control of trophic changes, putting the patient on crutches with splints and training him in walking—has a highly beneficial effect on the physical and psychological conditions of patients; it stimulates and motivates them to further work.

The preservation of the intact axons of the spinal cord is of great importance in the success of functional restoration. When the spinal cord stumps were separated by less than 2 mm, even a very small number of intact axons led to a considerable restoration of motor function (Ugryumov, 1956b). Three such cases have been reported from the Saratov Institute (Arkhangel'skii, 1956; Krasovskii, 1956). These facts were not accidental. Collier (1904) reported, from his own cases, the late restoration of motor function in a patient who appeared to have a complete transection of spinal cord. Lhermitte (1919) reported the reappearance of sensation after a lapse of 15–18 months in two patients where clinical signs of a complete transection of the spinal cord had been observed during that period. Duncan (1955) noticed that there was an excellent recovery of both motor and sensory function in cats following compression of the spinal cord, even when the ligature had been left partly obstructing the ventrolateral tracts. Trankvillitati (1960) reported the case of her patient Mrs. S., 14 months after the second lumbar vertebra was crushed by dislocation up to the fourth lumbar vertebra. There were no active movements in her lower extremities, including the lower part of her body. The lower abdominal and tendon reflexes were absent. The joints were less mobile. There was no sensation from below the L_2 segment. After six months of treatment, she could raise her legs from the hip joint, the tendon reflexes reappeared, and later she started responding to the application of pain and tactile stimuli. The patient was sent home on crutches, and she continued the physical therapy. After six years, active movements appeared in her ankle joints and it was possible for her to bear weight without the splints. At present she moves only with a cane.

Experiments on dogs confirmed that a *small number* of intact non-transected fibers of the spinal cord were capable of undertaking a large number of functions. Hence, in our experiments on two dogs, an area of about 7 percent of the cross section of spinal cord was preserved during a transection. This included fibers of the vestibulospinal and the olivospinal tracts of the right side. The transection was at the level of Th_{10}. Within three weeks after operation, coordinated function appeared in these animals but sensation was not restored. It was difficult to differentiate these animals from intact dogs by observing the nature of their movements (Fig. 54). Bernstein and Bernstein (1973) have reported neuronal alteration and reinnervation following axonal regeneration and sprouting in mammalian spinal cord.

The ability of the descending tracts of the spinal cord to provide a substitute function was unusually pronounced and a significant safety factor

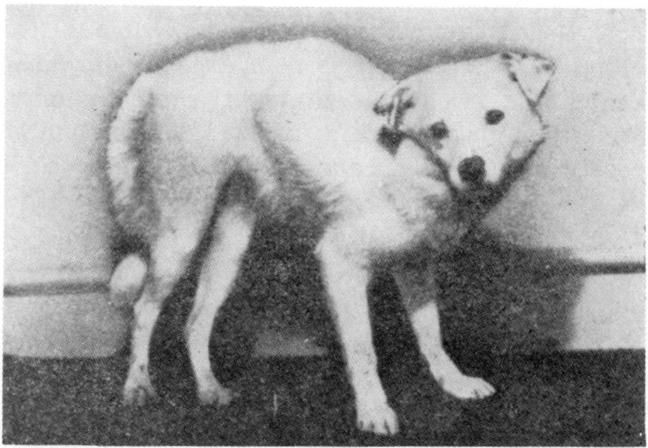

FIG. 54. A dog with incomplete transection of the spinal cord, one month after operation.

may be provided through additional impulse conduction even when only about one tenth of all the axons are preserved.

The possibility for the restoration of motor function through nerve recovery emphasized the necessity of a quick and definite diagnosis after injury. Early operative intervention could have a very beneficial effect, as decompression or removal of a bone splinter in patients could protect the intact fibers from further damage. Ugryumov and his colleagues paid great attention to examination of the nature of the injury. It was shown that the excitability of peripheral nerves and muscles was often preserved during trauma with reversible changes (Babichenko, 1956). In such patients, the abdominal reflexes were retained (Arkhangle'skii, 1953, 1955). The reflex evacuation of the urinary bladder after its filling is a sign of an incomplete transection of the spinal cord and is usually absent in patients with a complete spinal transection, especially in the initial phases of recovery (Ugryumova, 1956; Wischevsky & Livshits, 1973). Leukocytic changes in the peripheral blood below the level of injury might also be an indication of the absence of complete transection of the spinal cord since a sharp change in the number of leukocytes was not observed in patients with incomplete spinal section (Lobanova, 1956).

The general beneficial effect of operative intervention can be seen in individuals if the subdural space of the spinal cord is restored after operation. The functions of the internal organs, which were altered as a result of injury, can become more nearly normal (Blanskaya, 1956; Maiorov, 1956; Pryakhina, 1956; Suponitskaya, 1956; Ugryumov, 1956b). Reflex activity, weight-bearing, and locomotor function may be restored to varying degrees (Babichenko, 1963, 1965; Kruglyi, 1956; Ugryumov, 1956a; Ugryumov, Lubenskii, & Narodovol'tseva, 1967).

These investigations indicate that it is possible to restore the propagation of excitation along an intact nerve fiber of the spinal cord through the application of suitable methods of treatment, and as a result, significant development of motor function can be achieved. In other institutions where work with spinal patients has been carried out, the recovery of nerve conduction is considered the principal method for the restoration of motor function (Kogan, 1967; Livishits, Melamud, Plotnyagina, Shul'dyakov, Kireev, & Kózel, 1969).

The possible recovery of nerve conduction, even when the diagnosis of complete transection of the spinal cord was established by laminectomy, has been observed in some cases. This indicated the need for an extremely careful approach to surgical interference in the treatment of spasticity. The intrathecal administration of ethyl alcohol has been adopted in other countries (Guttmann, 1956; Guttmann & Robinson, 1955), but this abolishes the possibility of impulse conduction once and for all. Abramson and his colleagues recommended conservative treatment of spasticity by blocking the γ-efferents; and, apparently, this method may be highly effective in several types of spasticity (Abramson, 1962; Abramson & Hirschberg, 1951; Hirschberg & Abramson, 1951).

Compensatory Development of Substitute Functions

Complete transection of the spinal cord is considered one of the most serious injuries and, as a result, the patient is bedridden, often forever. The disability is further aggravated by trophic disorders which are inevitable due to changes of the normal tissue nutrition and the disturbance of pelvic organ function. The dystrophic processes develop not only in the spinal cord but also in other related organs, such as the nerve-muscle apparatus (Cherkasova, 1955, 1960; Maiorchik, 1947), the skeletal structures (Abramson, 1948), the internal organs and the sympathetic nervous system (Milyantsevich, 1956; Tayushev, 1965). In a number of investigations, it was found that the vegetative functions, such as thermoregulation, cardiovascular phenomena, intestinal functions, and the ratio of catecholamines in the blood plasma are sharply altered, particularly in the case of spinal transections above the level of Th_8 (Connell, Frankel, & Guttmann, 1963; Guttmann, Frankel, & Pacslack, 1965; Guttman, Munro, Robinson, & Walsh, 1963; Guttmann, Silver, & Wyndham, 1958; Hedeman & Sil, 1974; Hedeman, Shellenberger, & Gordon, 1974).

As a rule, treatment of patients with disrupted conduction is limited to the training of how to sit and move with the help of a wheelchair. In England, Czechoslovakia, and in a number of other countries, patients who were already capable of using a wheelchair were subjected to intensive training of the muscles of the shoulder girdle and the trunk. Such training could permit a patient to participate in the International Sports Festivals which are regularly organized for paraplegics (Guttmann, 1952; Jochheim & Strohkendi, 1972; Weiss & Beck, 1973). However, in most cases among the patients with a loss of conduction, walking is carried out by pulling one unflexed leg after the other by the activity of the muscles of the shoulder girdle and the wide muscles of the spine, innervated from the cervical region of the spinal cord (Guttmann, personal communication; Ugryumov, 1960). This type of walking has almost no practical value when the amount of labor it consumes is considered.

Many reports indicating the possibility of activation of reflex activity in the spinal cord are available from the literature. In spinal patients with a transection at the level of Th_4, Pool (1946) recorded electrical activity in the distal segment. Kuhn and his co-workers, working with spinal patients, concluded that the isolated spinal cord in a human being could provide reflex activity in a similar manner to that in the spinal cord of animals (Kuhn, 1950;

Kuhn & Macht, 1948). This would help in the restoration of function in patients. These authors attach particular importance to the development of extensor spasm in the leg muscles observed six months or more after trauma.

The possibility of the extremities developing complex movement during paralysis has been reported in patients with spinal trauma. Usually these movements involved the inclusion of a new group of muscles (Long & Lawton, 1955). It is a pity that these investigations were not pursued further so that the possibility of restoration of compensatory functions could be fully described. Guttmann and others failed to explain the inclusion of intercostal muscles during respiratory movements in a case where the spinal cord was severed at the level of C_1 (Guttmann & Silver, 1965).

At present, the treatment of spinal patients is being reconsidered in a number of medical institutions. Thus, Livishits reported that electrical stimulation of the urinary bladder muscles, which cause micturation, had a significant role in the act of restoration of the pelvic organs' functions (Livshits, 1969; Vishnevskii, Livshits, & Khoderov, 1965, 1967). Use of this method prevents the development of cystitis and also helps in the recovery from diseases of the urinary bladder which may have developed. Apart from this, electrostimulation was found to be a highly effective method for development of automatism in emptying the urinary bladder.

More recently, other new, successful applications of this method have been reported. Electrostimulation of abdominal organs promoted defecation which was made easy and automatic and could be related to a particular time of day. Another striking effect of electrostimulation was the normalization of trophic changes in the tissue. Bedsores were delayed, particularly in the region of the sacrum and buttocks, i.e., close to the area of stimulation.

For the last few years, a number of medical institutions have started attaching more importance to the application of physical therapy. An honored physician, Dr. A. N. Trankvillitati, achieved significant results in the restorative treatment of patients with spinal traumas. She worked out a method in which the passive movements of the lower extremities played an important role in the beginning of treatment. This was combined with active movement of the upper part of the body–the part which was not paralyzed. As a result of persistent exercise, the motor function of the lower extremities was partially restored even in patients with a loss of nerve conduction. In her treatment, as well as in treatment in other countries, great importance was paid to the care of patients immediately after receiving the injury. This method of treatment was further developed (Trankvillitati, 1965a, 1965b, 1966, 1967, 1969) and we shall describe it below in detail. Other specialists started to place more importance on the passive movements of the paralytic extremities during the treatment of patients with spinal trauma (Livshits et al., 1969). Bazilevskaya (1968) suggested that physical therapy should be started within the first few days of injury along with the preparation for movement of the paralytic extremities which might prevent various complications. Tension and stretching are utilized for treating the patient's muscles. They place more emphasis on these procedures, particularly for the lower parts of the long muscles of the trunk and the proximal joints of the extremities (Naidin, Shlykov, Zakharchenko, Komolova, Kudryavtsev, Perov, & Stolyarzh, 1969). In many hosptials and sanatoria, physical therapy is becoming one of the principal methods of restorative treatment (Slabyansk, Saki et al.)

Possible Sympathetic Nervous Involvement to Provide Compensatory Control of Motor Functions

The significance of the sympathetic nervous system in the recovery process after spinal cord injury is shown by its adaptive and trophic effects and by the possible utilization of indirect paths for the transmission of afferent impulses to the brain.

The adaptotrophic role of the sympathetic nervous system was reported by L. A. Orbeli and a group of his students. The essence of this study was to show that the sympathetic nervous system was capable of changing the functional characteristics of an organism by adapting them in the best possible manner to a given form of activity in particular concrete conditions, and also by setting up a new level of sensation and response in the individual organs (Orbeli, 1923, 1924, 1927, 1932, 1938).

The first investigation of this problem was conducted by Ginetsinskii (1923). He demonstrated that the transversely striated muscle of a frog, when fatigued by rhythmic nerve stimulation, returned to its original, or even greater amplitude of contraction, if the sympathetic nerve was also stimulated during the period of fatigue.

This effect was due to an improvement in neuromuscular conduction (Ginetsinskii, 1926a, 1926b) and also due to a rise in the excitability of the entire neuromuscular apparatus (Strel'tsov, 1926). Similar adaptotrophic effect of the sympathetic nervous system in an organism can be shown in warm-blooded as well as cold-blooded animals (Ginetsinskii, Nekhoroshev, & Tetyaeva, 1927). It has been shown in numerous investigations that this effect can be seen in all parts of the central nervous system, particularly with relation to the activity of the cerebral cortex (Asratyan, 1930).

The effect of the sympathetic nervous system on the spinal cord can be seen by changes in the rate of the reflex response (Tonkikh, 1925, 1927). Unilateral sympathectomy produces a change of threshold in a number of reflexes in the posterior extremities, according to the findings of Kunstman (1928). The motor excitation, which could normally be observed by stimulating at a rate of 180/min, cannot be reproduced after sympathectomy.

Extirpation of the abdominal sympathetic chain produces a disturbance in the reflex activity of those dogs having a partial transection of the spinal cord (Stefantsov, 1961). The effect of alteration of catecholamine levels after spinal cord trauma has been studied by Hedeman et al. (1974). Osterholm and Mathews (1972a, 1972b) have described the effect of norepinephrine synthesis on hemorrhagic necrosis following experimental spinal cord injury. A more extensive discussion of pathophysiological response to spinal cord injury has been presented by Osterholm (1974).

As can be seen from these reports, the underlying mechanism of the adaptotrophic effect of the sympathetic nervous system is probably due to facilitation in the transmission of excitation. This may happen as the result of an increase in the quantity of transmitter at the synapses (Lekhtman, 1969) or by increasing the post synaptic sensitivity (Galitskaya, 1956). A perfusion of proserine potentiates the effect of the sympathetic nerve on the fatiguability of the skeletal muscle in a frog, according to Lekhtman's findings. He suggests that this can be explained by the interaction of two systems–the nervous and the humoral. On one side, the transmission of excitation from nerve to muscle is improved due to the action of proserine and, on the other, the proserine facilitates sympathetic nervous system function by increasing the quantity of acetylcholine.

The interrelation between the sympathetic and the adrenal systems is beyond any doubt. A rise in activity of the sympathetic nervous system may be replaced, to a certain extent, by activation of the adrenaline liberating function of the suprarenals. The relation between these processes was first demonstrated by Ginetsinskii (1924). He produced strychnine convulsions in frogs after unilateral removal of the abdominal sympathetic chain and bilateral extirpation of the suprarenal glands. It was found that in these cases, the convulsions stopped much earlier on the sympathectomized side in comparison to the side with an intact sympathetic chain. When the suprarenals were not removed, the convulsions continued as long as in the control animals, i.e., as if the liberation of adrenaline stimulated by the administration of strychnine substituted for the action of the sympathetic nerves.

Experimental investigations directed at studying the interaction between the vegetative nervous system and the suprarenal glands showed that bilateral adrenalectomy decreased the efferent discharges in the vegetative nerves evoked by stimulation. Similarly, changes were observed in the character of both spontaneous and evoked afferent impulses of these nerves, indicating a decreased excitability of the receptor structures. In both cases, the use of hydrocortisone led to a complete restoration of the response, both in magnitude and form (Nozdrachev, 1969).

The close interrelation between the two systems definitely influences the activity of an animal's higher nervous system. In the case of removal of the superior cervical sympathetic ganglia and the medullary part of the surparenal glands, gross irregularities were observed both in the EEG and in the behavior patterns (Karamyan, 1958). In line with these findings, the importance of interaction between the two systems should be expected and this would affect the chances of restoration of impaired function.

The role of the sympathetic nervous system and its adaptotrophic effect on the compensatory mechanisms in an injured organism are unusually pronounced. Thus, the effect of extirpation of an abdominal sympathetic ganglion retards restoration of the functions which were impaired after the hemisection of a spinal cord (Stefantsov, 1961, 1964). If the sympathectomy is done as soon as the functions have been restored in an animal, then a temporary decompensation also occurs. In these conditions, the removal of the suprarenal considerably aggravates the changes produced by the hemisection and sympathectomy. The administration of adrenaline, on the other hand, helps in functional restoration (Urgandzhyan, 1962, 1967; Urgandzhyan & Bakhchieva, 1964).

Accordingly, the significance of the sympathoadrenal system and its interaction with other systems was important in explaining the adaptability and plastic properties of a living organism. A decrease in the function of the adrenal system, when observed in patients with spinal cord damage (Robinson & Munro, 1958), may prevent the recovery process due to a lowering of the adaptotrophic effect of the sympathetic nervous system. Hence, it is particularly necessary to find a means of increasing those functions which produce conditions favorable for the restorative processes, in a living organism where the integrity of the central nervous system has been lost.

Sympathetic Neurons in Alternate Pathways

The role of the sympathetic nervous system in the restoration of function is not only limited to its adaptotrophic effect. There may be some importance in the transmission of afferent impulses by an "indirect" path which bypasses the spinal cord. This is particularly important for "organizing" sensation in those parts of a body which have lost their connection with the central nervous system, particularly with the brain.

The presence of "indirect" connections between peripheral organs and the central nervous system was demonstrated in a number of physiological experiments. Tonkikh (1927, 1930) demonstrated long ago that Sechenov's inhibition could be produced by a sympathetic chain. A spinal motor reflex, produced by electrical stimulation of the hind limb in a cat with a doubly transected spinal cord, could be inhibited during the emotional excitement of an animal (Airapetyants & Balakshina, 1933). Painful interoceptive stimulation in spinal animals produces a prolonged inhibition of sympathetic reactions (Bobrova, 1959). Similar phenomena have been noticed by Berezina and

Rudashevskii (1950) in patients with transected spinal cords.

Golub (1949) reported that the sympathetic nervous system has the ability to connect the peripheral organs and tissues with the central nervous system as a result of its profuse branching, without involving the spinal cord. Transmission of an afferent impulse from the pelvic organs via the pelvic and vagus nerves was shown experimentally by the formation of "indirect" paths (Golub, Leontyuk, & Novikov, 1957). They stitched a part of the small intestine to the wall of the urinary bladder and noticed a change in the blood pressure and the rate of respiration in response to stimulation of the latter. Golub, Amvros'ev, Leontyuk, Novikov, Orlova, and Kheinman (1960) suggested that the transmission of afferent impulses along a sympathetic path may tend to normalize the activity of the internal organs in a spinal animal. Interoceptive reflexes have not been prevented by removing the thoracic region of the spinal cord; this applies particularly to the shaking movements of the head and the generalized movement of the anterior part of the body produced by inflating the urinary bladder or the rectum or by stimulating the skin of a hind limb (Bulygin, 1959; Bulygin & Shchannikova, 1958; Bulygin & Zorina-Tsikina, 1956; Kul'vanovskii, 1958; Yakimovich, 1958). Stimulation of the muscles of the posterior extremities after a complete transection of the spinal cord in a rabbit produced a change in the blood pressure and rate of respiration (Kolychev, 1959). In patients with transection of the spinal cord, Aronovich (1946) reported the presence of pain sensation from the testicles and Guttmann and Wittering (1947) noticed a rise in blood pressure during retention in the urinary bladder.

There are reports showing the interaction between the sympathetic reflexes produced by stimulation of the different afferent nerves (Franz, Evans, & Perl, 1966). The authors suggest that a spinal integration mechanism exists which controls the activity of the preganglionic neurons.

The significance of the cells of the spinal ganglia in the transmission of sensation was reported by Bulygin and Belorybkina (1959). They produced a motor response in an animal by stimulating the spinal ganglion during perfusion of the circulation. In their opinion, this suggests that the input to the ganglion cells may be mediated by the sensory endings of spinal neurons.

It is very likely that the nerves supplying the deeply situated blood vessels play an important role in the propagation of afferent impulses. Impulses from the skeletal muscle receptors may be propagated through nerves supplying the blood vessels (Fleisch, 1956). It has also been shown that the deep lying nerves supplying the vessels are the conductors of sensation since they often connect the organs with individual intersegmental ganglia or even with ganglia situated on the opposite side of the body (Levitskaya, 1956).

It is characteristic of the afferent innervation of animals that these fibers can be identified at a great distance from their own ganglion and that they enter into different segments of the spinal cord which may be distant from where they originated. Thus, Krokhina's (1960) investigations have shown that the afferent innervation of the large intestine in a cat consists of sensory fibers which enter the paravertebral ganglia at the level of Th_1-Th_5. Afferent fibers of the lumbar and thoracic segments of the spinal cord participate in the sensory innervation of vessels of the thigh, as was shown by removing the spinal ganglia (Orlova, 1956). The presence of somatic fibers going to a sympathetic chain along the spinal cord was also confirmed in a number of histological investigations (Leontyuk, 1956; Loiko, 1956; Ranson & Billigsley, 1918; Roux, 1900). The majority of the afferent fibers enter into the composition of a sympathetic chain in the lumbar region (Kalita, 1956).

Investigation into the embryogenesis of the vegetative nervous system demonstrated that the sproutings from cells of the spinal ganglia participate in the formation of a sympathetic chain both in chick and rat embryos (De Castro, 1923) and also in human and cat embryos (Golub & Kichina, 1956). In all probability, the somatic afferent fibers leaving the spinal ganglion cells enter a sympathetic chain and, in a number of cases, take part in its composition, until they reach the organ which they are to innervate. Considerable extension of the afferent innervation in a sympathetic chain has been stressed by the work of Il'ina (1960) who observed regeneration of the nerve fibers of spinal nature in the sympathetic chain situated at a distance which was far away from the site of the operation during operations for the fractional removal of paravertebral ganglia in different segments.

Thus, the sympathetic nervous system and the somatic nerve fibers accompanying it were capable of implementing the "indirect" propagation of afferent impulses to the cerebral cortex from all parts of the body by a pathway, bypassing the spinal cord. This is particularly important for spinal patients, because this produces the spatial orientation of the body, and may also help in the development of motor functions.

Stimulation of the Resorptive Processes in Patients with a Complete or Partial Transection of the Spinal Cord

The Role of Pyrogenic Preparation in the Treatment of Spinal Patients

The use of Piromen in patients with spinal traumas was explored by several physicians in the USA, but the results were not uniform. Rosner (1954), using it in small doses at a late stage after operation on several patients, obtained a positive therapeutic effect which was manifested by a considerable increase in the degree of movement. However, other investigators did not obtain positive results according to a report by Windle (1959).

In view of the experimental work with Pyrogenal in 1959, the Farmakomitet (Drug Control Authority) of the Ministry of Health (USSR) permitted the use of this preparation for therapeutic purposes in patients with a number of disabilities–in particular, those with injury of the spinal cord. On the basis of our physiological investigations, several physicians started using it in consultation with Prof. Kh. Kh. Planel'es and P. Z. Budnitskaya.

The results of the use of Pyrogenal were positive (Kogan, 1961; Trankvillitati & Nesmeyanova, 1961). The time required for treating patients was reduced 2-3 times with the administration of Pyrogenal and the restoration of motor functions was more complete (Trankvillitati, 1967). In all the patients, the size of the muscles increased considerably more, within a year, than with only the application of physical therapy without the use of Pyrogenal (Table 7). Similarly, there was considerable increase in the mobility of the joints (Trankvillitati, 1967).

The best results were obtained in cases involving the administration of Pyrogenal in early periods after the trauma (Kogan 1965a, 1965b). Treatment with Pyrogenal was particularly effective in the case of a knife injury which caused an incomplete transection of the spinal cord. The contiguity of the stumps gave the axons a chance to grow through the area of section. The administration of Pyrogenal resulted in an increase in the activity of the paralyzed muscles, a minimum change in their tone, an improvement in the propagation of excitation (Tkach & Kogan, 1965), and the normalization of the vegetative and motor disorders usually present in incomplete transections (Rasskazov, 1967). Positive results with Pyrogenal in the restorative treatment of spinal cord injuries were also noticed by others (Lubenskii, 1965; Lubenskii & Narodovol'tseva, 1964).

What could be the mechanism of Pyrogenal action by which it helped in

TABLE 7. Comparison of Increase in the Size of Muscles in Patients Having Injury and Transection of the Spinal Cord, after a Year of Treatment with Physical Therapy, as Compared to the Same Treatment Plus Administration of Pyrogenal

Groups of muscles	Part investigated	Increase in size of muscles in patients (in cm)	
		With Pyrogenal (6 persons)	Without Pyrogenal (6 persons)
Leg	Lower	3.0–5.0	0.5–1.0
Leg	Middle	6.0–9.0	1.0–2.0
Leg	Upper	4.0–7.0	0.5–1.0
Thigh	Lower	7.0–9.0	1.0–2.0
Thigh	Upper	9.0–12.0	2.0–3.0

recovery from different traumatic disturbances of nerve function and caused a generalized increase in muscle tone and vital activity of the patients?

As already mentioned, pyrogens activate the hypophysioadrenal system. The amount of corticosteroids and catecholamines in the blood and urine increases under the action of pyrogens, since these preparations also act on the suprarenal medulla (Brichant et al., 1960; Janches, Dendukas, Segal, & Galze, 1965; Shuster & Flynn, 1961; Siedek, Mostbeck, & Schnetz, 1959).

The mechanism of Pyrogenal action on the hypophysioadrenal system is not completely clear. Wexler (1963) has suggested that pyrogens increase the activity of the suprarenal cortex by directly acting on the hypophysis, or, in other words, the pyrogens are not considered a stress-producing agent and the action is specific. Japanese investigators (Takebe et al., 1966) also hold the same opinion. Veselkin (1965) considered that Pyrogenal is an extremely effective stimulator with an unusual character that has a number of properties which are common to ordinary stress-producing agents but differs from them by being a specific stimulator.

Planel'es (1965), who introduced Pyrogenal and worked with it for a number of years, suggested that the changes in concentration of catecholamine and serotonin and their ratio in the central nervous system have a definite role in the mechanism of its action (Planel'es & Popenenkova, 1965). This was also the opinion of other investigators (Kuruma, 1966; Kuruma & Takagi, 1964).

The ratio of concentration of serotonin and catecholamines has a great influence on the functional state of the physiological systems in the entire animal, as well as on its behavior. Changes in the concentration of catecholamines or serotonin in the brain are sharply reflected in an animal's behavior and its ability to develop conditioned reflexes.

Adrenaline and noradrenaline, when administered in small doses, excite the motor activities of animals (Bondarev, 1938; Kuz'menko, 1938; Pribytkova, 1936) and appreciably affect the conditioned reflexes in human subjects (Traugot, Balashov, & Kaufman, 1961).

The function of the suprarenal glands is altered in patients having a transection of the spinal cord (Razdol'skii, 1952). The concentration of adrenaline and noradrenaline in blood plasma is considerably decreased (up to 50 percent) when compared to normal, if the spinal cord is transected at the level of Th_6 or higher (Munro & Robinson, 1958, 1960; Robinson & Munro, 1958). A decrease in the concentration of blood catecholamines in spinal patients might reflect considerably on the tone of the central nervous system and of the organism as a whole, particularly when the normal balance is lost, with an alteration in the ratio of serotonin and noradrenaline in different parts of the brain. According to modern concepts, the catecholamines are indispensible for carrying out a chain of neurohormonal reactions through the hypothalamus (Tonkikh, 1964). One is led to consider whether Pyrogenal affects the metabolism inside the brain, in view of (1) the presence of an adrenergic substrate in the reticular formation of the brain (Vogt, 1957); (2) the ability of this system to produce catecholamines (Dell, 1960) from the precursors penetrating through the blood-brain barrier (Axelrod, Well-Malherbe, & Tomchick, 1959; Il'yuchenok, 1965); (3) the role of biogenic amines in the functional state of the central nervous system and of the whole organism. In fact, it was reported by Minchenko (1968) that a single administration of Pyrogenal to a dog, at a dose which produces a febrile reaction, led to a considerable rise in the concentration of biogenic amines in the midbrain reticular structures, in the cerebral cortex, and in the cerebellum. A change in the ratio of noradrenaline and serotonin was observed in this process, both in their free and bound forms. These changes inevitably produced several biochemical alterations which were followed by a number of physiological changes, among which are the following:

There is a stimulation of carbohydrate and phosphorus metabolism (Daudova, 1957; Neifakh & Zdrodovskaya, 1956; Veselkin, 1960; Zdrodovskaya, 1957) with pyrogen administration (Woods, Landy, & Shear, 1959; Woods, Landy, Whitby, & Burk, 1961). An animal receiving Pyrogenal shows stimulation of a number of systems, as a result of which the tone of the animal is increased and its functional status becomes altogether different. Activation of the hypophysioadrenal system with Pyrogenal enhances and prolongs the adaptotrophic effect of the sympathetic nervous system which had been lowered in patients due to a lesion in the spinal cord.

From these facts, it became clear how Pyrogenal helps spinal patients during restorative treatment. An improvement of the metabolic processes, an acceleration of the blood flow, and an intensification of the synthesis of nucleoproteins should lead to a normalization of tissue trophism and an increase in muscle size. A rise in the concentration of catecholamines in the brain and a normalization in the level of corticosteroids in the blood have a "toning up" effect on an organism and increase the potentialities for the formation of new reflex reactions. Apart from this, Pyrogenal promotes the regenerative process leading to the restoration of the impaired functions. Pyrogenal can be considered as a true stimulator of the restorative processes in an animal whose activity has been impaired as a result of injury or disease of the spinal cord.

Electromyographic Studies Showing Inclusion of Trunk and Leg Muscles in the Motor Activity of Patients with Spinal Cord Injury

The patients on whom we conducted electromyographic investigations were treated by Dr. A. N. Trankvillitati, using the method she worked out involving the administration of Pyrogenal (Goncharova, Nesmeyanova, &

Trankvillitati, 1969; Nesmeyanova, 1969, 1970, 1973, 1975; Nesmeyanova & Trankvillitati, 1970).

The 20 patients under investigation were provisionally divided into two groups: In the first group, 10 patients were included in which the diagnosis of spinal lesion at the level of mid or lower thoracic segments was established by laminectomy and where there was an *absence* of *spinal cord conduction* in the initial 1-2 years of treatment. Treatment was started on nine acute bedridden patients several months, or even a year, after the injury; in one patient, the treatment was started immediately after the trauma.

In the second group of 10 patients, diagnosis of a spinal lesion at various levels in some, and anatomical transection in others, was established by laminectomy. However, evidence for *conduction* of impulses during their spinal cord reappeared as early as the first few months of treatment. The treatment of two patients, using this method was started within a few days of the injury and in the remaining group after a lapse of several months, or even several years. The patients were either bedridden or were able to stand on their legs but unable to move.

We originally divided the patients into the first or second group, according to the diagnosis established either by laminectomy, or clinically without any operative interference. However, during the course of treatment it was possible, on the basis of the periodic observation of the neurologic status and the electromyographic data, to transfer some patients of the first group to the second when recovery began to appear. In future statements, we shall consider only those patients in the first group having a complete loss of spinal conduction and an absence of functional recovery as observed in the process of treatment. Summaries of the case histories of these patients are given in the appendix.

The physiotherapy which we employed consisted mainly of submitting the patient to repetitive passive movements of the legs, and massage as well as active movements of the upper part of the body including the hands. Treatment was administered in two stages: In the first stage (4-6 months), the exercises were done in a horizontal position; in the second stage (6-12 months), in a vertical position.

The muscular activity of the patient was developed by stretching the unflexed leg (lifting up) in a movement which is essential for the process of learning to walk, as well as attempting to flex and extend the leg at the knee joint, in a manner essential for the walking process.

Electromyograms were recorded, both from the muscles of the shoulder girdle, and from the upper and lower parts of the long muscles of the trunk as well as the gluteal, thigh, and leg muscles. The recording of muscle potentials was obtained using bipolar electrodes with a separation of 8 mm. These were fixed on the skin with adhesive tape. The muscle potentials were fed to a preamplifier (UBP 1-01) and were recorded by an oscillograph N_{102}.

Treatment

Pyrogenal was administered by injection in increasing doses usually on alternate days, according to the schedule worked out by Prof. Planel'es, although in several cases, it was given daily. The course of treatment was started with a minimum dose of 50 human MPD*, which was gradually increased by 25 MPD every second or fourth injection till it reached 300-500 MPD. This treatment was continued for one to two months and was then repeated after an interval of one to two months. With this gradual increase in dosage, the febrile reaction usually did not appear, though there were some changes in the hormonal environment and the hemopoietic system which produced a chain of metabolic alterations.

Partial restoration of motor function was observed in the lower extremities of all the patients. Before starting treatment, activity was recorded in the muscles of the shoulder girdle on the first group of patients during attempts to raise their leg while lying on their back. This muscle activity is shown in Fig. 55 and was found to be less pronounced in the upper parts of the long muscles of the trunk (Fig. 56). In the course of treatment, the amplitude of the potentials from muscles innervated by proximal segments of the spinal cord quickly increased. Gradually, the lower parts of these muscles, which were innervated from distal spinal segments, began to be included in the activity. Figure 57 is an electromyogram obtained from a patient belonging to the first group, two months after starting treatment. Activity was recorded from the upper and lower parts of the latissimus and longissimus dorsi and from the obliquus externus abdominis. Though the whole latissimus dorsi is innervated from the cervical region of the spinal cord, the activity in its lower parts usually appeared only after a short treatment. The amplitude of the potentials in the lower parts of the long muscles of the trunk was

*MPD–Minimum pyrogenic dose which approximately equals to 0.1 mg.

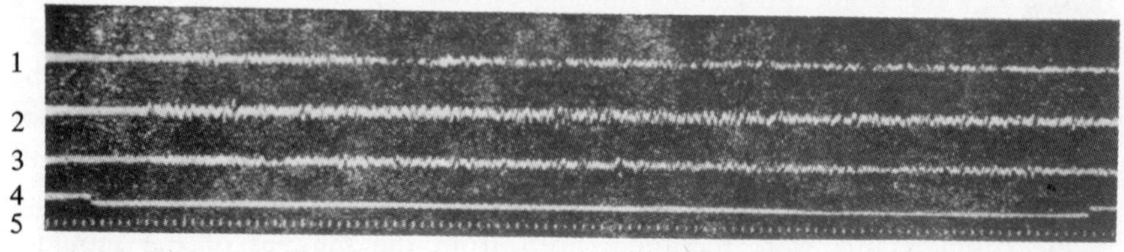

FIG. 55. Activity of the muscles of the shoulder girdle during an attempt to raise leg (lying on the back), before starting treatment.

1–pectoralis major; 2–trapezius; 3–deltoideus; 4–mark showing the signal for movement; 5–time, 20 msec.

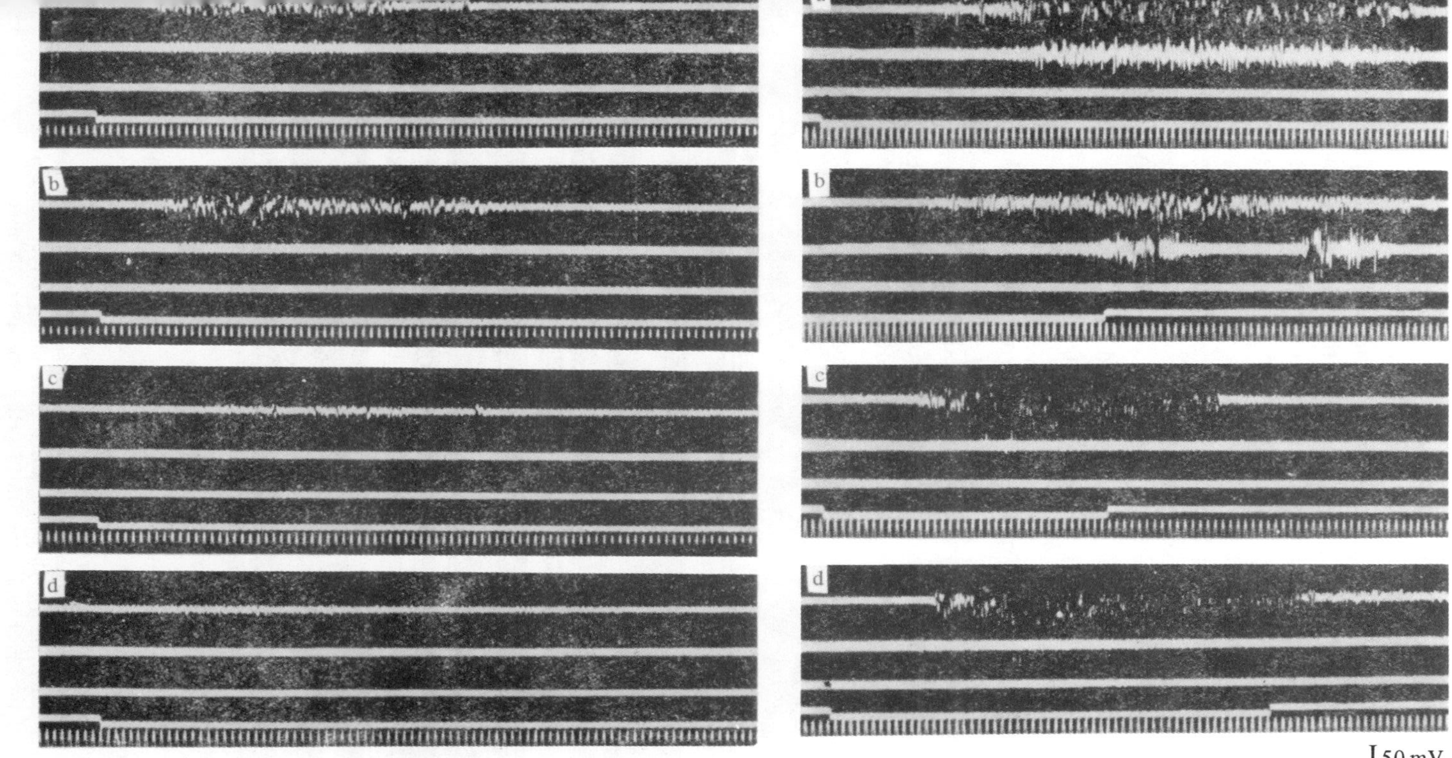

FIG. 56

FIG. 57

FIG. 56. Muscle activity of the trunk and extremity during a patient's attempt to raise leg (lying on the back) before start of treatment.

First three beams in the electromyograms a–d: a–upper and lower parts of the latissimus dorsi and gluteus maximus; b–upper and lower parts of the longissimus dorsi and vastus lateralis; c–upper and lower parts of the rectus abdominis and rectus femoris; d–upper and lower parts of the obliquus abdominis externus and gluteus medius; fourth beam–mark showing the signal for a movement; fifth beam–time, 20 msec.

FIG. 57. Muscle activity of the trunk and extremity when raising leg (lying on the back) two months after start of treatment.

First three beams in the electromyograms a–d: a–upper and lower parts of the latissimus dorsi and rectus femoris; b–upper and lower parts of the longissimus dorsi and gluteus maximum; c–upper and lower parts of the obliquus abdominis and gluteus medius; d–upper and lower parts of the rectus abdominis and gluteus medius; fourth beam–mark showing the signal for a movement; fifth beam–time, 20 msec.

considerably less than in the upper parts of these muscles and the potentials appeared with a delay of 1.0–1.2 sec greater than their time of appearance in the latter. In the obliquus abdominis externus, only isolated volleys with variable potentials were recorded and in the muscles of the extremity no activity was recorded as was the case before starting treatment.

After extensive treatment of the patient for a period of 5-7 months, activity was recorded in the upper and lower parts of all the muscles of the trunk, during lifting the leg by the patient into a vertical position (Fig. 58). The amplitude of these potentials was increased and their latency was reduced to 300-400 msec. With longer treatment, they were delayed by 30–70 msec, or even by as little as 20 msec.

After six to eight months of treatment with Pyrogenal, the muscles of the extremities and their proximal joints began to show evidence of motor activity. At first, the impulses from individual motor units or from several units worked synchronously; apart from this, short volleys of varying potentials were recorded which we termed group potentials (Fig. 59A). These

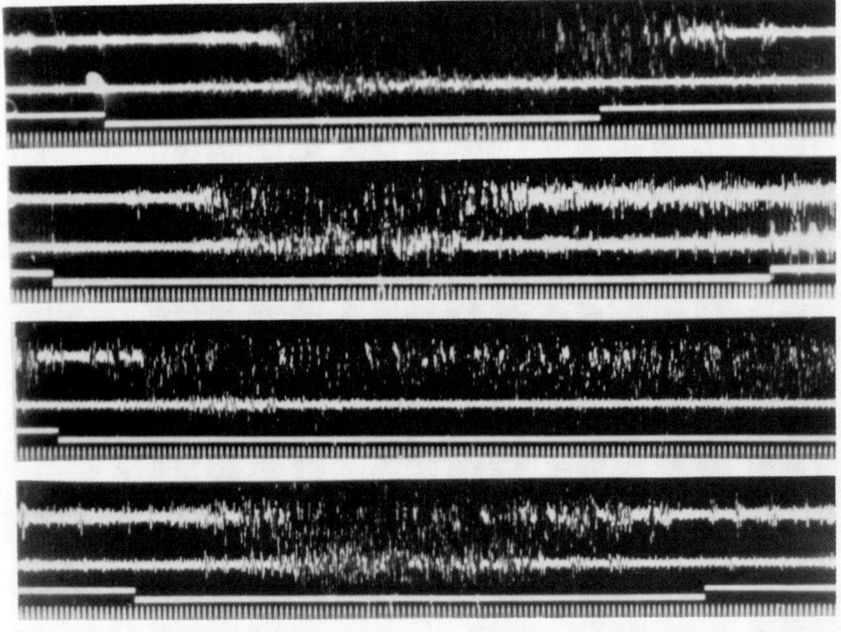

FIG. 58. Muscle activity of the trunk when raising leg (standing with crutches) 7½ months after start of treatment.

First two beams in the electromyograms a–d: a–upper and lower parts of the latissimus dorsi; b–upper and lower parts of the longissimus dorsi; c–upper and lower parts of the obliquus abdominis externus; d–upper and lower parts of the rectus abdominis; third beam–mark showing the signal to a movement; fourth beam–time, 20 msec.

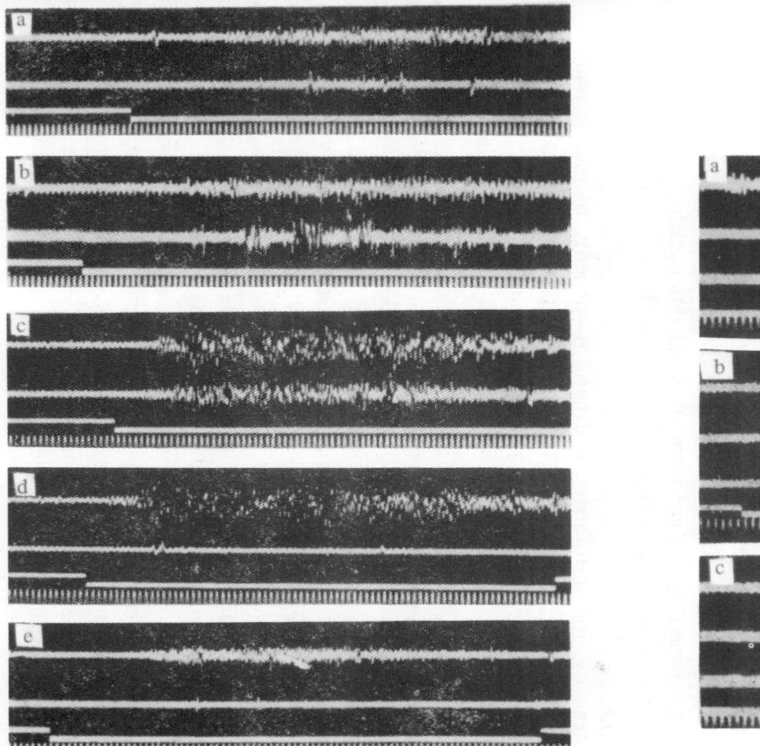

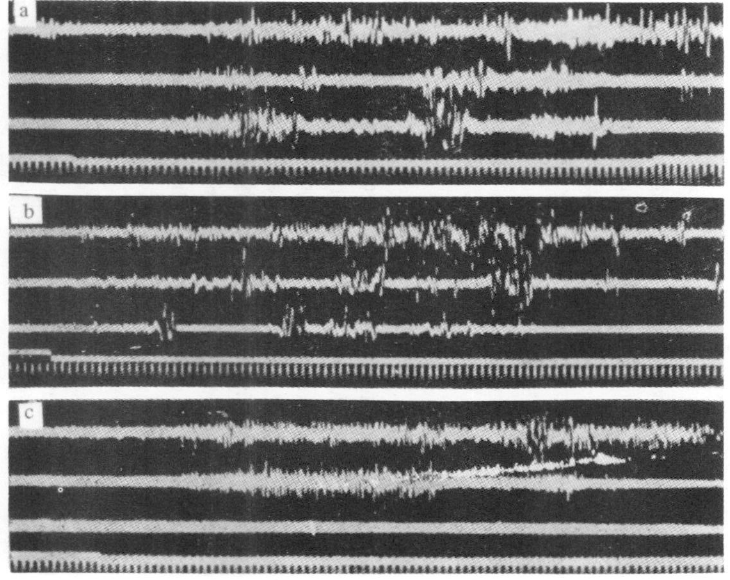

FIG. 59. Muscle activity of the trunk and lower extremities when raising unflexed leg (standing on crutches), eight months (A) and three years (B) after starting treatment with Pyrogenal.

A: First two beams in the electromyograms a–e: a—upper part of the latissimus dorsi and rectus femoris; b—upper part of the longissimus dorsi and vastus lateralis; c—upper part of the obliquus abdominis externus and gluteus medius; d—upper part of the obliquus abdominis externus and sartorius; e—upper part of the rectus abdominis and biceps femoris; third beam—mark showing the signal for a movement; fourth beam—time, 20 msec.

B: First three beams in the electromyograms a–e: a—upper and lower parts of the latissimus dorsi and gluteus medius; b—upper and lower parts of the longissimus dorsi and gastrocnemius; c—upper and lower parts of the recutus abdominis and biceps femoris; fourth beam—mark showing the signal for a movement; fifth beam—time, 20 msec.

were more delayed than the activity which appeared in muscles situated above the joint and were of small amplitude. During the course of treatment and training, a change was noticed in the nature of their activity. An interference (total) electromyogram was recorded in some muscles but the latency in its appearance was reduced (Fig. 59B). The delays in appearance of activity in the leg muscles which were observed in the course of treatment and training are presented in Table 8.

Training Patient to Learn How to Walk

In the beginning, movement in the vertical positon was executed by raising leg with the help of the trunk muscles and carrying it forward passively, resting the body on crutches. Gradually, the patient learned how to walk, during which he actively flexed his legs at the hip joints and then pulled them forward. He then learned to climb up and down a staircase.

In several muscles of the legs, when walking, an interference electromyogram was recorded, but in others, group potentials were seen (Fig. 60). Thus, a number of muscles of the extremities, particularly the gluteus medius, actively participated in the process of walking.

When muscle shortening was recorded by mechanogram simultaneously with an electromyogram from the hip joint, during the process of walking in two patients, it could be seen that the muscle activity which appeared during stepping was accompanied by a displacement of the joint angle by 15°, i.e., leg movement in the process of walking occurs with the involvement of the hip joint (Fig. 61).

The time necessary for restorative treatment in patients of the second group (having either a spinal lesion at various levels or anatomical lesion established by laminectomony) and the gradual inclusion of muscle activity of individual joints depended, in each case, on the degree and level of injury. It has been shown by electromyographic studies that activity in the muscles innervated by a distal segment of the spinal cord appears only after some treatment and training in the majority of cases (Bikushev, Manovich, & Novicova, 1974). Similarly, a greater latency was observed in the EMG of such cases when compared with time of appearance of electrical activity in the upper part of these muscles, i.e., initially, the recovery is of a compensatory type. However, activity in the muscles of the thigh and even of the leg appeared comparatively early—say, within a period of one to three months. During comparable damage to the spinal cord at the level of the cervical segments, the same phenomenon was noticed in the muscles of the upper extremities. The characteristic feature of patients belonging to this particular group appeared later during the course of treatment, when stable weight-bearing was restored in the lower extremities due to the development of tone in the antigravity muscles and at the same time voluntary movements

TABLE 8. Variations in the Delay (in msec) of the Appearance of Activity in the Muscles Situated before the Joints in Relation to the Muscle Situated above the Joints (Movement: Lifting Leg)

Name of patient and date of experiment	Position	Delays in the appearance of activity in the muscles							
		Latissimus dorsi lower part	Longissimus dorsi lower part	Obliquus abdominis externus lower part	Rectus abdominis lower part	Gluteus medius	Sartorius	Vastus lateralis	Biceps femoris
		in relation to the upper part of							
		Latissimus dorsi	Longissimus dorsi	Obliquus abdominis externus	Rectus abdominis	Obliquus abdominis externus	Obliquus abdominis externus	Longissimus dorsi	Rectus abdominis
I.P.									
Oct. 25, 1966	Lying on	No activity							
Oct. 25, 1966	back								
Nov. 27, 1966	”		No activity		2000				
Nov. 27, 1966	Standing on crutches	20	1160	1240	1200	1200	1200	1320	1200
Mar. 23, 1967	”	20	450	500	480	160	260	320	500
Apr. 14, 1968	”	20	60	120	240	40	–	40	No activity in biceps femoris
N.K.									
Nov. 3, 1966	”	20	70	80	150	100	100	320	460
Jan. 4, 1967	”	20	70	60	100	40	–	100	120
Mar. 17, 1967	”	20	70	30	20	20	–	40	120
P.B.									
Nov. 21, 1966	Lying on back	20	160	140	180	400	220	560	280
Feb. 9, 1967	Standing on crutches	20	100	120	100	300	200	400	200
Jan. 12, 1968	”	20	20	80	100	300	–	300	200

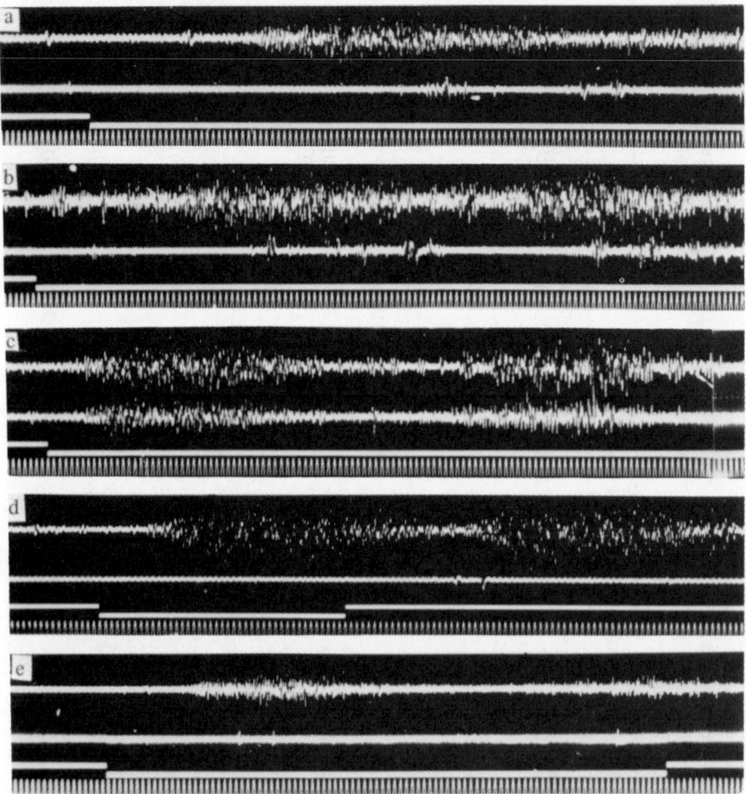

FIG. 60. Activity of the muscles of the trunk and lower extremities during walking in a patient belonging to the first group.

First two beams in the electromyograms a-d: a—upper part of the latissimus dorsi and rectus femoris; b—upper part of the longissimus dorsi and vastus lateralis; c—upper part of the obliquus abdominis externus and gluteus medius; d—upper part of the obliquus abdominis externus and sartorius; e—upper part of the rectus abdominis and biceps femoris; third beam—mark showing the signal for a movement; fourth beam—time, 20 msec.

appeared in the knee and ankle joints (Fig. 62). In the majority of cases, there was almost complete recovery of motor activity in the patients with a partial transection of the spinal cord, even in the cervical region.

Figure 63 shows that a high amplitude interference myogram, which is characteristic of a normal individual, was recorded from the leg muscles of a patient in the second group.

The application of intensive physical therapy within the first few days after injury prevented trophic changes and the development of hypertonicity of the flexor or extensor groups of muscles in our experiments on animals as well as

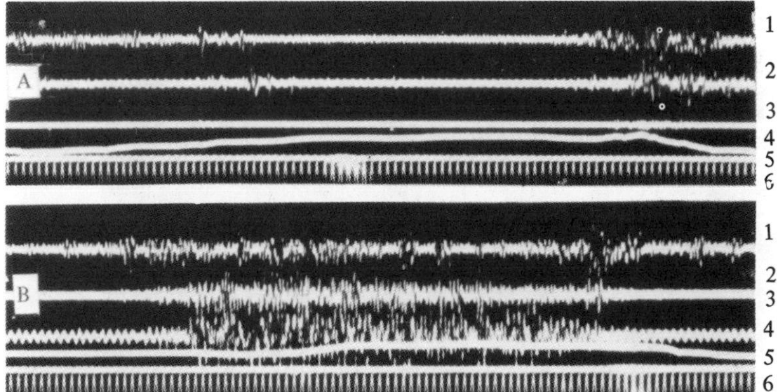

FIG. 61. Mechanogram and electromyogram recorded during walking in two patients of the first group.

A: 1–lower part of the longissimus dorsi; 2–gluteus medius; 3–biceps femoris. B: 1–upper part of the latissimus dorsi; 2–lower part of the latissimus dorsi; 3–gluteus medius; 4–mechanogram of the hip joint; 5–mark showing the signal for a movement; 6–time, 20 msec.

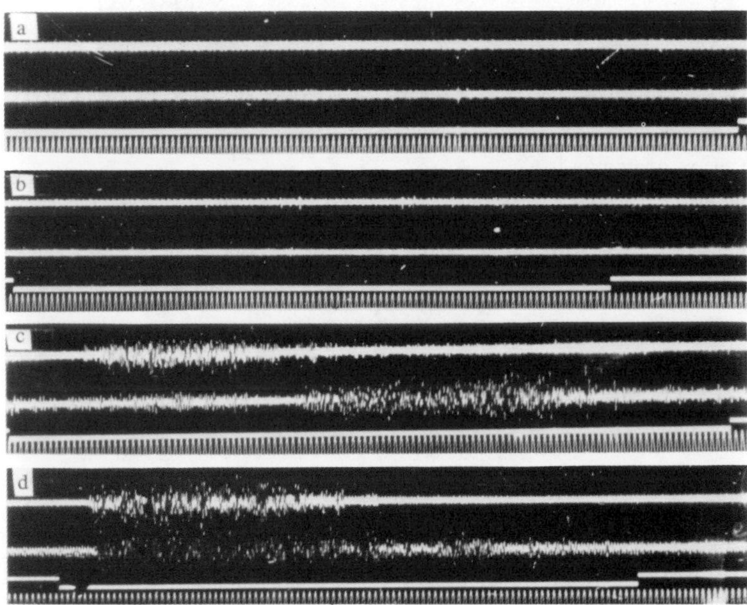

FIG. 62. Activity of leg muscles during an attempt at movement of an ankle joint.

A, b–in patients of the first group; c, d–in patients of the second group. First two beams in the electromyograms a-d: gastrocnemius and tibialis anterior; third beam–mark showing the signal for a movement; fourth beam–time, 20 msec.

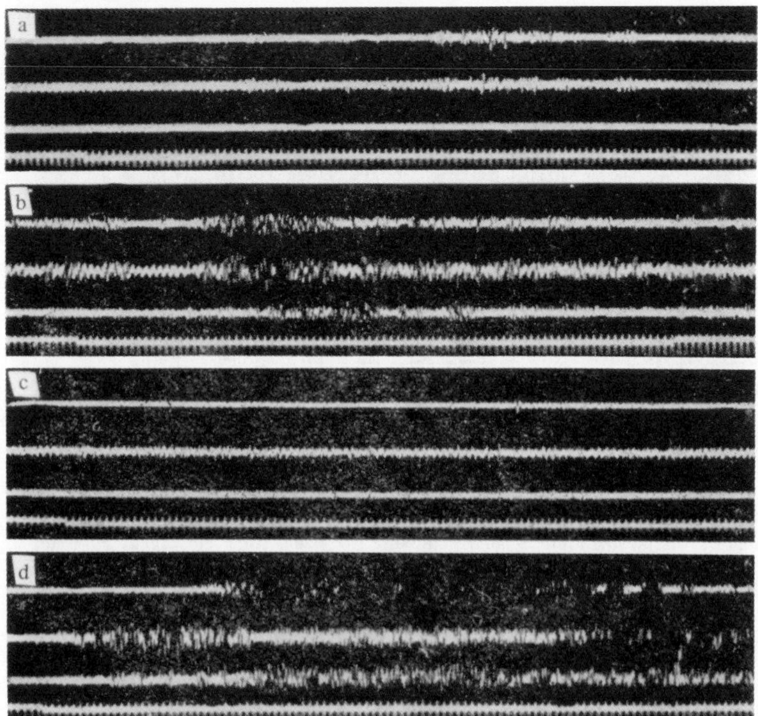

FIG. 63. Activity of the muscles of the trunk and extremities during walking in a patient belonging to the second group.

First three beams in the electromyograms a–d: a–upper and lower parts of the latissimus dorsi and gluteus maximum; b–upper and lower parts of the longissimus dorsi and rectus femoris; c–upper and lower parts of the obliquus abdominis externus and gluteus medius; d–gastrocnemius, tibialis anterior and peroneus longus; fourth beam–mark showing the signal for a movement; fifth beam–time, 20 msec.

in patients treated under the guidance of Dr. Trankvillitati. When treatment was started at a later stage after injury, the resulting trophic changes and the hypertonicity of the muscles were usually reduced and even disappeared completely. In the course of therapy, significant tone was developed in the extensor and flexor groups of muscles, whose behavior was close to normal, but the force was so inadequate that weight-bearing was impossible, depending on where the spinal cord was severed from its supraspinal influences. If the recovery of function occurred by reinnervation, the extremities recovered the ability to support stable weight-bearing.

It is quite possible that simultaneous appearance of activity in several muscles of the lower extremities could, partially, help in weight-bearing, as was demonstrated on dogs. It has recently been reported that the postural tone of muscles in the extremities depends on the tonic component of the knee jerk and this is provided by the lumbar region of the spinal cord (Babkin, 1967). These facts allow us to think that it might be possible to achieve the restoration of weight-bearing by the extremities in patients where there is a loss of conduction in the spinal cord.

In spinal dogs the majority of the trunk muscles which were responsible for the development of a pattern of unstable weight-bearing also participate in the process of weight-bearing in normal animals, as has already been mentioned. In patients with impaired conduction in the spinal cord (as opposed to a normal human being), activity was also recorded in many muscles of the trunk and extremities when the patient was standing. This phenomenon was observed even when the knee and ankle joints were fixed by splints (Fig. 64). This feature might help in the maintenance of weight-bearing to a certain extent.

Control of Long Muscles of the Trunk

It is surprising that during the treatment of spinal patients with a complete loss of conduction, there is the possibility of activating muscles innervated from a distal spinal segment during voluntary motor activity. How can the transmission of impulses from the proximal to the distal segment of the spinal cord be explained, when a patient belonging to the first group (having a lesion at the thoracic level) carries out an independent movement? Is there any nervous connection between the two segments of the cord? Let us see what is known about the innervation of the long muscles of the trunk.

It is an established fact that these muscles are innervated from a large number of spinal segments. For example, the whole latissimus dorsi is innervated from all the cervical segments of the spinal cord, the longissimus dorsi is innervated from the C_4 to S_2 segments, and the obliquus abdominis externus and the rectus abdominis receive their supply from the Th_5-L_1 segments (Vorob'ev, 1938). After transection in the thoracic or lumbar region of the spinal cord, the lower parts of the long muscles of the trunk are partially innervated by segments of the spinal cord above the lesion since each portion of these muscles is connected with a least two spinal segments. Due to this fact, the lower parts of the long muscles are comparatively easily reactivated during treatment and training. The movement of raising the leg without knee flexion (to which great significance has been attached in the development of the motor function of the lower extremities) is initially carried out exclusively by the contraction of the muscles of the shoulder girdle and of the upper parts of the long muscles of the trunk. After some time, the lower parts of these muscles participate in this movement. During

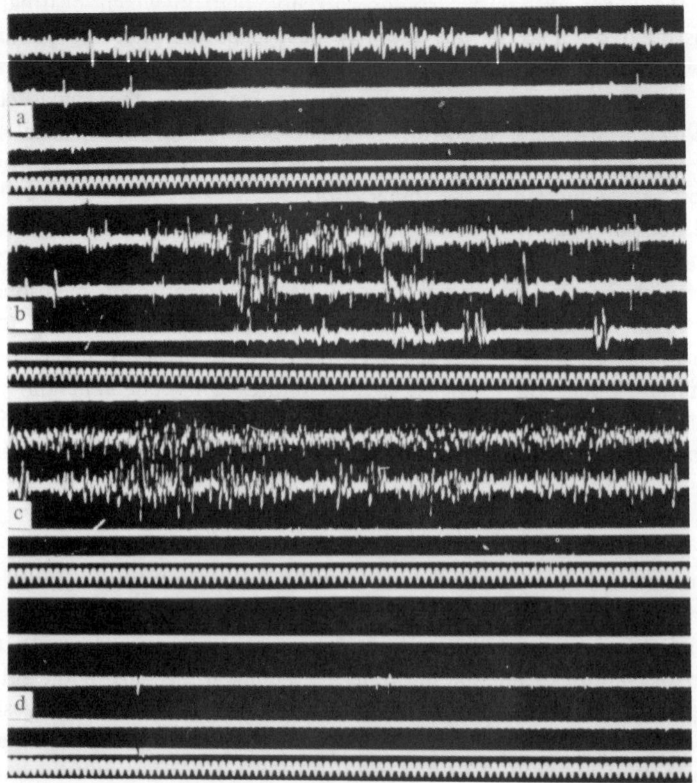

FIG. 64. Activity of muscles of the trunk and lower extremities during standing in patients of the first group when the knee and ankle joints were fixed with splints.

First three beams on a–d–electromyograms; a–m. latissimus dorsi, upper and lower regions of m. gluteus maxima; b–m. longissima dorsi, upper and lower regions of m. gastrocnemius; c–m. obliquus abdominis externus, upper and lower regions of m. gluteus media; d–m. rectus abdominis, upper and lower regions of m. gracilis; fourth beam–signal for movement; fifth beam–time 20 msec.

this leg movement, the skin over the gluteus medius may be displaced. It has been shown that stimulation of the skin or its displacement might facilitate the inclusion of muscles lying below it in the motor response by activating the gamma efferent fibers (Hagbarth, 1952; Eldred & Hagbarth, 1954). Likewise, our results indicated that cutaneous stimulation is an essential factor for the successful inclusion of muscles in motor activity (Nesmeyanova, 1968b). On the other hand, stretching a muscle excites the muscle spindle (Matthews, 1964) which, in turn, produces muscular contraction (see Fig. 20).

From these considerations it is possible that muscular and cutaneous receptors, whose impulses are considered to be initiators for muscular contraction, may play a primary role involving muscles which have previously been innervated by a distal segment of the spinal cord. Repeated passive flexion of the leg at the knee, or lifting the entire leg, produced gradual activation of the receptors in the quadriceps or the gluteus medius muscle which initially caused the contraction of isolated groups of fibers and subsequently a contraction of the whole muscle. These reactions can be seen easily even during mild stretching of the muscle or displacement of the skin over it. The latter may occur in some selected movements of the body. Activation of muscles in different parts of the body and in the joints of the extremities should appear in succession starting with the proximal muscles. Later, new groups of muscles might be involved in the activity due to the stimulation of related cutaneous and muscular receptors: Such stimulation would be completed with the stimulation of the motor nerve supplying the muscles involved in the movement.

This proposal was supported by conducting experiments on patients having a loss of conduction along the spinal cord. An electromyogram (Fig. 65) was taken in a patient with an injury of the spinal cord at the level of Th_5-Th_7 two years after treatment. The patient tried to bend her leg at the knee while lying on her side; this movement began by holding the pillow with her hands and ended with a mild movement of the leg flexing at the knee. In other words, it was a complex movement which started with activity of the muscles in the upper part of the body. The muscular activity involved in this movement first appeared in the upper part of the obliquus abdominis externus and then in its lower part. Subsequently, the gluteus medius and, later, the quadriceps and biceps femoris, and finally the leg muscles, were all included in the activity–as if a chain of reflex reactions appeared, where the contraction of one muscle produced the contraction of other muscles situated distal to the joint.

Flexion and extension movements of the leg at the knee in another patient were relatively localized and quite prominent for three years following treatment. It seemed that they were associated with a hand movement (Fig. 66). However, the electromyograms demonstrated that all the trunk muscles reacted in this movement as in the previous case. First, the upper parts of these muscles reacted, then, with a slight delay, the response also appeared in the lower parts. Subsequently, the gluteal and the thigh muscles reacted and this became considerably higher both in amplitude and frequency and showed a prolongation in the duration of the discharges (Fig. 67).

Thus, though this movement seemed to be localized, it was initiated in the upper part of the trunk muscles, as in the previous case. The apparent localization of movement was due to the fact that considerable excitation of the muscles of the extremity was correlated with a very slight movement of the hand or trunk. This is possibly due to the development of a reflex as a result of training.

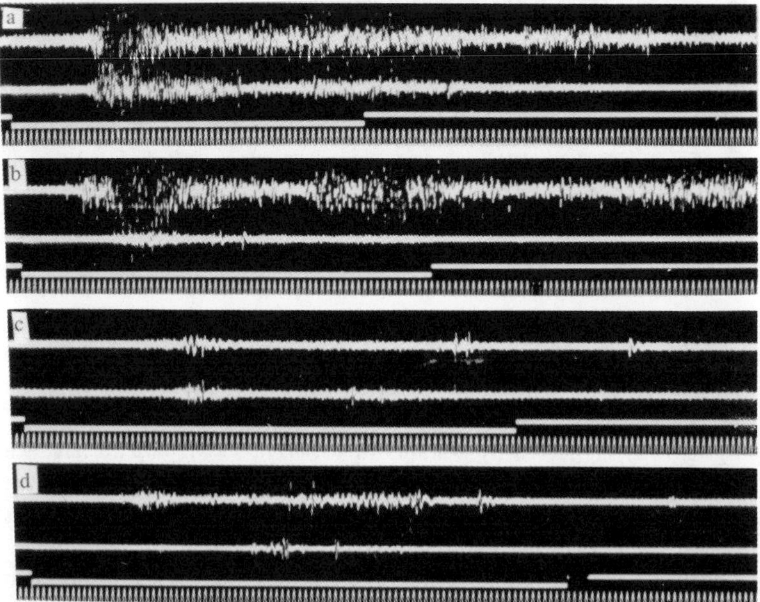

FIG. 65. Activity of the muscles of the trunk and lower extremities during flexion of the leg at the knee in a patient belonging to the first group, two years after starting treatment.

First two beams on a-d electromyograms: a—obliquus externus upper and lower regions; b—obliquus externus lower regions of gluteus media; c—gluteus media, vastus literalis; d—vastus lateralis, gastrocnemius; third beam—signal for movement; fourth beam—time, 20 msec.

Another patient, whose lesion was at Th_{12}-L_1, learned to walk nicely with canes, by standing with only the help of crutches and moving one leg forward, flexing it at the knee. It was found in an electromyogram, which was recorded during this movement, that in this case the upper part of the obliquus abdominis externus muscle was also stimulated first, followed by activation of its lower part. Later the gluteus medius and then the rectus femoris and the gastrocnemius were included in this activity (Fig. 68). In this case, the initiation of movement also took place from the upper part of the long muscles of the trunk and the shoulder girdle muscles which were innervated by the proximal segment of the spinal cord. The absence of a visible difference in the pattern of activity of the individual muscles innervated by either of the spinal segments is characteristic of the development of this type of local movement. The movements of the lower extremities in the other patients of the first group were carried out in the same manner and initiated with a voluntary contraction of muscles.

During the course of treatment, the activity of the muscles in patients with vertebral or spinal trauma was periodically investigated by taking an electromyogram. Certain changes in its character were observed, which can be seen from the electromyograms that have been presented. First, the nature of the activity depended on the innervation of the muscle; if the activity was even partially provided from the proximal spinal segment, an interference electromyogram was recorded in this muscle from the beginning of the treatment. Initially, these were of moderate amplitude but later the amplitudes increased. The terms "high," "moderate," and "low," which we used for expressing the

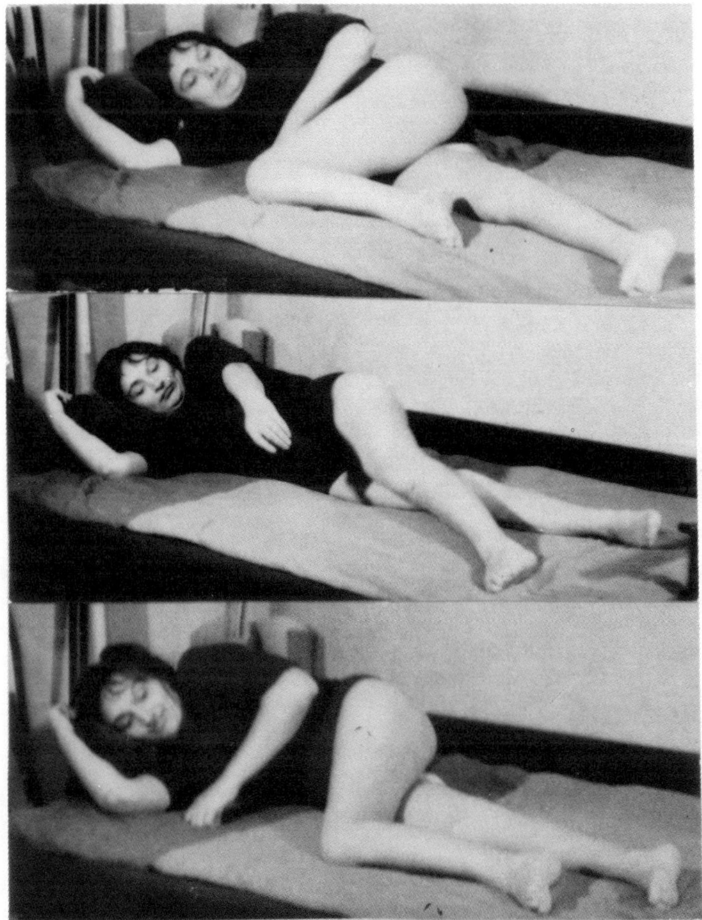

FIG. 66. Patient of the first group flexing and extending her leg at the knee, three years after start of treatment.

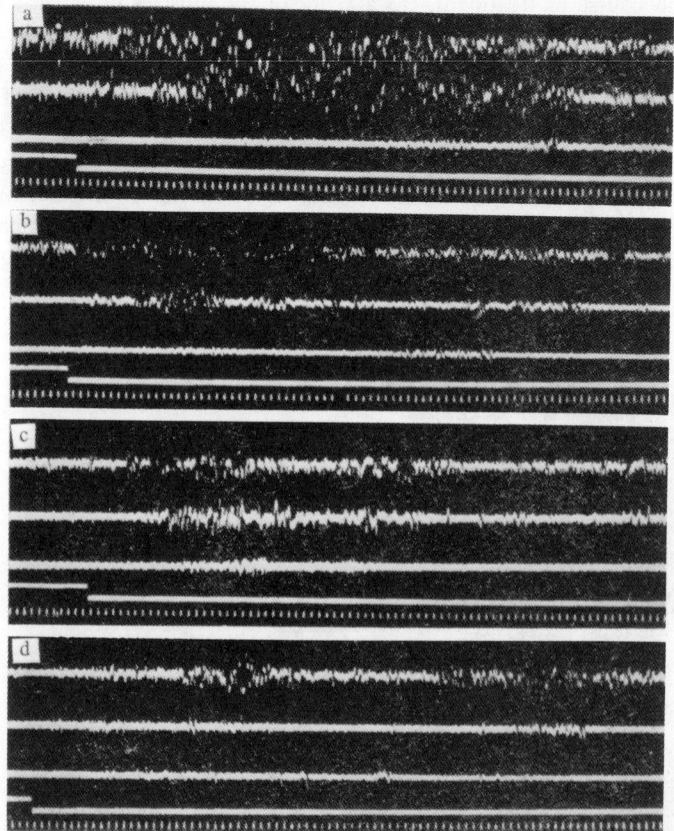

FIG. 67. Activity in muscles of the trunk and lower extremities during flexion of leg at the knee in a patient of the first group, three years after start of treatment.

First three beams in the electromyograms a–d: a—upper and lower parts of the latissimus dorsi and rectus femoris; b—upper and lower parts of the longissimus dorsi and gastrocnemius; c—gluteus medius; d—upper and lower parts of the rectus abdominis and tibialis anterior; fourth beam—time, 20 msec.

amplitude, are comparative terms since we utilized electrode placement where the distance between the electrodes was not always constant. In our experimental conditions, activity higher than 150 mV was considered to be a high amplitude, from 50-150 mV—a moderate amplitude—and less than 50 mV—a low amplitude.

The pattern of activity of the lower parts of the muscles, which were innervated from the distal spinal segment, was determined by the condition of the neuronal innervation of that particular reflex arc, especially in relation to the state of excitability of the receptors and the degree of development of that particular response. Therefore, during the course of treatment, an interference electromyogram with moderate amplitude, which later increased, usually appeared earlier in muscles of the proximal joints of the extremities. This was particularly true in the gluteus medius lying below the skin adjacent to that covering the obliquus abdominis externus, and this muscle was first included in the resulting response. Group potentials were recorded in the quadriceps heads and also those of the gluteus maximus, the sartorius and the adductor longus; and in several cases, at a later stage in the treatment, an interference electromyogram was also recorded. In the other muscles like the flexors of the thigh (biceps femoris, semitendinosus) and especially the leg muscles, the activity usually appeared late and was only recorded in the form of isolated potentials with varying amplitude or in small volleys with low or moderate amplitude. According to the classification of Yusevich (1958), electromyograms which had a variation of potentials appearing in groups or in small groups could be placed in this second category. This type of electromyogram is characteristic of a number of diseases of the peripheral nervous system. Such activity definitely cannot produce flexion of an ankle joint. In fact, as a rule, this movement does not occur during walking in patients of the first group. Walking is carried out by the activity of muscles situated proximal to the joints.

Thus, in spite of the absence of conduction along the spinal cord, there is partial restoration of motor function even after a complete interruption of

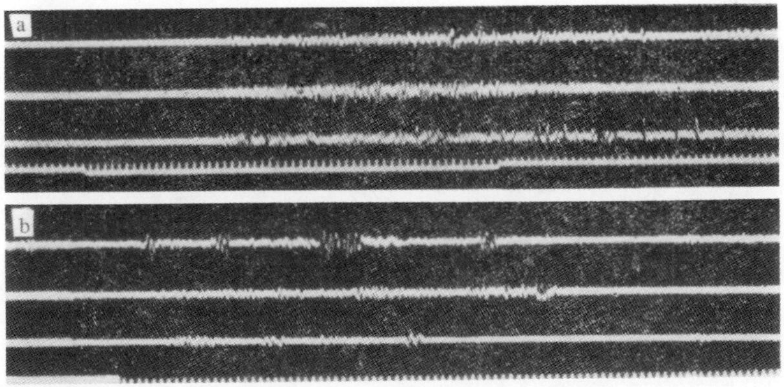

FIG. 68. Activity in muscles of the trunk and lower extremity of a patient of the first group during a leg movement initiated by flexing it at the knee.

First three beams in the electromyograms a–b: a—upper and lower parts of the obliquus abdominis externus and gluteus medius; b—gluteus medius, rectus femoris, gastrocnemius; fourth beam—mark showing the singal for a movement; fifth beam—time, 20 msec.

conductivity. The capacity for reorganization of motor function plays a leading role in the development of the compensatory processes. This is mainly dependent on the possibility of transmitting the neural excitation along a new reflex arc, preserving the traces of excitation for a prolonged period, and maintaining the neuronal apparatus of the spinal cord in a normal state with the help of physical training. The transmission of afferent impulses to the brain along the sympathetic nervous system, bypassing the spinal cord, might help to a certain extent in the development of motor functions of those patients with a complete loss of conduction. This afferent pathway helps to achieve a spatial reorientation of the body, i.e., the inclusion of muscles innervated by the distal segment of the spinal cord in such movement may be facilitated by the adaptotrophic effect of the sympathetic nervous system.

The use of the above method for treating patients with a partial loss of conduction provides a possibility of achieving a comparatively full-fledged recovery of motor function; this helps to obtain a restoration of conduction of excitation along intact fibers of the spinal cord (Jochheim & Strohkendi, 1973).

CONCLUSION

In summary, the evidence which has been presented indicates that partial restoration of motor function may occur even after complete transection of the spinal cord. The following may be the principal methods of recovery:

1. Compensatory development of alternative motor functions. This can occur due to movements carried out by muscles which do not usually participate in the injured motor activity and also by involving muscles of the extremities in activity innervated from the distal segment of the spinal cord.
2. Neural restitution, i.e., the restoration of conduction along intact axons other than those seriously injured fibers of the spinal cord.
3. Regeneration of the fibers in the spinal cord. In all cases, where propagation of impulses is restored through an injured area, it is probable that regenerated nerve fibers provide the additional connections.

In the present work, we have found that the characteristics of the spinal cord's reflex activity, when separated from the higher segments of the central nervous system, have helped in development of compensatory functions. These provide the possibility of developing new reflex motor reactions which spinal animals do not normally possess, as well as the stability of these atypical reactions and their possible inhibition.

The appearance of these properties in a transected spinal cord may be due to a revival of functions which have been lost in the course of phylogenetic development (Orbeli, 1949). One of the principal causes of these phenomena in the lower segments of the central nervous system is the gradual development of supraspinal control which results in suppression of functions that are characteristic of a spinal cord in the early stage of development in lower vertebrates. During development of the spinal cord, afferent input to the cord is progressively reduced and this will influence the organization of the spinal cord's neuronal apparatus which is essential for maintaining normal activity. In fact, we observed distinct changes in the neural organization of the cord when studying the effect of muscular disuse which appeared after transection. Within two weeks of operation, the dystrophic processes had already developed, involving mainly the interneurons and synapses of the motoneurons. These changes had considerably increased by the sixth month and were then associated with an impairment of reflex activity.

The addition of afferent stimuli, by the electrocutaneous excitation which evoked motor reflexes and by physiotherapy and massage, prevented the development of dystrophic processes in the neural elements of the spinal cord.

In the present work, we have shown that the functional peculiarities of the distal segment of the spinal cord reveal a high degree of plasticity in higher mammals and the ability to reorganize the motor functions when stimulated by reflex activity.

Is it possible to define whether any particular reflex elements are responsible for this plasticity or is this due exclusively to the integrated activity of the entire complex?

The survival of an organism when the function of its individual organs has been impaired, i.e., the ability to adapt to a changed condition, is carried out by the reorganization of central nervous system activity and this occurs mainly through participation of the cerebral cortex. Integration of central nervous system activity is very important here. However, even after a complete transection of the spinal cord there can be partial restoration of motor functions. It was often difficult to differentiate spinal dogs which had been treated, from intact ones when they were running, if their muscular tone was increased with a small dose of strychnine. Most surprising was the restoration of motor function in the lower extremities of patients following injury to the spinal cord which had resulted in failure of impulse conduction. We observed the activity of muscles of the extremities during the movement of trunk muscles in cases when these two groups were innervated by different segments of the spinal cord. This coordination helped these patients in carrying out their motor functions. It is improbable in these cases that the reorganization of function exclusively involved the cerebral cortex. We had the impression that the segmental apparatus of the transected spinal cord and the component parts of the spinal reflex arcs possess a high degree of plasticity.

Which of these elements determine the ability of the spinal cord to reorganize its functions? The flexibility of synaptic transmission has been suggested by modern physiology as the main cause of plasticity in the central nervous system, i.e., the capacity of individual synaptic connections to react to partial changes in the synaptic effect. The main cause of the appearance of synaptic plasticity is the post-synaptic reinforcement following application of tetanic stimulation to a presynaptic nerve fiber. This was studied mainly in the synapses of motoneurons, where the effect was distinct. The duration of this post-synaptic reinforcement was several times greater than the duration of the increased excitability, which is also of importance in the development of local excitation in the end plate. The mechanism of formation of atypical reflex reactions is well explained by the phenomenon of synaptic plasticity and the associated changes in the neurons. However, the reaction of different types of neurons in a spinal cord which is separated from its higher centers varied greatly. The degree and type of participation of internuncial and motor neurons in the reorganization of a motor function were not uniform. In addition, plasticity of the central nervous system was apparent not only through the reorganization of motor functions but also by the adaptation of neurons and their metabolism to a new level of activity involving the participation of the whole neuronal network, including the satellite cells.

Neurons Involved in Functional Recovery

A number of investigations, as well as our own, have given an opportunity for considering the participation of several types of neurons in the functional reorganization following different types of spinal injuries, particularly after cord transection.

The stability of the *α-motoneurons* is a characteristic feature of their activity in the intact spinal cord. Thus, in kittens, only 40 percent of the motoneurons acquired new functions after cross-suturing the nerves (Eccles, Eccles, & Magni, 1960). The stability of the structure and function of these motoneurons following disuse in a transected spinal cord were clearly demonstrated in our experiments. The size of the motoneurons was found to be practically normal following a period of disuse. Monosynaptic reflexes appeared regularly with a constant latent period even after three years after spinal transection. The nature of motor unit discharges, characterizing the activity of motoneurons in spinal and intact dogs, was similar when investigated in a relatively resting condition.

It is possible that the change in the activity of the motoneurons, which has been observed by a number of investigators after a spinal transection, can be explained by functional changes occurring in the interneurons which are reflected in the activity of the motor neurons.

We believe that the ability of motoneurons which produced motor activity is also related to the appearance of plasticity associated with that particular type of cell. In fact, releasing the stress or depriving the spinal cord of the constant tonic influence from higher centers does not appreciably affect the structure or function of the motor neurons. As a result, a rapid adaptation in the level of activity occurs in these big cells. They adapt to the new situation by increasing the oxidative processes and synthesizing nucleoproteins. The stability of the motor neurons not only maintained regular activity but also established the possibility of functional reorganization by the integrative action of the spinal cord.

The *interneurons* of the spinal cord and the synapses of the motoneurons have completely different characteristics. In contradistinction to the α-motoneurons, they are extremely sensitive to changes associated with their degree of activity. In the condition of disuse, when there are definite structural changes, a lowering in the synaptic function of such a particular reflex arc is observed. This is associated with an increase in function of the neighboring arcs which is possibly due to an increase in the number of synapses.

In a monosynaptic reflex arc, the synapses of the motoneurons are the first to suffer due to disuse; but in a polysynaptic arc, the interneurons are primarily affected. The possibility of development of new reflex reactions becomes a problem when polysynaptic reflexes have been impaired and consequently, the reorganization of motor function is much more difficult. Interneurons are present in large numbers in the structure of the spinal cord. They have wide neuronal connections, which gives them an opportunity to organize reflexes in many combinations and to assure the formation of new reflex pathways. When sensitivity of interneurons is altered, the regularity and stability of motoneuron activity might ensure constant motor activity in an animal.

Thus, the principal structures of the reflex network in the spinal cord—the internuncial and the motor nerve cells with their synaptic connections—are considered as being a single apparatus in which the participation of all individual elements is necessary for motor activity, particularly at the time of spinal development. The plasticity of the spinal reflex apparatus is ensured by a number of interrelated processes and afferent stimulation is considered to be one of its main components.

Restoration of motor function in the lower extremities of patients with spinal injury clearly demonstrates the presence of a high degree of plasticity in the distal spinal segment.

A question may be raised as to how an impulse can be transmitted from a proximal to a distal segment of a spinal cord in spinal patients who received treatment. In the course of treatment following injury, the lower parts of the long muscles of the trunk which are innervated from both segments of the spinal cord are activated relatively easily and quickly. Some of the gluteal muscles and subsequently the thigh muscles are, to some extent, included in this activity. The leg muscles are activated in the next stage of restorative treatment.

According to our concept, the muscular and cutaneous receptors, in which impulses are considered to be initiated during reflex muscular contraction, play a major role involving the muscles of the extremities. The passive flexion and extension of the extremities, the stretching of muscles and raising the leg straight without bending, are the main exercises in the beginning of restorative treatment for spinal patients. The impulses which appear in the muscle spindles at the time of skin displacement as a result of repeated movements serve as an initiator of muscular contraction. The patient was required to repeat movements which activated the muscle receptors. This was initially difficult in the trunk joints. Later, in the course of therapy, this movement was perfected and the muscular activity of the extremities increased. The delay required for the activation of the muscles of the extremities became gradually closer to the time of activation of the trunk muscles innervated by the proximal segment of a spinal cord. The maintenance of equilibrium by the patient was as important as the conduction of impulses in a distal segment of the spinal cord required for developing the walking process.

Now let us examine how treatment assured the maintenance of equilibrium during walking in patients with spinal transections. The function of the segmental apparatus is greater here than in an intact organism and this fact was observed in a number of investigations. However, it is necessary to remember that the process of development of the complex act of walking under conditions of spinal development may only occur in the presence of constant interaction of the neuronal apparatus of the proximal segments of a spinal cord, side by side with the corresponding area of the cerebral cortex. Maintenance of equilibrium is impossible in the initial stages of treating the patients, without participation of the visual system. Gurfinkel' and his associates (1965) clearly showed the importance of visual stimulation for the maintenance of posture in patients with impaired joint sense.

Proprioception from muscles innervated through the proximal part of a spinal cord may also play a significant role in the maintenance of equilibrium at the time of training a patient in walking and erect posture. Patients who had learned how to walk showed that they could determine the position of their body without seeing, although there was no sensation in their legs.

It is possible that, as a result of prolonged treatment, transmission of an afferent impulse along the sympathetic nervous system helps to determine the position of the body in relation to space and also helps to maintain its equilibrium.

Treatment

Restitution of function was demonstrable in several spinal patients when multiple restorative treatment consisting of physical therapy and Pyrogenal was applied. It was possible to observe this striking phenomenon in a number of the patients studied with a diagnosis of spinal transection after a lapse of several years following injury. In these cases, mild voluntary movements in all the joints of the extremities, the tone of the antigravity muscles and, in one case, even sexual functions were restored. Intensive treatment with the simultaneous application of Pyrogenal was the stimulus for development of all these functions which indicated recovery of impulse propagation through the injured area. It may be assumed that the structurally intact fibers of the spinal cord were not functioning in the initial period after injury, due to post-traumatic changes. Subsequently, the inactivity of the isolated spinal cord during complete paraplegia led to the development of dystrophic processes in its neuronal apparatus. Only properly directed intensive treatment, combined with the increased tone in a number of systems due to Pyrogenal, produced a condition favorable to restoration of the spinal neuron activity. When the inflammatory compression and hemorrhages were relieved, the intact fibers in the spinal cord were found to be capable of propagating impulses, and they probably took over additional functions. One can see here the phenomenon, reported earlier, whereby moderate activity helped to maintain the vital function of neurons which was found to be essential for the synthesis of nucleoproteins. Similarly, it appeared that changes in neuroglial proportions could play some role depending on the level of activity. This phenomenon was noticed in a number of investigations. The trophic function of neurons, including their protein synthesis, was observed to increase due to a rise in the number of satellite cells.

The Background for Regeneration

If integration of the activity of the central nervous system (which is possible due to its unique organization) is most essential for compensatory restoration, the property of high differentiation should mitigate against successful regeneration. Although the brain tissue possesses very good trophism, the abundant blood supply with its highly developed oxidative processes and the large number of satellite cells with their ability to transfer nutritive substances to a neuronal body, proved inadequate for restoration following damage to the nervous system. The growth potential of the central nervous system neurons was inadequate to develop a full-fledged regeneration.

However, a peripheral nerve, when transected and thereafter sutured, grows rapidly and its function is restored.

These differences in the conditions of functional restoration are further complicated by the process of evolution. The central nervous system is enclosed in a bony case which protects it from injuries. During its development, a large number of related activities become established, requiring an increasing number of neurons with complicated connections. As a result, no chances of implementing the restorative processes after injury of the central nervous system can be expected, but similar trauma to a peripheral nerve invariably led to the development of properties which accommodated and favored successful regeneration (Cook, 1973).

What are these properties? What is the difference in the processes involved during regeneration of central and peripheral neurons?

The main difference is found in the process which precedes regeneration, i.e., the degenerative process which follows sectioning of the fibers. In a peripheral nerve this process proceeds quickly; there is a disintegration of the axons and their myelin sheaths, the proteolytic enzymes are stimulated, a rise in the number of satellite cells is observed, and finally there is an acceleration of protein synthesis. The neuron provides the rapid supply of protoplasm to the injured area, i.e., the damaged end of the axon. Thus, the growth of axons and their myelination is continued and the propagation of impulses is restored. Similarly, a full-fledged synaptic connection is formed by the growing fibers. This regenerative process will progress successfully, if it is not prevented by a rapidly forming scar. It will happen either where continuity of the membranes is maintained or where they are interrupted and subsequently sutured. In contrast to this, the degenerating processes are sluggish and poorly developed in a CNS fiber. The disintegration and resorption of the degraded tissue proceeds very slowly. The proteolytic enzymes are not stimulated. No rise in the number of satellite cells is observed. The level of protein synthesis in the neurons remains unchanged. As a result, the regenerative process is much less well-developed. Is it possible to reorganize the regenerative processes subsequent to sectioning of the CNS fibers, so that they may resemble those found in a peripheral nerve?

Very hopeful results have been obtained by increasing the disintegrative processes and the dedifferentiation of tissue at the time of regeneration in mammals, as reported by Polezhaev.* One would expect that this general rule might also be applicable to the axons of the central nervous system.

Attempts to stimulate the processes which prolonged the duration of

*Editor's note: This concept involves the increase in proteosynthesis during tissue regeneration which is believed to result when the necessary precursors are available in greater amount due to enhanced breakdown during preceding degeneration.

disintegration in an injured area demonstrated that this was an effective approach. The administration of resorptive transplants in the gap of the spinal cord led to a rise in the number of glial cells and considerably accelerated the growth of axons. The important result was that these processes started earlier and, as a result, a comparatively profuse growth of axons was observed through the site of the lesion where the scar formation was taking place. Partial restoration of impaired function was observed in a number of animals. These experiments confirmed the hypothesis that restoration of the regenerating capability of the axons in the central nervous system is based on general rules which are similar for the regeneration of organs in vertebrates and tissues in mammals. They consist of an enhancement of initial tissue disintegration which leads to activation of the synthesis of RNA and this is the basis of the growth process.

It was found experimentally that there is stimulation of protein synthesis in the neurons during the final stage of these processes, preparatory to regeneration. Hence, it was important to test those substances influencing the synthesis of RNA in nerve cells for their ability to stimulate the regenerative process.

These substances were dinitryl malonic acid and pentoxyl. It was shown in preliminary experiments that these substances, in fact, had positive effects on the regeneration on intraspinal axons. Pentoxyl was found to be a relatively weak stimulator while dinitryl malonic acid produced a rapid and profuse growth of nerve fibers through the site of a spinal lesion in rats and the subsequent restoration of weight-bearing and locomotor functions in a dog which had been kept under observation for a prolonged period. Thus, this method of stimulating the synthesis of nucleoproteins and thus intensifying the regenerating capacity of the CNS fibers was shown to be not only possible but also probably effective.

By changing the character of the processes normally following sectioning of nerve fibers, it has been possible to stimulate their growth and obtain appreciably more regeneration. As a result, plasticity is manifested in a new form, i.e., the ability to reorganize the trophic functions of the central nervous system. According to the hypothesis developed by Parin (1966), these procedures can facilitate the integrated trophic functions simultaneously affecting a number of systems in an organism and provide a higher level of activity.

Scar Formation

The rapid formation of a dense scar in a traumatized spinal area is a serious hindrance to the successful regeneration of CNS fibers. For the last 20 years, many investigators have been involved with the problem of how to control the scar. The use of Piromen, Millipore, trypsin, and lidase prevents the development of a dense scar in the area of spinal trauma or the penetration of fibrous tissues in a spinal gap to varying degrees. We tried Pyrogenal, as this satisfies most of the requirements and seems to be an inhibitor of scarring when it is used at an early post-operative stage. The spinal scar, which formed under its influence, over a period of two years, differs considerably from the scar of control animals in respect to its friability. Pyrogenal inhibits the development of glial and collagenous scars. Its ability to stimulate the leukocytic enzymes, and start the reaction of depolymerization of the ground substance in connective tissue, changes the permeability and inhibits the maturation of the fibroblasts, leading to a sharp retardation of scar formation.

The action of Pyrogenal is not restricted to these effects. It has been shown that it stimulates the hyphophysioadrenal system, i.e., there is an overall increase in hormonal activity which results in an increase of metabolic activity. There is also a rise in the tone and volume of the muscles and an improvement in the blood supply. A rise in the concentration of catecholamines and serotonin in the brain produces an increased cerebral cortex tone. The effect of Pyrogenal mimics the action of sympathetic nerve stimulation which is usually reduced in patients with impaired conductivity in the spinal cord, particularly at the higher segmental levels. A spinal patient receiving Pyrogenal in our clinic was capable of moving himself, which was not otherwise possible, and this was extremely helpful at the time of the development of motor activity. Hence, Pyrogenal is considered to be a true stimulator of restorative processes in their different manifestations.

It may be concluded, on the basis of the material presented above, that the regeneration of neurons in the spinal cord and the compensatory development of motor functions after a complete interruption of conductivity are not impractical. For the former process, it is necessary to enhance the synthesis of nucleoproteins in neurons with transected axons and to prevent the rapid formation of a dense spinal scar. In the latter process, it is necessary to apply properly directed intensive physical therapy, including cutaneous stimulation. This will keep the neuromotor activity in normal condition and lead to the development of additional reflex reactions in the distal spinal segment. In this way, it is possible to develop activity in the muscles of the lower extremities.

One and the same process–an increase of the nucleoprotein synthesis in nerve cells–has been essential in order to achieve partial restoration of motor function in patients with an interruption of conductivity in the spinal cord. Similarly, the formation of new structures replacing degenerated ones in the processes of vital motor activity has facilitated the synthesis of structures essential for regenerating transected axons. The synthesis of nucleoproteins is the sole basis of life in the body of an animal, starting from the formation of an embryo from a template according to a genetic code which consists of selecting particular nucleic acids in strict sequence and ending with the reparative processes in an injured organism.

An elevation in the level of synthesis of nucleoproteins can be achieved with an increase of motor activity, on the one hand, and the use of pharmacological agents, on the other. Under these conditions, a high degree of plasticity is maintained in the central nervous system, particularly in the spinal cord following its separation from the higher centers.

APPENDIX

CASE HISTORIES OF SELECTED PATIENTS WITH SPINAL CORD INJURIES

P. P., female, born in 1939

In August, 1963, this patient received an injury of the vertebral column including the spinal cord. Laminectomy done at the level of T_5-T_7. Soon after trauma, the patient received Pyrogenal and physical therapy and then Pyrogenal and lidase; she was nevertheless completely bedridden till spring 1966. Application of Pyrogenal and physical therapy, but without an instructor, started again from April 1966. From September, 1966, patient practiced once a day with an instructor and thrice independently.

Neurologic status on December 27, 1966, 2½ years after injury and 4 months after start of treatment with restorative method: spastic paraplegia. Increased muscle tone and clonic twitching of muscles. Compensatory flexion with maximum stretching at the level of scapulae. No atrophy of muscles of the extremities. Pathological reflexes: signs of Babinski, Rossolimo and Gordon positive on both sides. Tendon reflexes–knee and ankle clonus exaggerated by stimulation. Patient could sit and crawl with or without assistance, and, if placed on leg splints, could stand erect and learn to walk.

Electromyographic investigation conducted at the beginning of treatment demonstrated that activity was only recorded in the upper parts of long muscles of the trunk at the time when the leg was being raised.

Electromyographic investigation on December 27, 1966: low amplitude interference electromyogram in the lower parts of long muscles of the trunk and in several muscles of extremities; low amplitude potentials appeared either in groups or in an isolated manner when the legs were being raised and the patient was in a vertical position.

Sensation: a zone of anesthesia at the level of T_4, hyperesthesia from T_5-L_2. All types of sensation–pain, temperature, touch, pressure, and muscle-joint senses–absent below this level. Function of pelvic organs not restored.

Neurologic status on March 24, 1969, 5½ years after trauma and 3 years after start of treatment: spastic paraplegia. Increased tone of muscles, more on the right side. Knee and ankle jerks–clonic type; pathological reflexes on both sides. Abdominal reflexes present except for the lower part of the right side–could move on crutches with splints, and go up and down stairs. Lying on side, could flex and extend the leg from the knee with the help of trunk muscles.

Electromyographic investigation: interference myogram with several volleys having high amplitude in both segments of long muscles of the trunk at the time of walking (and other movements). Also volleys of interference electromyogram or group potentials with moderate amplitude were recorded in a number of muscles of the extremities.

Sensation: at the level of T_4-T_5–zone of anesthesia; then from T_6-T_8–hyperesthesia; and T_9-T_{10}–hypoesthesia, followed by anesthesia. Discrimination of superficial touch and pain present on the right thigh, could recognize movement of right large toe. Involuntary micturition with an automatism at an interval of 1½ to 2 hours.

N. K., female, born in 1942

On August 7, 1961, received spinal injury resulting in a compression fracture of T_{12} and partial damage of L_1. Laminectomy on August 15, 1961 revealed spinal cord injury covering a length of about 3 cms with damage to dura matter. Spinal cord was almost completely destroyed and the debris washed out. From January, 1963, patient treated by Dr. Trankvillitati and received Pyrogenal. Initially, she had difficulty in following instructions and could only move on crutches when assisted. However, in the middle of February, 1963, patient began to walk up and down stairs.

Neurological status on January 4, 1967, 5 years after injury and 3 after start of treatment: flaccid paraplegia, decreased tone of leg muscles. Knee and ankle jerks absent on both sides. During stress and excitement, fibrillar twitchings noted in muscles, particularly in gluteus. She could walk on crutches with splints or with cane on a flat surface, or move up and down stairs.

Electromyographic investigation demonstrated an interference electromyogram with high amplitude in upper parts of the long muscles of the trunk and low amplitude in lower parts when raising the leg (or during other movements). In muscles of the extremities, these potentials appeared either alone or in a low amplitude group. Disturbance of all types of sensation from T_{12}, except the lateral part of the right thigh where there was a zone of hyperesthesia. Functions of the visceral organs in the pelvic cavity automatic.

Neurologic status on March 20, 1969, about 7½ years after injury and one year after withdrawal of instructor: decreased tone of muscles without any pronounced atrophy. Passive movements fully present in both knee and hip joints; movements in ankle joints only with difficulty, R > L. Knee jerks absent on both sides; ankle jerks present, a distinct clonus noted on the left but short-lasting on the right. Rossolimo and Mendel-Bekhterev signs prominent on both sides. She could move on crutches with splints or with cane for a prolonged period, placing the legs in turn and moving up and down a staircase up to the fourth floor.

Electromyographic investigation revealed an interference electromyogram with moderate amplitude in the upper and lower parts of trunk muscles and in muscles of the lower extremities when walking (or during other movements) involving lower extremities. No significant changes in the character and distribution of sensation.

P. B., male, born in 1925

On August 29, 1962, received an injury in the vertebral column–fracture of T_{10}-T_{11} with compression over the spinal cord. Laminectomy on September 3, 1962, revealed a lesion of the spinal cord with debris washed out. The patient was in hospital up to October, 1963. Treatment consisted of several massages to improve general condition of patient; discharged in bedridden condition. From April, 1965, received Pyrogenal and commenced physical therapy with instructor, and then, independently in a health resort as suggested by Dr. Trankvillitati.

Neurologic status on February 9, 1967, about 4½ years after beginning of physical therapy: flacid paraplegia, decreased muscle tone, foot drop. Knee reflexes present, $R > L$; ankle reflex distinct on the right and absent on the left. Pathological reflexes: Babinski, Rossolimo and Mendel-Bekhterev signs positive on both sides. Patient moved on crutches with splints.

Electromyographic investigation: high amplitude interference electromyogram in the trunk muscle when trying to move and in a number of muscles of the extremities–isolated or group potentials. Decrease in all types of sensation from the level of T_{10}-T_{11}; a zone of hyperesthesia at the approximate level of T_{10}. Functions of pelvic organs were not restored.

Neurologic status on March 21, 1969, about 5½ years after injury: no change in condition of reflexes. Improvement in movements: patient could sit, stand and move, placing legs in turn; could move other leg when standing only with a cane, flexing it at the knee.

Electromyographic investigation: high amplitude interference electromyogram when walking and during other movements in all muscles of the trunk and extremities. No change in sensation. Automatism developed in functions of pelvic organs.

N. S., male, born in 1937

On April 16, 1964, received an injury of the vertebral column with a spinal cord injury due to fall from a height. Laminectomy on April 17, 1964; vertebral process of T_{11} removed and 1.5-cm gap in spinal cord detected. Diagnosis: multifragmented compression fracture of T_{11} with dislocation of T_{12}. Gap of spinal cord at this level. Cystotomy performed.

Neurologic status on May 15, 1964: flaccid paralysis of lower extremities with an absence of all types of sensation from the level of T_{12}. Knee and ankle jerks absent. Abdominal reflex present in the right upper quadrant. Examined by Dr. Trankvillitati on March 29, 1965. Active movement not seen in a single joint. Patient was unable to turn in bed without assistance. From April to October, 1965, received Pyrogenal ATP, massage and physical therapy with instructor. Later, another course of Pyrogenal repeated and physical therapy applied independently. By June, 1965, patient was able to stand on crutches with splints and began to learn to walk. In September, started to ascend a staircase; catheter was removed in November. Sexual functions reappearing, becoming practically normal in September 1966 (see Jackson, 1972). Patient married in December 1966.

Neurologic status on March 6, 1967, about 3 years after injury and 2 years following start of treatment: spastic paralysis, active flexion possible in hip and knee joints, more pronounced in the left leg. Knee reflexes present, $L > R$; ankle reflex–clonic type on the right and absent on the left. Babinski, Rossolimo and Mendel-Bekhterev signs positive on both sides. During this period, patient was found to be capable of standing on the left leg and, thereafter, also on right leg without cane; there was an increased tone of the extensor muscles.

Electromyographic investigation demonstrated an interference electromyogram with high and moderate amplitude in muscles of the trunk and in several leg muscles, when moving; group potentials with moderate amplitude were seen in other leg muscles. Altered sensation on the ventral surface from the level of T_{12} and in the back from L_1-L_2. Zone of hyperesthesia in the lateral side of thighs: patient responds to pain, pressure and cold on both sides; pain sensation more pronounced on the left.

T. M., female, born in 1939

Received a brain concussion with a compression fracture of the vertebral column (together with an open fracture of the right leg) during a landslide on August 29, 1963. Immediately developed flaccid paralysis with functional impairment of pelvic organs. Laminectomy on September 10, 1963 revealed anatomical section of the spinal cord at the level of T_{11}-L_1. Repeated laminectomy on July 10, 1964 in connection with a pain syndrome. Scar tissue removed from traumatic area; pain disappeared but only temporarily. From September 1964 to July 1965, patient treated at the Institute of Orthopedics, where leg fracture was corrected and suprapubic tube removed. Because ischial osteomyelitis developed in May 1966, it was not possible to commence restorative treatment. In February 1967, an operation was performed for osteomyelitis; after recovery, she began to practice physical therapy under guidance of Dr. Trankvillitati (from December 1968).

Neurologic status on April 3, 1969, about 5½ years after injury and 4 months after start of physical therapy: flaccid paralysis. Decreased muscle tone. Contracture of right foot. Knee and ankle jerks and also pathological reflexes, absent. No abdominal reflexes. Patient moved easily on crutches with splints, placing the legs in turn; could sit and turn in bed and also crawl.

Electromyographic investigation demonstrated an interference electromyogram in shoulder muscles and in long muscles of the trunk when raising the leg. The amplitude increased during similar movements in a vertical position. Of all the muscles of the extremities, only the gluteus media was included in the activity. All types of sensation absent from the level of T_{12} downward; an indistinct zone of hypoesthesia at the level of T_{11}. Pelvic organs: micturition restored.

Neurologic status on November 13, 1969, about 6½ years after injury and 11 months after beginning of physical therapy: general condition of patient–good. Moved on crutches with splints, freely placing the legs in turn. Decrease in all types of sensation from the level of T_{12}. Sensation indistinct, not always appearing at the time of application of strong pressure in the region of a vascular bundle. Occasionally, during a passive foot movement, patient could localize the side, R > L. Lying on back, raised the leg straight; lying on side, easily flexed leg at the knee. Abdominal reflexes present on both sides of the upper and middle and absent in the lower parts. Ankle and knee jerks present on both sides. Pathological reflexes absent.

Electromyographic investigation demonstrated that muscles of the extremities began to be included in the activity; an interference electromyogram in the gluteus media, in both standing and lying positions; group potentials with low amplitude in a number of other muscles of the extremities. Sensation: pain, tactile and temperature sensations absent from T_{12} downwards on both sides; an indistinct zone of hyperesthesia at the level of T_{11}. Variation in cutaneous temperature present, R > L. Could distinguish a prolonged strong pressure in the vascular bundle, more distinct on the right.

I. M., female, born in 1941

Due to fall from a height on August 31, 1968, received a vertical injury with a compression fracture of T_8-T_{12}. Immediately developed a flaccid paralysis with functional impairment of pelvic organs. Two laminectomies within first few days of the trauma: first–at the level of T_{12}-L_5, second after 3 days–T_5-T_{12}. From the first days of treatment, received Pyrogenal and practiced physical therapy with an instructor under guidance of Dr. Trankvillitati.

Neurologic status on March 27, 1969, about 6 months after injury and start of physical therapy: tone of muscles in the right leg decreased and in the left, increased. Complete absence of active movements; passive movements on left knee and hip limited due to restricted mobility. The volume of muscles of thigh and leg: L > R. Knee jerks: R > L; ankle jerk distinct on the right, and clonic type on the left. Pathological reflexes: Babinski, Rossolimo, Mendel-Bekhterev signs present on both sides, more distinct on the left. Electromyographic investigation demonstrated activity only in the shoulder muscles and in upper parts of the long muscles of the trunk when attempting to raise the leg when lying on the back. All types of sensation absent along the distribution of T_9. No hyperesthesia. Urinary bladder automatic.

Neurologic status on September 13, 1969, about 14 months after injury and after start of physical therapy: patient began to move on crutches with splints or corset, easily placing the legs in turn. Unsteady. Mobility of left hip and knee restricted. Volume of muscles of thigh and leg: R > L. Knee jerks present; ankle jerks also present on both sides but of clonic type on the left. Pathological reflexes present on both sides.

Electromyographic investigation demonstrated an interference electromyogram in shoulder girdle muscles and in upper parts of the long muscles of the trunk during a leg raising movement, lying on the back. Low amplitude group potentials in lower parts of the trunk muscles. Pressure over the left rectus femoris caused activity to appear in it; moreover, muscle potentials appeared in the gastrocnemius and tibialis anterior of the ipsilaternal extremity. This phenomenon was less distinct on the right. During an attempt to turn on her side, some activity appeared in the gluteus maximus. Decrease in all types of sensation from T_{12}. Sensation indistinct and did not always appear when strong pressure was applied in the region of a vascular bundle. She could occasionally localize the side, R > L during a passive foot movement.

T. Ts., female, born in 1940

Received a skull injury with a compression fracture of the vertebral column on April 19, 1961. Immediately developed a flaccid paralysis with functional alteration of pelvic organs. Fracture of T_{12} and lesion of dura mater with damage to the spinal cord established by laminectomy. Bedridden without movement for 8 years. In April 1969, following a consultation with Dr. Trankvillitati, patient commenced physical therapy and also received Pyrogenal.

Neurologic status on April 7, 1969, about 8 years after injury and just before start of physical therapy: bed sores over sacrum in the regions of hip, knee and ankle joints. Mobility of knee joints restricted, right metatarsophalangeal joints deformed. Knee and ankle jerks absent. No pathological reflexes. Abdominal reflexes retained in upper parts on both sides. Movements completely absent: patient could not turn independently, could neither sit nor raise her legs.

Electromyographic investigation demonstrated no activity in trunk muscles during first attempt to raise her leg, but during a second attempt, potentials with small amplitude were recorded in upper parts of the long muscles. During the fifth attempt, isolated potentials in lower parts of the same muscles were recorded. Pain and tactile sensations absent from T_{12}. Could clearly distinguish strong pressure from both thighs, R > L. Pelvic organs not functioning properly.

Neurologic status on November 4, 1969, about 6 months after start of physical therapy: patient moved 200–300 m on crutches with splints, but movement was unsteady; could turn in bed without assistance, crawl and sit. Bed sores present only in the region of knee joints. Tone of muscles decreased and movement of knee and ankle joints restricted. Right ankle joint was found to be deformed. Knee reflexes absent; ankle reflex on the left, absent, and on the right, of clonic type. Babinski and Rossolimo signs positive. Abdominal reflexes present in upper parts on both sides.

Electromyographic investigation demonstrated an interference electromyogram in shoulder muscles and in upper parts of the long muscles of the trunk; when raising leg, amplitude was much lower in the lower parts of these muscles. Muscles of the leg inactive. Decrease of all types of sensation from T_{12}. Prolonged strong pressure along the course of a vascular bundle very easily distinguished in the right thigh but not always in the left. A distinct variation in the cutaneous temperature observed, R > L. Impairment of functions of pelvic organs.

Neurologic status on February 26, 1970, about 9 months after start of physical therapy: patient moved on crutches with splints and strolled on walkers; could sit without help and put her hands up when seated. Condition of the reflexes–same as noted earlier. Electromyographic investigation demonstrated group potentials of low amplitude in several muscles of the extremities during a leg movemnt, lying on the back, and also during walking.

Sensation: as noted earlier; derangement in the function of pelvic organs retained.

I. L., female, born in 1924

In June 1964, sustained a compression fracture of T_{12} and fragmentation of L_1 with dislocation of vertebrae; fracture of right third rib and pubic and ischial bones of both sides, double fracture of right femur with fragmentation, separation of cocyx, concussion of brain. Patient in deep shock, thus laminectomy not performed. Clinical diagnosis of complete transection of spinal cord established. Under supervision of Dr. Trankvillitati from the first few days after the injury. Pyrogenal therapy started from the sixth day and continued for 5 months; physical therapy began after the seventh day following injury. Patient could easily flex her legs at the ankle joints after 1½ months; functions of pelvic organs were restored after 7 months; she was placed in a corset on crutches after 8 months and began to learn to walk.

Neurologic status on December 8, 1966, about 2½ years after injury residual spastic paralysis. Increased tone of muscles, R > L. Movements restricted in the right ankle joint. Knee reflexes present, L > R; clonici movement of both feet, R > L. Patient could sit freely, stand, and move without cane.

Electromyographic investigation demonstrated an interference electromyogram, appearing in all the muscles of the trunk and legs under investigation when raising her leg and when stepping. Deep sensation altered on both sides; decrease of pain sensation in the region of thigh; tactile sensation preserved in the legs. Complete restoration of functions of pelvic organs.

Neurologic status on March 28, 1967, 2 years and 9 months after the injury: full movements in hip and knee joints, L > R; movements restored in the left ankle joint, restricted in the right. Muscle power: L > R; increased tone, R > L. Knee reflexes present, L > R; clonic movements of both feet, R > L. Pathological reflexes present.

Electromyographic investigation during movement of feet and phalanges demonstrated an interference electromyogram only in muscles which normally ensured such movements. Sensation: slight decrease in sensation from T_{12}. Tactile sensation restored, joint-muscle sense reappeared, hyperesthesia in knee regions and decreased sensation on both sides below the knee.

T. B., female, born in 1935

Periodic attacks of acute pain in the left hand and in the left scapular region from February 1965; gradually developed a general weakness and tremors in right leg; pain gradually increased. Laminectomy on May 26, 1965 at the level of C_3–C_5, in connection with an osteochondritis of C_5. Complete failure of conductivity of the spinal cord from the level of C_5–C_7 on the second day after operation. Second laminectomy at the level of C_6–L_1 on June 11, 1965 with removal of a large subdural neuroma. After operation, movements were restored in the left hand but spasticity increased in the lower extremities–developed a spastic paralysis with disturbance of sensation from the level of T_4, along with a disorder of pelvic organs. Motor functions and sensation not restored until 1966. Patient could turn in bed with difficulty. From March 1966, following consultation with Dr. Trankvillitati, patient began to receive Pyrogenal and vitamins, as well as massage and physical therapy. After 2 months, she was able to walk, using a cane, crutches or a walker. The sensation threshold was lowered and the functions of pelvic organs restored. Considerable improvement was noted due to continued treatment.

Neurologic status on December 29, 1966, about 1½ years after operation and 10 months after the beginning of treatment: patient moved using only a cane without splints, could step up and down a staircase. Unrestricted movements in both hands; muscle power good; muscle tone unchanged. Spastic paralysis. Movements restricted in knee and ankle joints. Knee reflexes positive with a widening of zone, L = R; clonicity of both feet. Babinski sign positive on the right; Rossolimo, Gordon, and Oppenheim signs present on both sides. Abdominal reflexes absent.

A. Sh., male, born in 1921

Vertebral column and spinal cord at the level of T_{11}–L_1 injured in 1962 during an air crash. Laceration of spinal cord established by laminectomy and the debris washed out. Application of Pyrogenal and physical therapy started one month after the injury following a consultation with Dr. Trankvillitati. Patient was able to stand and began to walk with a cane or on crutches after 10–11 months.

Neurologic status on May 14, 1967, about 5 years after injury and start of treatment; flaccid paralysis, decreased muscle tone in the lower extremities. Moderate atrophy of thigh and leg muscles. Unrestricted movement of hip joints; in the knee joints, nearly full flexion and in the ankles, restricted on the right and dorsiflexion on the left. Power of muscles innervated from the proximal spinal segments. Abdominal reflexes: unaltered in the left upper and middle parts and absent in the right. Knee and ankle jerks absent. No pathological reflexes. Movement possible with a stick in a single splint on the right leg.

Electromyographic investigation demonstrated a high amplitude interference electromyogram in muscles of the trunk and legs at the time of voluntary movement. During movement of the left foot, group potentials in the leg muscles. During movement of the right foot, no activity in leg muscles. All types of sensation retained up to the upper third of the leg from where the pain, temperature, and pressure sensations were less pronounced; tactile sensation on the legs present but joint-muscle sense absent. Functions of pelvic organs and sexual functions restored.

Neurologic status on April 1, 1968, about 6 years after the injury: muscle power good; practically no restriction in active flexion of hip and knee joints; flexion in ankle joints possible only at the time of weight-bearing. Movement possible with the help of a stick without splints. Knee and ankle jerks absent on both sides. No pathological reflexes.

During flexion of left leg at the knee and ankle joints, electromyographic investigation demonstrated an interference electromyogram in muscles that normally participate in this movement. In the right extremity, no activity was recorded in muscles of the ankle joint during movements. Sensation remained at the same level as noted earlier.

T. M., male, born in 1946

Due to a fall from a height on April 5, 1968, patient received a severe brain concussion with a compression fracture of the vertebral column at the level of T_{10}-T_{11}. Immediately developed flaccid paralysis with impairment of functions of pelvic organs. No spinal gap detected by laminectomy. From February to May 1969, received Pyrogenal and practiced physical therapy under the guidance of Dr. Trankvillitati.

Neurologic status on March 18, 1969, about a year after the injury and one month after start of physical therapy: flaccid paralysis. Knee and ankle jerks absent. No pathological reflexes. Abdominal reflexes unaltered in the upper and middle parts on both sides. Could move on crutches with splints with great difficulty; could sit and turn from prone to supine position and vice versa.

Electromyographic investigation demonstrated that at the time of raising his leg very slowly, when lying on the back, activity appeared in both parts of the trunk muscles. This was absent in the leg muscles. Sensation disturbed along the distribution of T_{10}-T_{11}. A zone of hyperesthesia from T_{12}-L_1, and absence of all types of sensation below this level. Suprapubic drainage tube was removed 7 months after operation and bladder became automatic.

Neurologic status on May 8, 1969, about 3 months after starting physical therapy: could move on crutches with splints, placing the legs in turn; tried to turn on one side and flex the right leg at the knee. Electromyographic investigation demonstrated activity in the trunk muscles during movement; isolated potentials appeared in several leg muscles, particularly in the ankle joint muscles. Impairment of sensation was at the same level. Patient could accurately localize the area where strong pressure was applied, and also localize the flexion of the right foot more distinctly. Later, functions of pelvic organs as well as sexual functions were restored.

BIBLIOGRAPHY

Abercrombie, M. & M. L. Johnson. The outwandering of cells in tissue cultures of nerves undergoing Wallerian degeneration. *J. Exper. Biol.*, **19**, 2, 1942, 266–283.

Abramson, A. S. Bond disturbances in injuries to the spinal cord and cauda equina (paraplegia). *J. Bone and Joint Surg.*, **30A**, 1948, 982–987.

Abramson, A. S. Changing concepts in the management of spasticity. In *Basic Research in Paraplegia.* Springfield, Ill.: Charles C. Thomas, 1962, 205–207.

Abramson, A. S. & G. G. Hirschberg. The role of the contracture of certain muscle groups and the effect of its elimination on the overall spasticity in patients with transverse spinal cord lesions. *Bull. Hosp. Joint Dis.*, **13**, 1951, 164–172.

Acadi, A. M., T. F. Dougherty & I. Cohran. The electron microscopic study of the ground substances of connective tissue. *Nature,* **178**, 1956, 1061–1062.

Afelt, Z. Variability of reflexes in chronic spinal frogs. In *Central and Peripheral Mechanisms of Motor Functions.* Prague: Czech. Acad. Sci., 1963, 37–41.

Afelt, Z. The plasticity problems of spinal reflexes in frogs. In *Tsentral'nye i Perifericheskie Mekhanizmy Dvigatel'noi Devatel'nosti Zhivotnykh i Cheloveka.* Moscow: Nauka, 1964, 9–10.

Afelt, Z. Locomotor reactions in chronic spinal preparation of the frog. *Acta. Biol. Exper.*, **25**, 3, 1965, 161–172.

Afelt, Z. The plasticity problem of spinal reflexes in frogs. In *Nervnye Mekhsnizmy Dvigatel'noi Deyatel'noisti.* Moscow: Nauka, 1966, 58–64.

Afelt, A. & N. V. Weber. Posttetanic potentiation of the reflex reactions in a chronically isolated spinal cord. In *Materialy Nauchnoi Konferentsii Fiziologov, Biokhimikov, Patofiziologov i Farmakologov.* Makhachkala: 1970, 11–16.

Agduhr, E. Uber die plurisegmentelle Innervation der einzelnen quergestreiften Muskelfasern. *Anat. Anz.*, **52**, 1919, 272–291.

Airapetyants, E. Sh. & V. L. Balakshina. Two cases of associated inhibition in case of dominant. *Tr. Leningradskogo Ob-va Estestvoispytatelei*, **62**, 1–2, 1933, 141–145.

Aleksandrovskaya, M. M. Neirogliya pri Razlichnykh Psikhozakh (Neuroglia in various psychoses). Moscow: Medgiz, 1950.

Aleksandrovskaya, M. M. Sosudistye Izmeneniya v Mozgu pri Razlichnykh Patologicheskikh Sostoyaniyakh (Vascular changes in the brain under various pathological conditions). Moscow: Midgiz, 1955.

Aleksandrovskaya, M. M., F. A. Brazovskaya, Yu. Ya. Geinisman, P. B. Kazakova, V. N. Larina & V. N. Mats. Morphological reorganization of neuroglia in the condition of increased activity of the nerve centers. *Dokl. AN SSSR*, **180**, 3, 1968, 719–722.

Aleksandrovskaya, M. M., Yu. Ya. Geinisman & V. N. Mats. Morphological findings of glio-neuronal correlation during increased activity of neurons. *Zhurn. Nevropatol. i Psikh. im. Korsakova*, **65**, 2, 1965, 161–167.

Alnaes, E., J. Yansen & T. Rudjord. Fusimotor activity in the spinal cat. *Acta Physiol. Scand.*, **63**, 3, 1965, 197–212.

Anderson, F. D. Morphology of a chronically isolated segment of the cat spinal cord. *Anat. Rec.*, **133**, 1959, 243.

Angeletti, P. U., D. Gandini-Attardi, G. Toschi, M. L. Salvi & R. Levi-Montalcini. Metabolic aspects of the effect of nerve growth factor on sympathetic and sensory ganglia. *Biochem. et Biophys. Acta*, **95**, 1960, 111–120.

Anokhin, P. K. Plastika Nervov pri Voennoi Travme Perifericheskoi Nervnoi Sistemy (Plasticity of the peripheral nervous system in war injuries). Moscow: Medgiz, 1944.

Anokhin, P. K. Theory of functional system as a basis for understanding the compensatory processes in an organism. *Uch. Zap. MGU, Psikhologiya*, **2**, 1947, 32–40.

Anokhina, A. P. Morpho-physiological study of regeneration of nerve fibers in a transplant. Doctoral dissertation, Moscow: 1953.

Anson, M. L. The estimation of pepsin, trypsin, papain, and cathepsin with hemoglobin. *J. Gen. Physiol.*, **22**, 1938–39, 79–80.

Arend, I. E. Regulating mechanisms for connective tissue development in experimental wounds. *Arkh. Anat. Gistol. i Embriol.*, **63**, 2, 1972, 26–33.

Arkhangel'skii, M. S. Some peculiarities in the restoration of reflex activity in the late phase of the spinal trauma. In *Tezisy Dokladov Soveshchaniya po Voprosam Patofiziologii i Terapii Travmaticheskikh Povrezhdeniy Spinnogo Mozga.* Saratov: 1953.

Arkhangel'skii, M. S. Changes in reflexes after spinal cord injury. Doctoral dissertation, Saratov: 1955.

Arkhangel'skii, M. S. The changes in some reflexes in a late phase of the traumatic disease of the spinal cord and the nature of their restoration. In *Voprosy Eksperimental'nogo i Klinicheskogo Izucheniya Posledstvii Travmy Spinnogo Mozga.* Moscow: 1956, 98–102.

Arnautova, E. N. & T. N. Nesmeyanova. Restoration of conduction in the reflex arc after transection and regeneration of the posterior root fibers of the spinal cord in rats. *Dokl. AN SSSR*, **157**, 6, 1964, 1486–1489.

Arnautova, E. N. & T. N. Nesmeyanova. Conduction of excitation in the spinal reflex arc transection and regeneration of the posterior root fibers. *Fiźiol. Zhurn. SSSR*, **102**, 12, 1966, 1434–1440.

Aronovich, G. D. Testicular pain sensation in the traumas of spinal cord. *Khirurgiya*, **1**, 1946, 35–39.

Arteta, J. L. Research on the regeneration of the spinal cord in the cat submitted to the action of pyrogenous substances of bacterial origin. *J. Compar. Neurol.*, **105**, 2, 1956, 171–177.

Asboe-Hansen, G. Hormonal effects on connective tissue. *Physiol. Rev.*, **38**, 3, 1958, 446–462.

Ashby, P., M. Verrier & E. Lightfoot. Segmental reflex pathways in spinal shock and spinal spasticity. *J. Neurol. Neurosurg. & Psychiat.*, **37**, 12, 1974, 1352–1360.

Asratyan, E. A. Effect of extirpation of superiorcervical sympathetic ganglia on the food conditioned reflexes of a dog. *Arkh. Biol. Nauk.*, **30,** 1930, 243–265.

Asratyan, E. A. Cerebral cortex and plasticity of the nervous system. *Usp. Sovrem. Biol.*, **5,** 5, 1936, 803–821.

Asratyan, E. A. Cerebral cortex and plasticity of the nervous system. *Usp. Sovrem. Biol.*, **6,** 3, 1937, 451–468.

Asratyan, E. A. Fiziologiya Tsentral'noi Nervnoi Sistemy (Physiology of CNS). Moscow: AN SSSR, 1953, 247–267.

Asratyan, E. A. Protective role of inhibition in the spinal cord. *Zhurn. Vyssh. Nerv. Deyat.*, **5,** 2, 1955, 187–197.

Attardi, D. G. & R. W. Sperry. Preferential selection of central by regenerating optic fibers. *Exper. Neurol.*, **7,** 1, 1963, 46–64.

Austin, G. (Ed.), The Spinal Cord. Springfield, Ill.: Charles C. Thomas, 1972.

Austin, G. & M. Sato. Repetitive firing of single dorsal root ganglion cells and motoneurons. In *Basic Research in Paraplegia.* Springfield, Ill.: Charles C. Thomas, 1962, 107–127.

Avtsyn, A. & L. Il'ina. Neurology. In *Bol'shaya, Med. Entsiklopedia,* **20.** Moscow: 1961.

Axelrod, J., H. Well-Malherbe, & R. Tomchick. The physiological disposition of ^{3}H-epinephrine and its metabolite metanephrine. *J. Pharmacol. and Exper. Therap.*, **127,** 4, 1959, 251–256.

Babichenko, E. I. The functional status of peripheral nerve-muscle apparatus in patients as a consequence of trauma to the spinal cord. In *Voprosy Eksperimental'nogo i Klinicheskogo Izucheniya Posledstvii Travmy Spinnogo Mozga,* Moscow: AN SSSR, 1956, 149–146.

Babichenko, E. I. Restorative treatments following a damage to the vertebral column and spinal cord. In *Lechenie Zabolevanii i Povrezhdenii Pozvonochnika.* Novosibirsk: 1963, 135–136.

Babichenko, E. I. Surgical treatments of the injuries to the vertebral column and spinal cord and their complications. In *Tezisy Ob'yedinennoi Nauchnoi Konferentsii Neirokhirurgov.* Leningrad: 1965, 9–14.

Babkin, P. S. Physiological types of human proprioceptive and exteroceptive reflexes. Doctoral dissertation, Krasnoyarsk: 1967.

Bakulev, A. N. Traumatic cysts of the brain. *Nevropatologiya i Psikhiatriya,* **5,** 12, 1935, 1965–1970.

Bammer, H. & A. von Muralt. Qualitative Untersuchungen über die Absorption motorischer Vorderhornzellen im Ultraviolettliort nach Einwirkung vin succinodinitril. *Pflugers Arch.*, **258,** 2, 1953, 90–94.

Bammer, H. & A. von Muralt. Der Einfluss von Succinodinitril auf das Ultraviolett-absorptionsspektrum in Nucleolus und Cytoplasma motorischer Vorderhornzellen von Kaninchen. *Pflugers Arch.*, **260,** 1955, 216–224.

Barakina, N. F. Distribution of ribonucleic acids in cells during the regeneration of extremities in axolotl. *Dokl. AN SSSR,* **79,** 6, 1951a, 1049–1052.

Barakina, N. F. Distribution of ribonucleic acids during regeneration in tail-less amphibians. *Dokl. AN SSSR,* **81,** 2, 1951b, 293–296.

Barakina, N. F. Concentration of ribonucleic acids in the cells during an artificially-induced regeneration of an organ. *Dokl. AN SSSR,* **86,** 5, 1952a, 1053–1055.

Barakina, N. F. Distribution of ribonucleic acids in the cells during regeneration in an amputated extremity in albino mice. *Dokl. AN SSSR,* **83,** 6, 1952b, 917–919.

Barnard, J. W. & W. Carpenter. Lack of regeneration in spinal cord of rat. *J. Neurophysiol.*, **72,** 3, 1950, 223–229.

Barnes, C. D. Gamma motor system in spinal shock. *Arch. Internat. Physiol et. Biochim.*, **72,** 5, 1964, 871–878.

Baron, M. Histo-physiological study of heterogenous regeneration in pericellular apparatus (synapses). *Trudy Per. Mos. Gos. Med. In-ta.*, **1,** 1935, 1–2.

Barr, M. & E. G. Bertram. The behaviour of nuclear structures during depletion and restoration of nissl material in motor neurons. *J. Anat.*, **85,** 1951, 171.

Barron, D. H. Structural changes in anterior horn cells following central lesions. *Proc. Soc. Exper. Biol. and Med.*, **30**, 1933, 1327–1329.

Barsegyan, R. O. & G. N. Krivitskaya. The restoration of locomotor function and morphological regeneration in the spinal cord after a complete transverse section in dogs. In *Materialy Desyatoi Ob'yedinennoi Yubileinoi Nauchnoi Konferentsii Fiziologov Pedagogicheskikh Vuzov Respublik Zakavkaz'ya'.* Erevan: AN Arm. SSSR, 1967, 7–11.

Baru, A. V. Temporary connections in cyclostomata fishes. In *Voprosy Sravnitel'noi Fiziologii i Patologii Vysshei Nervnoi Deyatel'nosti.* Leningrad: Medgiz, 1955, 92.

Bassett, C. A. L. & J. B. Campbell. Spinal cord regeneration within micro-filter sheaths. In *Basic Research in Paraplegia.* Springfield, Ill.: Charles C. Thomas, 1962, 12.

Bassett, C. A. L., J. B. Campbell & J. Husby. Peripheral nerve and spinal cord regeneration: factors leading to success of a tubulation technique employing Millipore. *Exper. Neurol.*, **1**, 1959, 386–388.

Batkin, A. A., G. T. Petrov & S. F. Frolov. Use of pyrogenal in the operative treatment of fractures with cicatrical contractures and for grafting skins with burn injuries. In *Pirogenal.* Moscow: Meditsina, 1965, 213–216.

Bazanova, I. S. Electrophysiological study of adaptation in the central part of a somatic reflex arc by adequate stimulation of the propriceptors. In *Elektrofiziologiya Nervnoi Sistemy.* Rostov-on-the Don, 1963, 33–34.

Bazanova, I. S. Adaptation in a somatic reflex arc. *Fiziol. Zhurn. SSSR.*, **50**, 1, 1964, 87–94.

Bazanova, I. S., L. I. Ershova, O. S. Merkulova & V. P. Chernigovskii. Phenomenon of "adaptation" in vaso-motor and somato-motor centers duirng a prolonged stimulation of afferent nerves. In *Materialy Nauchnoi Konferentsii po Probleme Funktsional'nykh Vzaimootneshenii mezhdu Razlichnymi Sistemami Organizma.* Ivanovo: 1962, 5–12.

Bazilevskaya, Z. V. Results of treatment of injuries to the vertebral column and spinal cord. In *Voprosy Travmatologii i Ortopedii pedii.* Irkutsk: 1968, 4–13.

Beeson, P. B. Tolerance to bacterial pyrogens. I. Factors influencing its development. *J. Exper. Med.*, **86**, 1947a, 29–38.

Beeson, P. B. Tolerance to bacterial pyrogens. II. Role of reticuloendothelial system. *J. Exper. Med.*, **86**, 1947b, 39–47.

Belen'kii, V. E., V. S. Gurfinkel' & E. I. Pal'tsev. Elements controlling the voluntary movements. *Biofizika,* **12,** 1, 1967, 135–141.

Bénes, V. Stav a perspeetivy lečenimistniho poraneni. *Českosl. Neurol.*, **21**, 2, 1958, 115–123.

Bennett, I. L. & E. Cluff. Bacterial pyrogens. *Pharm. Rev.*, **9**, 4, 1957, 427–475.

Beránek, R. & P. Hnik. Long-term effects of tenotomy on spinal monosynatptic response in the cat. *Science,* **130,** 3381, 1959, 981–982.

Beránek, R. & P. Hnik. The problem of plasticity of spinal synapses. In *Tsentral'nye i Perifericheskie Makhanizmy Dvigatel'noi Deyatel'nosti Zhivotnykh.* Moscow: AN SSSR, 1960, 352–356.

Beránek, R., P. Hnik, L. Vyklicky & Y. Zelena. Facilitation of the monosynaptic reflex due to longterm tenotomy. *Physiol. Bohemoslovenica,* **10,** 6, 1961, 543–551.

Berezina, M. P. & S. E. Rudashevskii. Associated inhibition of reflex responses in man with a transection of the spinal cord. *Uch. Zap. LGU., Biol.*, **22,** 1950, 229–238.

Bernstein, J. J. & M. E. Bernstein. Neuronal alteration and reinnervation following axonal regeneration and sprouting in mammalian spinal cord. *Brain Behav. Evol.*, **8,** 1973, 135–161.

Bernstein, M. E. & J. J. Bernstein. Regeneration of axons and synaptic complex formation rostral to the site of hemisection in the spinal cord of the monkey. *Int. J. Neurosci.*, **5,** 1, 1973, 15–26.

Bernstein, J. J. & L. Guth. Nonselectivity in establishment of neuromuscular connections following nerve regeneration in the rat. *J. Exper. Neurol.*, **43,** 1961, 262–275.

Bete, A. The plasticity (adaptability) of the nervous system. *Usp. Sovrem Biol.*, **3,** 1, 1934, 82–93.

Bier, A. Beobachtungen über Regeneration beim Menschen. *Dtsch. Med. Wochenschr.*, **43,** 1917, 705; **44,** 1918, 729; **45,** 1919, 4.

Bier, A. Über Knochenregeneration über Pseydoartrosen und über Knochentransplantation. *Arch. Klin. Chirurgie.*, **127,** 1923, 1-136.

Bigland, B. & O. Lippold. Motor unit activity in the voluntary contraction of human muscle. *J. Physiol.*, **123,** 1954, 214-227.

Bikels, G. Über das Verhalten des proximalen Teiles der hinteren Wurzeln bei Degeneration und Regeneration. *Neurol. Zbl.*, **20,** 1907, 951-968.

Bikuschev, S., Z. H. Manovich & W. P. Novikova. Stimulational electromyography and electroneurography in the clinic of nervous diseases. Moscow: Medgiz, 1974.

Bishop, P. O., D. Jeremy & J. W. Lance. The optic nerve properties of a central tract. *J. Physiol.*, **121,** 2, 1953, 415-432.

Black, P., R. S. Markowitz, S. M. Cianei & J. E. Dunn. Recovery of Function after Spinal Cord Injury in Monkeys. St. Louis, Mo.: American Association of Neurological Surgeons, 1974.

Bobrova, M. V. Effect of interoceptive and exteroceptive painful stimulating on the reflex activity of spinal cord. Doctoral disseration, Leningrad: 1959.

Bodian, D. Nucleic acid in nerve cell regeneration. *Soc. Exper. Biol.*, **1,** 1947, 163-174.

Bogdanovich, Yu. I. & G. S. Palamarchuk. Use of pyrogenal in the treatment of traumatic iridocyclitis. In *Pyrogenal.* Moscow: Meditsina, 1965, 254-260.

Bolton, B. The blood supply of the human spinal cord. *J. Neurol. and Psychiatry,* **41,** 1939, 659-677.

Bondarev, N. I. Effect of adrenaline and thyroxine on the excitability of cerebral cortex. *Fiziol. Zhurn. SSSR,* **25,** 6, 1938, 926-929.

Boroyskii, M. L. Experimental and morphological analysis of the changes in the central and in peripheral nervous system and in several tissues of an organism following a lesion and compensation of its functions in case of homotransplantation of nerve. In *Annotatsiya Nauchnykh Rabot ANN SSSR.* Moscow: Medgiz, 1958a, 87.

Boroyskii, M. L. Peculiarities of the structural changes of an organism in case of ensuring functions by an altered and compensated trophism. In *Soveremennye Voprosy Nervizma v Fiziologii i Patologii.* Moscow: Medgiz, 1958b, 375.

Brachet, J. The control of protein synthesis. *New Biol.*, **31,** 1960, 25-38.

Bragin, A. M. Electrophysiological study of immediate effects of dorsal hemisection and complete transverse section of the spinal cord in cats and dogs. Doctoral dissertation, Moscow: 1966.

Brattgard, S. O., J. E. Edström & H. Hydén. The chemical change in regenerating neurons. *J. Neurochem.*, **1,** 1957, 316-325.

Brattgard, S. O., H. Hydén & J. Sjostrand. Incorporation of ^{14}C-orotic acid and ^{14}C-lysine in regenerating single nerve cells. *Nature,* **182,** 1958, 801-802.

Braude, A. I., G. E. Vaisberg, T. I. Afanas'eva & N. I. Givental'. The effects of bacterial polysaccharides on the experimental regeneration of tissues. *Byull. Eksperim. Biol. i Med.*, 7, 1961, 107-109.

Brazovskaya, F. A. Morphological characteristic of neurons during an active and relatively resting state. In *Tezisy VII Syezda Anatomov, Gistologov i Embriologov.* Tbilisi: 1967, 288-289.

Brazovskaya, F. A. Qualitative changes in the glioneuronal complex during a change in the degree of afferentation. *Dokl. AN SSSR,* **178,** 4, 1968, 968-970.

Brazovskaya, F. A., E. N. Iordanskaya & T. N. Nesmeyanova. Stimulation of the regenerative process in the transected spinal cord of a dog. In *Tezisy Dokladov IX Vsesoyuznogo Syezda Fiziologov, Biokhimikov i Farmakologov,* **1,** Moscow: AN SSSR, 1959, 98.

Brazovskaya, F. A., T. N. Nesmeyanova & E. N. Arnautova. Condition of the neuronal apparatus of transected spinal cord depending on the degree of its activity. In *Nervnve Mekhanizmy Dvigatel'noi Deyatel'nosti,* Moscow: Nauka, 1966, 49-57.

Brazovskaya, F. A., T. N. Nesmeyanova & E. N. Iordanskaya. Scar formation in the central nervous system under the action of pyrogênal. *Byull. Eksperim. Biol. i Med.*, **11,** 1960, 121-123.

Brazovskaya, F. A., T. N. Nesmeyanova & E. N. Iordanskaya. Scar formation in the central nervous system of a dog. *Vopr. Neirokhirurgii,* **3,** 1962, 6-9.

Brichant, J., E. Engel., J. C. Demanet, & A. M. Riondel. Modifications pharmacodynamiques de la response corticosurrenale et de la fibronolyse du caillot à l'administration d'un pyrogene chez homme. *Rev. Franc Etudes Clin. Et. Biol.*, **5**, 1960, 464–470.

Brodskii, V. Ya. Cytospectrophotometric investigation of the synthesis of RNA in the nuclei of the retinal ganglionic cells. *Dokl. AN SSSR*, **130**, 1960, 189–192.

Brodskii, V. Ya. The neuronal RNA in different functional states of the nervous system. In *Nukleinovye Kisloty i Nukleoproteidy.* Moscow: AN SSSR, 1961, 204–108.

Brodskii, V. Ya. Trofika Kletki (Cell trophism). Moscow: Nauka, 1966.

Brodskii, V. Ya., A. S. Aref'eva & L. P. Kuznetsova. Destructive phase of the physiological regeneration of neuron. *Tsitologiya*, **8**, 5, 1966, 662–664.

Brodskii, V. Ya. & N. V. Nechaeva. Dependance between the qualitative changes of RNA, intensity of activity and the tropism of neuron. *Dokl. AN SSSR*, **123**, 1958, 756–759.

Brodskii, V. Ya. & N. V. Nechaeva. Qualitative changes in the protein contents of the mucosal cells by inhibiting the synthesis of ribosomal RNA with gold. *Dokl. AN SSSR*, **166**, 5, 1966, 1211–1213.

Bromlei, N. V. & V. N. Orekhovich. Proteolysis in a malignant growth and regeneration. *Usp. Sovrem. Biol.*, **3**, 6, 1934a, 660–675.

Bromlei, N. V. & V. N. Orekhovich. Proteolysis in the regenerating tissues. Autolysis of normal and regenerating tissues. *Dokl. AN SSSR*, **3**, 1934b, 44–47.

Bromlei, N. V. & V. N. Orekhovich. Tissue hydrolytic property of the regenerating blast cells. *Dokl. AN SSSR*, **1**, 4, 1934c, 930–932.

Brown, J. O. & G. F. McCouch. Abortive regeneration of the transected spinal cord. *J. Compar. Neurol.*, **87**, 1947, 131–137.

Brown-Sequard, C. E. De la regeneration de la moelle epiniere d'après l'experimentation et des faits clingues. *Arch. Physiol. Normal et Pathol.*, **5**, 4, 1892, 410–413.

Buchthal, F., C. Guld & P. Rosenfalck. Multielectrode study of the territory of a motor unit. *Acta Physiol. Scand.*, **39**, 1957a, 83–104.

Buchthal, F., C. Guld & P. Rosenfalck. Volume conduction of the spike of the motor unit potential investigated with a new type of multielectrode. *Acta Physiol. Scand.*, **38**, 1957b, 331–354.

Buchwald, J. S., E. S. Halas & S. Schramm. Progressive changes in efferent unit response to repeated cutaneous stimulation in spinal cats. *J. Neuro-Physiol. Scand.*, **39**, 1965, 83–104.

Budnitskaya, P. Z. The method of obtaining pyrogenal from the cultures of *Ps. aeroginosa. Patol. Fiziol. i Eksperim. Terapiya*, **5**, 1960, 69–73.

Budnitskaya, P. Z. Isolation, chemical characteristics and several biological properties of pyrogenal. In *Eksperimental'nye Issledovaniya i Klinicheskoe Primenenie Pirogenala.* Moscow: Medgiz, 1961, 8–23.

Budnitskaya, P. Z. The chemical nature of the pyrogenic substance in pyrogenal. *Byull. Eksperim. Biol. i Med.*, **3**, 1962, 53–56.

Budnitskaya, P. Z. Isolation, chemical characteristic and several biological properties of pyrogenal. Doctoral dissertation, Moscow: 1963.

Budnitskaya, P. Z. The chemical characteristics of pyrogenal P and T. In *Pirogenal.* Moscow: Meditsina, 1965, 17–24.

Bueker, E. B., I. Schenkein & J. I. Bane. The problem of distribution of a nerve growth factor specific for spinal sympathetic ganglia. *Cancer Res.*, **20**, 1960, 1220–1223.

Bulygin, I. A. Issledovanie Zakonomernostei i Mekhanizmov Interotseptivnykh Refleksov (Investigation of factors and mechanism of interoceptive reflexes). Minsk: 1959, 229–244.

Bulygin, I. A. & D. Z. Shchannikova. Interoceptive conditioned reflexes from urinary bladder after the removal of the spinal cord in the thoracic region. *Trudy In-ta Fiziologii, AN BSSR*, **2**, 1958, 178.

Bulygin, I. A. & K. F. Zorina-Isikina. Interoceptive reflexes from urinary bladder after the transection of the spinal cord. *Trudy In-ta Fiziologii AN BSSR*, **1**, 1956, 129–143.

Cajal S. Ramon. Notes preventives sobre la degeneration y regeneration de las vias nervisas centralis. *Trav. Lab. Invert. Biol.*, **4**, 1906, 295–301.

Cajal S. Ramon. Degeneration and Regeneration of the Nervous System. London: 1928.

Campbell, I. F., C. A. L. Bassett, Y. Husby & C. R. Noback. Axonal regeneration in transected adult feline spinal cord. *Surg. Forum.*, **8**, 1957a, 528.

Campbell, I. F., C. A. L. Bassett & C. R. Noback. Regeneration of adult mammalian spinal cord. *Science*, **126**, 1957b, 929.

Campbell, J. B., V. Crescito, J. J. Tomasula, H. D. Demopoulos, E. S. Flamm & J. Ransohoff. Experimental treatment of spinal cord contusion in the cat. *Surg. Neurol.*, **1**, 1973, 102–106.

Campbell, J. B. & W. F. Windle. Relation of Millipore to healing and regeneration in transected spinal cord of monkeys. *Neurology*, **10**, 1960, 306–311.

Cannon, W. B. & H. Haimovici. The sensibilization of motoneurons by partial "denervation." *Amer. J. Physiol.*, **126**, 1, 1939, 731–740.

Cannon, W. B. & A. Rosenblueth. Pavyshenie Chuvstvitel'nosti Denervirovannykh Struktur (Increasing sensitivity of denervated structures). Moscow: IL, 1951.

Cannon, W. B., A. Rosenblueth & Ramos J. Carsia. Sensibilization de les neuronas espinales por denervation parcial. *Arch. Inst. N. Cardial Max.*, **15**, 1945, 327–348.

Carrel, A. & A. Ebeling. Trephones embryonnaires. *Compt. Rend. Soc. Biol.*, **89**, 1923, 1266–1268.

Carrel, A. & A. Ebeling. Role des trephones leucocytaires et de cellules epitheliales. *Compt. Rend. Soc. Biol.*, **90**, 1924, 29–36.

Cass, D. T. & R. F. Mark. Reinnervation of axolotl limbs. I. Motor nerves. *Proc. Roy. Soc. London*, **B 190**, 1098, 1975, 45–58.

Castro, F. de. Evolucion de los ganglios sympaticos vertebrales y prevertebrales conexiones y citoarguitechtonic de algunos grupos de ganglios en el neno y nombre adulto. *Trab. Lab. Invest. Biol.* Madrid: 1923.

Cate, J. ten. Zur innervation der Fortbewegung der Haifische. *Arch. Neurl. Physiol.*, **18**, 1933, 15–23.

Chambers, W. W. Structural regeneration of the mammalian central nervous system in relation to age. In *Regeneration in the Central Nervous System.* Springfield, Ill.: Charles C. Thomas, 1955, 135.

Chance, M. R. A., A. J. Lucas & J. A. H. Waterhouse. Changes in the dimensions of the nuclei with activity. *Nature.*, **177**, 4519, 1956, 1081–1082.

Cherkasova, T. I. Functional status of long muscles of the back after compression fractures of the vertebral column. *Ortopediya, Travmatologiya i Protezirovanie*, **6**, 1955, 39–46.

Cherkasova, T. I. Altered functions of the nerve muscle apparatus after the trauma to the vertebral column and spinal cord. In *Problema Kompensatornykh Prisposoblenii.* Moscow: AN SSSR, 1960, 25–31.

Chumak, B. A. Effect of pentoxyl on the regeneration of transverse striated muscle. *Nauchnye Trudy Rostovskogo Medinstituta*, **10**, 1959, 158–162.

Chumak, B. A. Effect of pentoxyl on the tissue reparative processes. In *Materialy k Nauchno-Prakticheskoi Konferentsii Khirurgov Rostovskoi Oblasti.* Rostov-on-Don, 1960, 122–123.

Clark Le Gros, W. E. The problem of neuronal regeneration in the central nervous system. *J. Anat.*, 77, 1942, 20–48.

Clark Le Gros, W. E. The problem of neuronal regeneration in central nervous system. II. The insertion of peripheral nerve stumps into the brain. *J. Anat.*, **77**, 1943, 251–259.

Clemente, C. D. Penetration of brain by regenerating peripheral nerve fibers. *Anat. Rec.*, **112**, 1952, 319.

Clemente, C. D. Structural regeneration in the mammalian central nervous system and the role of neuroglia and connective tissue. In *Regeneration in the Central Nervous System.* Springfield, Ill.: Charles C. Thomas, 1955, 147–161.

Clemente, C. D. The regeneration of peripheral nerves inserted into the cerebral cortex and the healing of cerebral lesions. *J. Compar. Neurol.*, **109**, 1, 1958, 123–151.

Clemente, C. Neuronal degeneration and regeneration. In *Regenerative Phenomena in the CNS.* Los Angeles: UCLA Brain Information Service, 1972.

Clemente, C. D., W. W. Chambers, L. Greene, S. D. Mitchell & W. F. Windle. Regeneration of the transected spinal cord of adult cats. *Anat. Rec.*, **109**, 1951, 280.

Clemente, C. D. & W. F. Windle. Regeneration of the transected nerve fibers in the spinal cord of adult cats. *J. Compar. Neurol.*, **101**, 3, 1954, 691–731.

Cohen, S. Purification and metabolic effects of a nerve growth promoting protein from snake venom. *J. Biol. Chem.*, **234**, 5, 1959, 1129–1131.

Cohen, S. & R. Levi-Montalcini. A nerve growth stimulating factor isolated from snake venom. *Proc. Nat. Acad. Sci.*, **42**, 1956, 571–574.

Cohen, S., R. Levi-Montalcini & V. Hamburger. A nerve growth stimulating factor isolated from sarcoma 37 and 180. *Proc. Nat. Acad. Sci.*, **40**, 9, 1954, 1014–1018.

Collier, J. The effects of total transverse lesion of the spinal cord in man. *Brain*, **27**, 1904, 38–63.

Connell, A. M., H. Frankel & L. Guttmann. The mobility of the pelvic colon following complete lesions of the spinal cord. *Paraplegia*, **1**, 2, 1963, 98–115.

Cook, A. W. Regeneration in the CNS. *Lancet*, **(817)**, 1973, 1442–1443.

Culler, E. A. Recent advances in some concepts of conditioning. *Psychol. Rev.*, **45**, 1938, 134–163.

Culler, E. & F. A. Mettler. Observations upon the conduct of a thalamic dog. Hearing and vision in decorticated animals. *Proc. Soc. Exper. Biol.*, **31**, 1934, 607–609.

Curtis, D. R. Pharmacological investigation upon inhibition of spinal motoneurons. *J. Physiol.*, **145**, 1959, 175–192.

Danilov, I. V. An American's attempt to understand the teaching of I. P. Pavlov. *Fiziol. Zhurn. SSSR.*, **38**, 3, 1952, 368–376.

Danilov, I. V. Summation phenomena in spinal centers frog Communication I. *Byull. Eksperim. Biol. i Med.*, **5**, 1953, 8–11.

Danilova, K. M. Controversial problem of origin and functional significance of mast cells. *Arkh. Patologii*, **1**, 1958, 3–9.

Danilova, K. M. Action of pyrogenal on connective tissue. *Patol. Fiziol. i Eksperim. Terapii*, **5**, 1961, 24–30.

Daudova, G. M. Effect of temperature on some aspects of metabolism. In *Ezhegodnik IEM AEM SSSR.* Vilnius: 1957, 219–211.

Davidoff, L. M. Regeneration in the spinal cords of cats and dogs. *Arch. Neurol. and Psychiatry*, **65**, 1951, 261–262.

Davidoff, L. M. & J. Ransohoff. Absence of spinal cord regeneration in the cat. *J. Neurophysiol.*, **11**, 1, 1948, 9–11.

Deekcke, L. & C. H. Tator. Neurophysiological assessment of afferent and efferent conduction in the injured spinal cord of monkeys. *J. Neurosurg.*, **39**, 1973, 65–74.

Deese, J. & W. N. Kellogg, Some new data on the nature of "spinal conditioning." *J. Compar. Physiol. and Psychiatry*, **42**, 3, 1949, 157–160.

Dell, P. Intervention of an adrenergic mechanism during brain stem reticular activation. In *Drug Action on Adrenergic Mechanism.* London: Ciba Foundation, 1960, 303–409.

Deryabin, L. N. Inborn movement of rabbit hind limbs in early post-natal period. *Fiziol. Zhurn. SSSR*, **50**, 7, 1964, 820–828.

Deryabin, L. N. Post-natal development of natural rhythmic movements in rabbit extremities by stimulating the skin. *Byull. Eksperim. Biol. i Med.*, **7**, 1966, 18–22.

Diamond, M. C., F. Law, H. Rhodes, B. Lindner, M. R. Rosenzweig & D. Krech. Increases in cortical depth and glia number in rat subjected to enriched environment. *J. Compar. Neurol.*, **128**, 1, 1966, 117–125.

Di Giorgio, A. M. Modificazioni funzionali del midollo spinale per effecto di impulsi asimmetrici cerebrali e cerebellary. *Arch. Fisiol.*, **47**, 1948a, 154–267.

Di Giorgio, A. M. Sui rapporti cerebello spinali; asimmetric cerebellari dopo deafferentazione e sezione del midollo spinale. *Arch. Nerve de Physiol.*, **28**, 1948b, 446–474.

Dinken, H. War injuries of the vertebral column and the spinal cord with special reference to physical treatment. *Med. Clin. North America*, **27**, 1943, 1077–1090.

Dmitriev, V. D. Importance of cerebral cortex in the development of compensatory processes following the damages to the spinal cord. Doctoral dissertation, Leningrad: 1951.

Dmitrieva, E. V. Distribution of nucleic acids in the skeletal muscle fibers during regeneration. *Dokl. AN SSSR*, **98**, 1954, 653–656.

Droz, B. Dynamic condition of proteins in the visual cells of rats and mice as shown by radioautography with labelled amino acids. *Anat. Rec.*, **145**, 1963, 157–167.

Droz, B. & C. Leblond. Migration of proteins along the axons of the sciatic nerve. *Science,* **137**, 1962, 1047–1048.

Druckman, R. Review of structural evidence of regeneration of nerve fibers in injury to the human spinal cord. In *Regeneration in the Central Nervous System.* Springfield, Ill: Charles C. Thomas, 1955, 241–246.

Duncan, D. Additional observations on hyperstaining myelin and alterations of neuroglia induced by restricting the growth of the spinal cord. *Anat. Rec.*, **119**, 1954, 296.

Duncan, D. Experimental compression of the spinal cord. In *Regeneration in the Central Nervous System.* Springfield, Ill.: Charles C. Thomas, 1955, 247–258.

Duncan, D. & N. Y. Bellegie. Penetration of an experimental sarcoma by nerve fibers from the spinal cord. *Texas Repts. Biol. and Med.*, **6**, 1948, 461–469.

Dykman, R. A. & P. S. Shurrager. Successive and maintained conditioning in spinal carnivors. *J. Compar. and Physiol. Phychol.*, **49**, 1, 1956, 27–35.

Dzheksenbaev, O. On the mechanism of pyrogenal action. *Patol. Fiziol. i Eksperimen. Terapiya,* **4**, 1959, 49–55.

Dzheksenbaev, O. S. & N. A. Ozeretskovskii. The adrenal system pitutary–the febrile reaction and the interaction between them during the administration of pyrogenal to guinea pig. In *Tezisy Simposimma po Rezul'tatam Eksperimental'nogo Izucheniya i Klinicheskogo Primeneniya Pirogenala.* Moscow: 1964a.

Dzheksenbaev, O. S. & N. A. Ozeretskovskii. Effect of pyrogenal on suprarenal cortex. *Byull. Eksperim. Biol. i Med.*, **5**, 1964b, 31–33.

Eccles, J. C. The Neurophysiological Basis of Mind. Oxford: Clarendon Press, 1935.

Eccles, J. C. Fiziologiya Nervnykh Kletok (Physiology of nerve cells). Moscow: IL, 1959.

Eccles, J. C. The effects of use and disuse on synaptic function. In *Brain Mechanisms and Learning.* Oxford: 1961, pp. 335.

Eccles, J. C. Fiziologiya Sinapsov (Physiology of synapses). Moscow: IL, 1966.

Eccles, J. C. Physiological problems in paraplegia. In *Regenerative Phenomene in the CNS.* Los Angeles: UCLA Brain Information Service, 1972.

Eccles, J. C. & A. K. McIntyre. The effects of disuse and of activity on mammalian spinal reflexes. *J. Physiol.*, **121**, 1953, 492–516.

Eccles, R. M. & R. A. Westerman. Enhanced synaptic function due to excess use. *Nature,* **184**, 1959, 460–161.

Eccles, J. C., R. M. Eccles & F. Magni. Monosynaptic excitatory action on motoneurons regenerated to antagonistic muscles. *J. Physiol.*, **154**, 1, 1960, 68–88.

Eccles, J. C., P. G. Kostyuk, & R. F. Schmidt. The effect of electric polarization of the spinal cord on central efferent fibres and of their excitatory synaptic action. *J. Physiol.*, **162**, 1962a, 138–150.

Eccles, J. C., P. G. Kostyuk & R. F. Schmidt. Presynaptic inhibition of the spinal cord on central afferent fibres and on their excitatory synaptic action. *J. Physiol.*, **161**, 1962b, 237–257.

Eccles, R. M., W. Kozak & A. R. Westerman. Enhancement of spinal monosynaptic reflex responses after denervation of synergic hindlimb muscle. *Exper. Neurol.*, **6**, 1962, 451–464.

Eccles, J. C., K. Krnjevic & R. Miledi. Delayed effect of peripheral severance of afferent nerve fibres on the efficacy of their central synapses. *J. Physiol.*, **145**, 1, 1959, 204–220.

Eccles, J. C., B. Libet & R. R. Young. The behavior of chromatolyzed motoneurons studied by intracellular recording. *J. Physiol.*, **143**, 1, 1958, 11–40.

Eccles, J. C., R. F. Schmidt & W. D. Willis. Depolarization of central terminals of group Ib afferent fibers of muscles. *J. Neuro-Physiol.*, **26**, 1963, 1–27.

Edds, M. Collateral regeneration in partially reinnervated muscles of the rat. *J. Exper. Zool.*, **129**, 2, 1955, 225–232.

Edström, J. E. Effects of increased motor activity on the dimensions and the staining properties of the neuron soma. *J. Compar. Neurol.*, **107**, 2, 1957, 295–304.

Egyhazi, E. & H. Hydén. Experimentally induced changes in the base composition of the ribonucleic acids of isolated nerve cells and their oligodendroglia cells. *J. Biophys. and Biochem. Cytol.*, **10**, 1961, 403–410.

Eichenberger, E., M. Schmidhauser-Kopp., H. Hurni, M. Frisay & O. Westphal. Biologische Wirkungen eines hochgereinigten Pyrogens (Lippolysaccharides) aus Sal. abortus. *Schweiz. Med. Wochenschr.*, **50**, 1955a, 1213-1218.

Eichenberger, E., M. Schmidhauser-Kopp., H. Hurni, M. Frisay & O. Westphal. Biologische Wirkungen eines hochgereinigten Pyrogens (Lipopolysaccharide) aus Sal. abortus. *Schweiz. Med. Wochenschr.*, **49**, 1955b, 1190-1196.

Eic-Nes, K., J. Demertrion, Y. Mayne & R. Jones. Isolation of cortisone from guinea pig bile. *Proc. Soc. Exper. Biol. and Med.*, **96**, 1957, 409–411.

Eldred, E., R. Granit & P. A. Merton. Supraspinal control of the muscle spindles and its significance. *J. Physiol.*, **122**, 1953, 498-523.

Eldred, E. & K. E. Hagbarth. Facilitation and inhibition of gamma efferents by stimulation of certain skin areas. *J. Neurophysiol.*, **17**, 1, 1954, 59–65.

Engle, E., J. Brichant, J. P. Delmer, A. Vernet & A. M. Riondel. Influence de la pyretotherapie sur la response surrenalienne et lactivité fibrinolytique on plasma chez l'homme. *Helv. Med. Acta.*, **24**, 1957, 459–462.

Essman, W. B. Effect of tricyanoaminopropane on the amnesic effect of electroconvulsive shock. *Psychopharmacologia,* **9**, 1966, 426–433.

Exner, S. Zur Kenntnis über die intermittierene Wirkung der Erregungen in der Zentralnervensystem. *Pflugers Arch.*, **28**, 1882, 487-506.

Falin, L. I. Nekotorye Spornye Voprosy Morfologii i Fiziologii Vtorichnoi Degeratsii Perifericheskikh Nervov (Disputable issues in morphology of secondary degeneration of peripheral nerves). Moscow: Medgiz, 1954.

Falin, L. I. The regeneration of nerve and the problem of restoration of its functions. *Arkh. Ant. Gistol. i Embriol.*, **42**, 5, 1962, 3-13.

Fedorov, B. G. Problems of the regeneration of synapses. *Byull. VIEM,* **2**, 1934, 24-34.

Fedorov, B. G. Mechanism of the regeneration of intraneuronal synapses. *Arkh. Anat. Gistol. i Embriol.*, **14**, 1, 1935a, 5-7.

Fedorov, B. G. Some data on ramification of a peripheral sprout in the sensory types of neurons inside ganglion. *Byull. VIEM,* **8**, 1935b, 20-29.

Fedotov, D. M. Effect of cartilage hydrolyzates on the development of organs in axolotl. *Dokl. AN SSSR,* **38**, 1, 1943, 52-54.

Feringa, E. K., J. S. Wendt & R. D. Johnson. Immunosuppressive treatment to enhance spinal cord regeneration in rats. *Neurology,* **3**, 1974, 287-293.

Fickler, A. Experimentelle Untersushungen zur Anatomia der trawmatischen Degeneration und der Regeneration des Rückenmarke. *Deutsch. Zeit. Nervenheilkunde.*, **29**, 1905, 1-56.

Filatov, V. P. Tkanevaya Terapiya. Uchenie o Biogennykh Stimulyatorakh (Tissue therapy. Study of biogenic stimulators). Moscow: Znanie, 1953.

Finikov, A. N. The treatment on bullet injuries to the spinal cord. In *Yubileinyi Sbornik v Chest' XXV-Letiya Nauchnoi Deyatel'nosti Prof. I. I. Grekova.* Moscow: 1921, 389.

Fischer, J., Z. Lodin & J. Kolousek. A histoautoradiographic study of the effect of section of the facial nerve on the uptake of ^{35}S-methionine by the cells of the ficial nerve nucleus. *Nature,* **181**, 1958, 341-342.

Fitzgerald, L. A. & R. F. Thompson. Classical conditioning of the hind limb flexion reflex in the acute spinal cat. *Psychol. Sci.*, **8**, 5, 1967, 213-214.

Fleisch, A. La regulation de la circulation peripherique. *Acta Neuroveget.*, **14**, 1956, 1–4; 88-93.

Foerster, O. Symptomologie der Erkrankungen des Rückenmarkes. *Handbuch der Neurologie,* **5**. Berlin, 1936, 206.

Frank, K. & M. G. F. Fourtes. Presynaptic and postsynaptic inhibition of monosynaptic reflexes. *Federat. Proc.*, **16**, 1957, 39–40.

Franz, N., M. Evans & H. Perl. Characteristics of viscerosynaptic reflexes in the spinal cat. *Amer. J. Physiol.*, **211**, 6, 1966, 1292-1298.

Franzisket, L. Gewohunheitsbildung und bedingte Reflexe bei Rücken-marksfroschen. *Z. Vergl. Physiol.*, **33**, 2, 1951, 142-178.

Franzisket, L. Untersuchungen zur sperifitat und kumulierung der Erregungsfahigkeit und zur Wirkung einer Erumudung in des Rückenmarksfroschen. *Z. Vergl. Physiol.*, **34,** 1953, 525-538.

Freeman, L. W. The metabolism of calcium in patients with spinal cord injuries. *Ann. Surg.*, **129,** 2, 1949a, 193-205.

Freeman, L. W. Treatment of paraplegia resulting from trauma to the spinal cord. *J. Amer. Med. Assoc.*, **140,** 1949b, 949-958; 1015-1022; **141,** 275.

Freeman, L. W. Return of function after complete transection of the spinal cord of the rat, cat, and dog. *Ann. Surg.*, **136,** 2, 1952a, 193-205.

Freeman, L. W. Discussion of paper by W. F. Windle, C. D. Clemente, D. Scott, and W. W. Chambers. *Arch. Neurol. and Psychiatry*, **67,** 1952b, 553.

Freeman, L. W. Return of spinal cord function in mammals after transecting lesions. *Ann. New York Acad. Sci.*, **58,** 5, 1954, 564-568.

Freeman, L. W. Functional recovery in spinal rats. In *Regeneration in the Central Nervous System.* Springfield, Ill.: Charles C. Thomas, 1955, 195-207.

Freeman, L. W., J. C. Finneran & D. M. Schlegel. Regeneration of spinal cord of the rat. *Amer. J. Physiol.*, **159,** 1949, 568-569.

Freeman, L. W., J. McDougall, C. C. Turbes & D. E. Bowman. The treatment of experimental lesions of the spinal cord of dog with trypsin. *J. Neurosurg.*, **17,** 2, 1960, 259-265.

Friede, R. L. Uber die trophische function der glia. *Virchow's Arch.*, **324,** 1953, 15-26.

Friede, R. L. Enzyme histochemistry of neuroglia. In *Progress in Brain Research,* **15.** Amsterdam: Elsevier, 1956, 35-47.

Friede, R. L. & M. Knoller. Proximodistal increase of enzyme activity in the dorsal spinal tracts. *J. Neurochem.*, **11,** 1964, 679-688.

Fudema, T. T., T. A. Fizzell & E. M. Nelson. Electromyography of experimentally immobilized skeletal muscles in cats. *Amer. J. Physiol.*, **200,** 1961, 963-967.

Fuks, B. B. Gistokhimiya i Morfologiya Normal'nogo i Povrezhdennogo Nerva (Histochemistry and morphology of normal and damaged nerve). Novosibirski: AN SSSR, 1959.

Fulton, C. P., F. L. Maynard, I. F. Riley & G. B. West. Humoral aspect of tissue mast cells. *Physiol. Rev.*, **37,** 2, 1957, 221-223.

Galitskaya, N. A. Acetylcholine sensitivity of the skeletal muscle during stimulation of sympathetic ganglion and cerebellum. *Materialy po Evolyutsionnoi Fiziologii,* **1,** 9, 1956, 1-97.

Galkin, V. A. Comparative evaluation of the different methods of preventing the post-operative peritoneal adhesions. Doctoral dissertation, Leningrad: 1966.

Galkin, V. A. & A. V. Sorokin. Effect of pyrogenal on the formation of peritoneal adhesions in rabbits. *Patol., Fiziol. i Eksperim. Terapiya.*, **3,** 1966, 56-57.

Gamble, H. & B. Jha. An effect of pyronin upon the rate of maturation of injured peripheral nerve fibers. *J. Anat.*, **93,** 2, 1959, 195.

Garcin, R. Considerations generales sur les maladies du collagene. *Rev. Neurol.*, **92,** 6, 1955, 419-428.

Geimanovich, Z. N. Voenno- travmaticheskie Porazheniya Pozvonochnika i Spinnogo Mozga (Injuries of the vertegral column and spinal cord). Tyumen: *Izd. Ukr. Psikhonevrol. In-ta,* 1943.

Gelfan, S. Neurone synapse population in the spinal cord; indication of their role in total integration. *Nature,* **198,** 4, 1963, 876.

Gelfan, S. Effect of spinal cord asphyxiation. In *Progress in Brain Research,* **12.** Amsterdam: 1964, 280-303.

Gelfan, S. Altered spinal motoneurons in dogs with experimental hind limb rigidity. *J. Neurophysiol.*, **29,** 4, 1966, 583-611.

Gelfan, S. & A. F. Rapisarda. Synaptic density on spinal neurons of normal dogs and dogs with experimental hind limb rigidity. *J. Compar. Neurol.*, **123,** 1964, 73-95.

Gelfan, S. & I. M. Tarlov. Interneurons and rigidity of spinal origin. *J. Physiol.*, **146,** 1959, 594-617.

Gelfan, S. & I. M. Tarlov. Altered neuronal population in L_7 segment of dogs with experimental hind limb rigidity. *Amer. J. Physiol.*, **205,** 606-616.

Gel'fand, I. M., V. S. Gurfinkel', Ya. M. Kots, M. L. Tsetkin & M. L. Shik. Synchronization of motor units and model concepts connected with it. *Biofizika,* **8,** 4, 1963, 475–497.

Gerard, R. W. & R. R. Crinker. Regenerative possibilities of the central nervous system. *Arch. Neurol. and Psychiatry,* **26,** 1931, 469–484.

Gerard, R. W. & T. Kappani. Studies on spinal cord regeneration in the rat. *Amer. J. Physiol.,* **76,** 1926, 211–212.

Gerard, R. W., T. J. Chamberlain & G. H. Rothschild. RNA in learning and memory. *Science,* **140,** 1963, 3565, 381.

Giaguinto, S. & O. Pompeiano. Generalized inhibition of spinal reflexes induced by cutaneous nerve stimulation in unrestrained cats. *Experientia,* **19,** 12, 1963, 653–654.

Gibson, W. C. Degeneration and regeneration of sympathetic synapses. *J. Neurophysiol.,* **3,** 3, 1940, 237–247.

Gilev, V. P. Effect of repeated damages on the regeneration of skeletal muscle in rats. *Dokl. AN SSSR,* **96,** 1954, 865.

Ginetsinskii, A. G. Effect of the sympathetic nervous system on the function of transverse striated muscle. *Russk. Fiziol. Zhurn.,* **6,** 1923, 3–6.

Ginetsinskii, A. G. Participation of the sympathetic nervous system in the strychnine convulsion. *Russk. Fiziol. Zhurn.,* **7,** 1924, 1–6; 226–232.

Ginetsinskii, A. G. Effect of sympathetic nerve on fatigued skeletal muscle under anaerobic conditions. *Russk. Fiziol. Zhurn.,* **9,** 1926a, 93–98.

Ginetsinskii, A. G. Influence of sympathetic nervous system on a motor nerve end plate. *Russ. Fiziol. Zhurn.,* **9,** 1926b, 99–105.

Ginetsinskii, A. G. Effect of electrostimulations on denervated muscle. In *Probelmy Sovremennoi Fiziologi Nervnoi i Myshechnoi Sistemy.* Tbilisi: 1956, 409–417.

Ginetsinskii, A. G., N. P. Nekhoroshev & M. B. Tetyaeva. Effect of the sympathetic nerve on the skeletal muscles in a warm-blooded animal. *Russk. Fiziol. Zhurn.,* **10,** 6, 1927, 483–495.

Ginger, L. C. & W. F. Windle. Studies on the chemistry and physiological action of bacterial pyrogens. In *Résumé Commun. II Internat. Congress of Biochem.,* **28.** Paris: 1952, 445–446.

Gintsburg, G. I. Removal of skull defects in adult rats and dogs. *Dokl. AN SSSR,* **87,** 1952, 869–871.

Gintsburg, G. I. Removal of bone defects of skull in mammals. *Trudy IMZh,* 11, 1954, 158.

Glees, P. Terminal degeneration within the central nervous system as studied by a new silver method. *J. Neuropathol. and Exper. Neurol.,* **5,** 1, 1946, 54–59.

Glees, P. Factors promoting regeneration of spinal neurons: Positive influence of nerve growth factor. In *Progress in Brain Research,* **13.** Amsterdam: Elsevier, 1964, 149.

Gokay, H. & L. W. Freeman. Drugs and spinal cord regeneration. *Quart. Bull. Indiana Univ. Med. Center,* **14,** 4, 1952, 67–69.

Goldberger, M. E. Restitution of function in the CNS. The pathological grasp in Macaca mulatta. *Exp. Brain Res.,* **15,** 1972, 79–96.

Goldberger, M. E. Restitution of function and collateral sprouting in the cat spinal cord: the deafferented animals. *Anat. Rec.,* **175,** 1973, 329.

Goldberger, M. E. & J. H. Growdon. Pattern of recovery following cerebellar deep lesions in monkeys. *Exp. Neurol.,* **39,** 1973, 307–322.

Golden, H. T. Effective treatment for traumatic and inflamed lesions using trypsin. *Clin. Med.,* **2,** 1955, 583.

Golub, D. M. Role of the sympathetic nervous system and the indirect innervation of organs and tissues. In *Voprosy Morfologii Perifericheskoi Nervnoi Sistemy.* Minsk: AN BSSR, 1949.

Golub, D. M., A. P. Ameros'ev, A. S. Leontyuk, I. I. Novikov, B. L. Orlova & F. B. Kheinman. Formation of new afferent paths of urinary bladder and of the large intestine. *Arkh. Anat. Gistol. i Embriol.,* **38,** 1, 1960, 3–19.

Golub, D. M. & M. B. Kishina. Formation of the sympathetic trunk and the anterior spinal plexus during embryogenesis in man and animal. In *Voprosy Morfologii Perifericheskoi Nervnoi Sistemy.* Minsk: ANBSSR, 1956, 11–34.

Golub, D. M., A. S. Leontyuk & I. I. Novikov. Artificial indirect pathways of afferent innervation of the pelvic organs. In *Materialy Nauchnoi Sessii, Posvyashchennoi 40-Letiyu Velikoi Oktyabr'skoi Sotsialisticheskoi Revolyutsii.* Minsk: 1957, 84.

Goncharova, L. S. Alteration and restoration of motor functions following local damages in cerebellum. Doctoral dissertation, Moscow: 1959.

Goncharova, L. S., T. N. Nesmeyanova, & A. N. Trankvillitati. Restorative processes in patients with spinal cord trauma with the application of physical therapy and pyrogenal. In *Reabilitatsiya Bol'nkkh s Posledstviyami Povrezhdenii Pozvonochnika i Spinnogo Mozga.* Kiev: Zdorov'e, 1969, 111–113.

Gorinevskaya, V. V. Travmy Pozvonochnika (Vertebral injuries). Moscow: Medgiz, 1933

Gorinevskaya, V. V. Osnovy Travmatologii (Principles of traumatology). Moscow: Medgiz, 1938.

Gorodinskaya, R. S. & O. P. Minut-Sorokhtina. Regeneration of the spinal cord. *Trudy Khabarovskogo Med. In-ta.*, **9**, 1948, 25.

Granit, R. Elektrofiziologicheskoe Issledovanie Retseptsii (Electrophysiological investigation of reception). Moscow: IL, 1957.

Granit, R. & B. Holmgren. Tonic and phasic ventral horn cells differentiated by post-tetanic potentiation in cat extensors. *Acta Physiol. Scand.*, 37, 1, 1955, 114–126.

Granit, R., C. Lob, & B. R. Kaada. Activation of muscle spindles. *Acta Physiol. Scand.*, **27**, 1952, 161–168.

Greene, L. C., R. G. Stuart & Y. Joralemon. Survival study of thermally injured rats treated with Piromen. *Proc. Soc. Exper. Biol. and Med.*, **82**, 1, 1953, 39–42.

Gurden, G. G. & E. R. Feringe. Effects of Sympatholytic Agents on CNS. Regeneration, Cystic Necrosis after spinal cord transection. *Neurology*, **2**, 1974, 187–191.

Gurfinkel', V. S. The posture of healthy individuals and those with prosthetic appliances after amputation of lower extremities. Doctoral dissertation, Moscow: 1961.

Gurfinkel', V. S., Ya. M. Kots & M. L. Shik. Regulyatsiya Pozy Cheloveka (Regulation of human posture). Moscow: Nauka, 1965.

Gurfinkel', V. S. & E. I. Pal'tsev. Effect of the condition of the spinal segmental apparatus in response to a simple motor reaction. *Biofizika*, **10**, 5, 1965, 855–860.

Guth, L. Regeneration in the mammalian peripheral nervous system. *Physiol. Rev.*, **36**, 4, 1956, 441–478.

Guth, L. Neuromuscular function after regeneration of interrupted nerve fibers into partially denervated muscle. *J. Exper. Neurol.*, **6**, 2, 1962, 129–141.

Guth, L. The problem of selectivity between nerve and end-organ following nerve regeneration. In *The Effect of Use and Disuse on Neuromuscular Function.* Prague: 1963, 135–142.

Guth, L. M. & W. F. Windle. Enigme of CNS regeneration. *Experimental Neurol.* Suppl. 5, 1970.

Guth, L. M. & W. F. Windle. Physiological, molecular and genetic aspects of CNS regeneration. *Experimental Neurol.* **39**, 3, 1973, 3–16.

Gutman, E. Ractors affecting recovery of motor function after nerve lesions. *J. Neurol. and Psychiatry*, **5**, 1942, 81–86.

Gutmann, E. Die funktionelle Regeneration der peripheren Nerven. Berlin: Akademie Verlag, 1958.

Gutmann, E. Trophic function of the nervous system. *Usp. Sovrem. Biol.*, **53**, 3, 1962, 323–346.

Gutmann, E., L. Guttmann, P. B. Medawar & L. Z. Young. The rate of regeneration of nerve. *J. Exper. Biol.*, **19**, 1942, 14–21.

Gutmann, E. & J. Holubar. The degeneration of peripheral nerve fibers. *J. Neurol. Neurosurg. and Psychiatry*, **13**, 2, 1950, 89–105.

Gutmann, E., B. Jakoubek, I. Hajek, V. Rohlicek & J. Skaloud. Effect of age on proteosynthesis in spinal motoneurons following nerve interruption as shown by histoautoradiography ^{35}S-labelled methionine. *Physiol. Bohemosl.*, **11**, 5, 1962, 437–442.

Gutmann, E. & F. K. Sanders. Recovery of fibre numbers and diameters in the regeneration of peripheral nerves. *J. Physiol.*, **101**, 1943, 489–518.

Guttmann, L. Rehabilitation after injuries to the central nervous system. *Proc. Roy. Soc. Med.*, **35**, 1942, 305.

Guttmann, L. Rehabilitation after injury to the spinal cord and cauda equina. *Brit. J. Physiol. and Med.*, **9**, 130, 1946, 162.

Guttmann, L. On the way to an international sports movement for the paralyzed. *Cord.*, **5**, 3, 1952, 7.

Guttmann, L. Studies on reflex activity of the isolated cord in the spinal man. *J. Nervous and Mental Diseases,* **116,** 1953, 957.

Guttmann, L. The absorption of ethyl alcohol in complete lesions of the spinal cord following intrathecal injection. *Excerpta Medica,* VIII, **8,** 9, 1956, 862.

Guttmann, L. The problems of spina bifida cystica. *Proc. Roy. Soc. Med.*, **50,** 1957, 10.

Guttmann, L. The regulation of rectal function in spinal paraplegia. *Proc. Roy. Soc. Med.*, **52,** 2, 1959, 86–89.

Guttmann, L. Spinal Cord Injuries Comprehensive Management and Research. Oxford: Blackwell, 1973a.

Guttmann, L. Sport and recreation for the mentally and physically handicapped. In *Conference on Sport for All.* London: Royal Soc. of Health, 1973b.

Guttmann, L. & H. Frankel. The value of intermittent catheterization in the early management of traumatic paraplegia and tetraplegia. *Paraplegia,* **4,** 2, 1966, 63–84.

Guttmann, L. & R. Robinson. The absorption of ethyl alcohol following intrathecal injection in spinal paraplegia. *Proc. Second Internat. Congress of Neuropathol.* London: 1955, 579–583.

Guttmann, L. & J. R. Silver. Electromyographic studies on reflex activity of the intercostal and abdominal muscles in cervical cord lesions. *Paraplegia,* **3,** 1, 1965, 1–22.

Guttmann, L. & D. Wittering. Effects of bladder distension on autonomic mechanisms after spinal cord injuries. *Brain,* **70,** 4, 1947, 361–404.

Guttmann, L., H. Frankel & V. Pacslack. Cardiac irregularities during labor in paraplegic women. *Paraplegia,* **3,** 2, 1965, 144–151.

Guttmann, L., J. Silver & C. H. Wyndham. Thermoregulation in spinal man. *J. Physiol.*, **142,** 406–419.

Guttmann, L., O. F. Munro, R. Robinson & J. J. Walsh. Effect of tilting on the cardiovascular responses and plasma catecholamine levels in spinal man. *Paraplegia,* **1,** 1, 1963, 4–18.

Haberland, G. Uber cellteilunggormone und ihre Beziehungen zur Wundeeilung, Befruchtung, Partenogenezis und Adventivembrionie. *J. Biol. Zbl.*, 1922, 4.

Haddad, A., S. Jucif & A. Cruz. Synthesis of RNA in neurons of the hypoglossal nerve nucleus, after section of the axon, in mice. *J. Neurochem.*, **16,** 6, 1969, 865–868.

Hagbarth, K. E. Excitatory and inhibitory skin areas for flexor and extensor motoneurons. *Acta Physiol. Scand.*, **26,** Suppl., 94, 1952, 2–57.

Hedeman, L. S., M. K. Shellenberger & J. H. Gordon. Studies in experimental spinal cord trauma. I. Alterations in catecholamine levels. *J. Neurosurg.*, **40,** 1974, 37–43.

Hedeman, L. S. & R. Sil. Studies in experimental cord trauma. II. Compression of treatment with steroinds, low molecular weight dextran, and catecholamine blocade. *J. Neurosurg.*, **40,** 1974, 55–51.

Heller, H. & S. Hesse. Substrate utilization by stimulated nerve, with particular reference to the Schwann cell. *Exper. Neurol.*, **4,** 1961a, 83–90.

Heller, H. & S. Hesse. Substance in peripheral nerve which influences oxygen uptake. *Science,* **133,** 1961b, 1708.

Hernandez Peon, R. & H. Brust-Carmona. Functional role of subcortical structures in habituation and subcortical structures in habituation and conditioning. In *Brain Mechanism and Learning.* Oxford: Blackwell, 1961, 393–412.

Hess, A. Ground substance of the developing central nervous system. *Anat. Rec.*, **118,** 1954a, 310.

Hess, A. Reaction of mammalian fetal tissue to injury. *Anat. Rec.*, **119,** 1954b, 35–52.

Hess, A. Discussion of failure of regeneration in the mammalian fetus. In *Regeneration in the Central Nervous System.* Springfield, Ill.: Charles C. Thomas, 1955, 176.

Hess, A. Reaction of fetal spinal cord, spinal ganglions and brain to injury. *J. Exper. Zool.*, **132**, 2, 1956, 349.

Hild, W., J. J. Chang & I. Tabaki. Electrical responses of astrocytic glia from the mammalian central nervous system cultivated "in vitro." *Experientia*, **14**, 6, 1958, 220.

Hirschberg, G. C. & A. S. Abramson. Effect of neostigmine studies on spasticity of skeletal muscle in upper motor neuron lesions. *Arch. Phys. Med.*, **32**, 1951, 575.

Hnik, P. The change of motor functions after deafferentiation. In *Tsentral'nye i Perifericheskie Nekhanizmy Dvigatel'noi Deyatel'nosti Zhivotnykh.* Moscow: AN SSSR, 1960, 234-240.

Hnik, P., L. Beránek, L. Vyklický & I. Zelená. The effect of long term tenotomy upon the function of muscle proprioceptors. In *Central and Peripheral Mechanisms of Motor Functions.* Prague: 1963, 93-96.

Hoffman, H. Rate of interrupted nerve-fibres regenerating into partially denervated muscles. *Austral. J. Exper. Biol. and Med. Sci.*, **29**, 1951, 211-219.

Hoffman, H. Acceleration and retardation of the process of axon-sprouting in partially denervated muscles. *Austral. J. Exper. Biol. and Med. Sci.*, **30**, 4, 1952, 541-566.

Hoffman, H. Axoplasm–its structure and regeneration. In *Regeneration in the Central Nervous System.* Springfield, Ill.: Charles C. Thomas, 1955, 112-126.

Hoffman, H. & P. Springell. An attempt at the chemical identification of "Neurocletin" (substance evoking axon-sprouting). *Austral. J. Exper. Biol. and Med. Sci.*, **29**, 1951, 417-424.

Holtzer, H. Comments on regeneration as opposed to neogenesis of amphibian neurons. In *Regeneration in the Central Nervous System.* Springfield, Ill.: Charles C. Thomas, 1955, 81-83.

Hooker, D. & J. E. Nicholas. The effect of injury to the spinal cord of rats in prenatal stages. *Amer. J. Physiol.*, **82**, 2, 1927, 503-515.

Hooker, D. & J. E. Nicholas. Spinal cord section in rat fetuses. *J. Compar. Neurol.*, **50**, 1930, 413-467.

Horrocks, L. A., A. Toews, D. Yashon & D. E. Locke. Changes in myelin following trauma of the spinal cord in monkeys. *Neurobiology*, **3**, 1973, 256-263.

Houlihan, R. & J. P. Da Vanzo. Nerve growth-promoting properties of 1,1,3-tricyano-2-amino-1-propane. *J. Exper. Neurol.*, **10**, 2, 1964, 183-189.

Howe, H. A. & D. Bodian. Refractoriness of nerve cells to poliomyelitis virus after interruption of their axones. *Johns Hopkins Hosp. Bull.*, **69**, 1941, 92-132.

Howitt, W. M. & I. M. Turnbull. Effect of hypotermia and methysergide on recovery from experimental paraplegia. *Can. J. Surg.*, **15**, 1972, 179-186.

Hunt, C. C. The reflex activity of mammalian spinal nerve fibres. *J. Physiol.*, **115**, 1951, 456-469.

Hunt, C. C. & S. W. Kuffer. Stretch receptor discharges during muscle contraction. *J. Physiol.*, **113**, 1951, 298-315.

Hunt, C. C. & A. Paintal. Spinal reflex regulation of fusimotor neurones. *J. Physiol.*, **143**, 1958, 195-212.

Hydén, H. Protein metabolism in the nerve cell during growth and function. *Acta. Physiol. Scand.*, **S-17**, 1943, 1-36.

Hydén, H. Protein and nucleotide metabolism in the nerve cell under different functional conditions. In *Symposium Sociétè Experimental Biologie*, **1**, 1947, 152-163.

Hydén, H. Biochemical changes in glial cells and nerve cells at varying activity. *IV. Internat. Congress of Biochem.*, **3**, 1959, 64-89.

Hydén, H. The neuron. In *The Cell*, **4.** New York: Academic Press, 1960, 215.

Hydén, H. The metabolic and functional interaction between the neurons and its glia. In *The Effect of Use and Disuse on Neuromuscular Functions.* Prague: 1963a, 184-196.

Hydén, H. Biochemical and functional interplay between neuron and glia. In *Recent Advances in Biological Psychiatry*, **6**, 1963b, 31-54.

Hydén H. Neuron. In *Functional'naya Morfologiya Kletki.* Moscow: 1963c, 235.

Hydén, H. The satellite cells in the nervous system. In *Strucktura i Funktsii Kletki.* Moscow: Mir, 1964, 116.

Hydén, H. & H. Eguhazi. Changes in RNA content and base composition in cortical neurons of rats in a learning experiment involving transfer of hardedness. *Proc. Nat. Acad. Sci.*, **52**, 4, 1964, 1031–1055.

Hydén, H. & C. Hamburger. Production of nucleo-protein in vestibular ganglion. *Acta Otolaringol.*, **75**, 1949, 53–81.

Hydén, H. & H. Hartelius. Stimulation of the nucleo-protein production in the nerve cells by malononitrile and its effect on psychic functions in mental disorders. *Acta Psychiatr. Neurol.*, **S-48**, 1948.

Hydén, H. & A. Pigon. A cytophysiological study of functional relationship between oligodendroglial cells and nerve cells of Deiters nucleus. *J. Neurochem.*, **6**, 1960, 57–72.

Ikeda, K. & J. B. Campbell. Dorsal root regeneration verified by injection of leucine-3H into the dorsal root ganglion. *Exper. Neurol.*, **30**, 1971, 379–388.

Il'ina, V. I. On the morphology of the sympathetic chain. In *Stroenie i Peaktivnye Svoistva Afferentnykh Sistem Vnutrennikh Organov.* Leningrad: 1960, 243.

Illis, L. Changes in spinal cord synapses and a possible explanation for spinal shock. *Exper. Neurol.*, **8**, 1963, 328–335.

Illis, L. Spinal cord synapses in the cat: The reaction of the bouton's termineaux at the motoneurone surface to experimental denervation. *Brain*, **87**, 3, 1964, 555–569.

Illis, L. S. Experimental model of regeneration in the CNS. I. Synaptic changes. *Brain*, **96**, 1973b, 47–60.

Illis, L. S. Regeneration in the CNS. *Lancet*, **1**, 1973a, 1035–1037.

Illis, L. S. Experimental model of regeneration in the CNS. II. The reaction of glia in the synaptic zone. *Brain*, **96**, 1973c, 61–68.

Il'yuchenok, R. Yu. Neirogumoral'nye Mekhanizmy Retikulyarnoi Formatsii Stvola Mozga (Neurohumoral mechanisms of reticular brain stem formation). Moscow: Nauka, 1965.

Inoue, S. On the proliferation stimulating nature of the regenerating nerve fibers. *Endocrinol. Japon*, **5**, 3, 1958, 217–219.

Iordanskaya, E. N. & T. N. Nesmeyanova. Effect of pyrogenal on the permeability of skin capillaries. In *Tezisy Dokladov Konferentsii po Rezul'tatam Eksperimental'nogo Izucheniya i Klinicheskogo Primeneniya Pirogenala.* Moscow: 1960, 5.

Iordanskaya, E. N. & T. N. Nesmeyanova. The change of tissue permeability with pyrogenal. In *Eksperimental'noe Izuchenie i Klinicheskoe Primenerie Pirogenala.* Moscow: 1961, 30–40.

Ivanova, S. N. Role of cerebral hemispheres in compensatory adaptations after the transection of the lateral half of the upper segments of the spinal cord in dogs. Doctoral dissertation, Moscow: 1953.

Jackson, R. W. Sexual rehabilitation after cord injury. *Paraplegia*, **10**, 1972, 50.

Jacob, F. & J. Monod. Genetic regulatory mechanisms in synthesis of proteins. *J. Mol. Biol.*, **3**, 1961, 318–356.

Jacoby, R. K., X. C. Turbes & L. W. Freeman. The problem of neuronal regeneration in the central nervous system. *J. Neurosurg.*, **17**, 1960, 385–393.

Jakoubek, B., T. Gutmann, I. Hajek & I. Syrovy. Changes in protein metabolism of peripheral nerve during functional activity. *Physiol. Bohemosl.*, **12**, 6, 1963, 553–561.

Janches, M., R. Dendukas, L. Segal & F. A. Galze. Effects of bacterial pyrogen on the elimination of urinary 17-hydroxycorticosteroids in normal subjects. *J. Clin. Endocrinol. and Metabol.*, **25**, 1965, 17–19.

Jankowski, K. & Z. Afelt. Degeneration and regeneration in the chronic spinal preparation of *Rana Esculenta. Acta Biol. Exper.*, **24**, 1, 1964, 3–11.

Jao Yhu Shu. The morphology and distribution of the oligodendroglia in the central nervous system of the rabbit. *Acta Anat. Sinica.*, **1**, 2, 1964, 64–172.

Jarstedt, J. Functional localization in the cerebellar cortex studied by quantitative determinations of Purkinje cell RNA. I. RNA changes in rat cerebeller Purkinje cells after proprio- and exteroceptive and vestibular stimulation. *Acta Physiol. Scand.*, **67**, 2, 1966, 243–252.

Jent, M., B. Koechlin, A. Muralt & Th. Wagner-Jauregg. Der neuroregenerative Wuchsstoff "NR". *Schweiz. Med. Wochenschr.*, **75**, 1945, 317–327.

Johnston, B. T., J. E. Schrameck & R. F. Mark. Re-innervation of axolotl limbs. II. Sensory nerves. *Proc. Roy. Soc.*, **B 190,** 1098, 1975, 59–75.

Joster, F. A. & M. B. Boche. Manipulation therapy for back conditions. In *Principles and Practices of Physical Therapy,* **3,** 23, 1941, 1–59.

Kaiser, H. K. & W. B. Wood. Studies on pathogenesis of fever: X. The effect of certain enzyme inhibitors on the production and activity of leukocytic pyrogen. *J. Exper. Med.*, **115,** 1, 1962, 37–47.

Kalita, T. N. Formation of human lumbar sympathetic trunk. Communication II. In *Voprosy Morfologii Perifericheskoi Nervnoi Sistemy,* **3.** Minsk: AN BSSR, 1956, 56–70.

Kandel, E. R. & L. Tauc. Heterosynaptic facilitation in neurones of the abdominal ganglion of *Aplysia Depilans. J. Physiol.*, **181,** 1, 1965a, 1–27.

Kandel, E. R. & L. Tauc. Mechanisms of heterosynaptic facilitation in the giant cell of the abdominal ganglion of *Aplysia Depilans. J. Physiol.*, **181,** 1, 1965b, 28–47.

Kao, C. C., Y. Shimizu, L. C. Perkins & L. W. Freeman. Experimental use of cerebellar cultured cortical tissue to inhibit the collagenous scar following spinal cord transection. *J. Neurosurg.*, **33,** 1970, 127–139.

Karamyan, A. I. On the compensatory activity of the central nervous system. Report III. *Izv. AN SSSR,* **2,** 1947, 227–235.

Karamyan, A. I. Effect of the sympatho-adrenal system on the reflex activity in the higher segments of the central nervous system. *Fiziol. Zhurn. SSSR,* **44,** 4, 1958, 316–326.

Kawai, J. & K. Sasaki. Effects of strychnine upon supraspinal inhibition. *Japan. J. Physiol.*, **14,** 3, 1964, 309–314.

Kawakami, M. Training effect and electromyogram. I. Spatial distribution of spike potentials. *Japan. J. Physiol.*, **5,** 1, 1955, 1–8.

Kazakova, P. B. Morphological changes in the cerebral cortex of the experimental animals during the compensation of altered functions. *Byull. Eksperim. Biol. i Med.*, **8,** 1966, 103.

Kazakova, P. B. Compensatory glioneuronal changes in the cerebral cortex of animals after lateral spinal hemisection. In *Vosstanovlenie Funktsii pri Porazheniyakh Tsentral'noi i Perifericheskoi Nervnoi Sistemy.* Leningrad: 1967, 89–91.

Kazakova, P. B. Morphological manifestations in the central nervous system during compensation of altered functions in dogs. *Arkh. Patologii.*, **8,** 1968, 32–37.

Kazakova, P. B. & T. N. Nesmeyanova. Influence of afferent stimuli on the function and structure of neurons of the transected spinal cord. *Fiziol. Zhurn. SSSR,* **58,** 1972, 40–45.

Kaznacheev, V. P. Principal enzymatic processes in the etio-path ogenesis of rheumatism. In *Trudy Novosibirskogo Gos. Med. In-ta.* Novosibirski: 1960, 36.

Kaznacheev, V. P. Heparin and the hemostasis. In *Voprosy Fiziologii i Patologii Geparina.* Novisibirsk: Nauka, 1965, 113–147.

Kaznacheev, V. P. & V. P. Lozovoi. Heparin, histamine and hyaluronic acid–hyaluronidase system. In *Materialy V'torogo Plenuma Sibirskogo Filiala Obshchestva Patofiziologov.* Chita: 1958, 153–155.

Kedrovskii, B. V. The macrophage system and its fate in healthy organism. *Usp. Sovrem. Biol.*, **20,** 1, 1945, 41–60.

Kellogg, W. N. A method for maintenance of chronic spinal animals. *J. Exper. Psychol.*, **36,** 1946, 366–370.

Kellogg, W. N. Is "Spinal Conditioning" is conditioning? *J. Exper. Psychol.*, **37,** 1947, 263–265.

Kellogg, W. N., J. Deese & N. H. Pronko. Behavior of lumbospinal dog. *J. Exper. Psychol.*, **36,** 1946, 503–511.

Kellogg, W. N., J. Deese, N. H. Pronko & M. Feinberg. An attempt to condition the chronic spinal dog. *J. Exper. Psychol.*, **37,** 2, 1947, 99.

Khoroshko, V. K. Trauma of the spinal cord and vertebral column. *Klinicheskaya Meditsina,* **16,** 4–5, 1938, 441–452.

Khoroshko, V. K. Physiotherapy of traumas of the spinal cord and vertebral column. *Fizioterapiya v Travmatologii,* **10,** 1941, 30–61.

Khrushchev, G. K. Sources of leukocytic trephones. *Byull. Eksperim. Biol. i Med.,* **18,** 6, 1944, 30–33.

Khrushchev, G. K. Rol' Leikotsitov Krovi v Vosstanovitel'nykh Protsessakh v Tkanyakh (Role of peripheral leukocytes in tissue restoring processes). Moscow: AN SSSR, 1945.

Khrushchev, G. K. Modes of participation of peripheral leukocytes in tissue processes. In *Tezisy Dokladov VI Vsesoyuznogo S'ezda Anatomov, Gistolov i Enhriologov,* 1958, 353.

Khrushchev, N. G., M. G. Skurskaya & L. N. Zontak. Mechanism of action of antileukocytic serum. In *Osnovnye Usloviya Regeneratsii Organov i Takanei u Zhivotnykh.* Moscow: 1966, 311–314.

Khurina, A. S. Restoration of motor and sensory functions in patients following the trauma to the spinal cord. In *Voprosy Eksperimental'nogo i Klinicheskogo Izucheniya Posledsvii Travmy Spinnogo Mozga.* Moscow: AN SSSR, 1956, 182–186.

Kimmel, D. L. Discussion of regeneration in spinal nerve roots. In *Regeneration in the Central Nervous System.* Springfield, Ill.: Charles C. Thomas, 1955, 173.

Kinderling, W., O. Wöhler & O. Westphal. Experimentalle Untersuchungen zur Differenzierung der therapeutischen wirkungen von bakterieller vaccine, reinem Polysaccharid. Pyrogen und acetylierten polysaccharid-Derivaten aus gram negativen Bakterien. *Arch. Exper. Pathol. und Bacteriol.,* **217,** 1, 1953, 293–311.

Kirkendall, W. M., R. E. Hodges & L. E. Jannary. The ACTH-like effect of fever in man. *J. Lab. and Clin. Med.,* **37,** 5, 1951, 771–775.

Kirsche, W. Regeneration in Zentralnervens system. *Forschen und Wirker,* **2,** 1960, 407–438.

Klyle, L., C. Arnold & H. S. Kupperman. The therapeutive effectiveness of trypsin in the treatment of thrombophlebitis. *Ann. N. Y. Acad. Sci.,* **68,** 1, 1957, 178–183.

Koechlin, B. A. The neuroregenerative factor "NR". In *Regeneration in the Central Nervous System.* Srpingfield, Ill.: Charles C. Thomas, 1955, 127–134.

Kogan, O. G. Use of pyrogenal in the treatment of patients with traumatic damage to the spinal cord. In *Eksperimental'nye Issledovaniya i Klinicheskoe Primenenie Pirogenala.* Moscow: 1961, 142–147.

Kogan, O. G. Comparative study of the effects of pyrogenal and several other therapeutic agents on the restoration of functions in spinal cord lesions in rats. In *Pirogenal.* Moscow: Meditsina, 1965a, 117–124.

Kogan, O. G. Therapeutic efficacy of pyrogenal in spinal cord injuries. In *Pirogenal.* Moscow: Meditsina, 1965b, 217–225.

Kogan, O. G. Mechanisms of the restoration of functions in patients with spinal cord lesions. In *Vosstanovlenie Funktsii pri Porazheniyakh Tsentral'noi i Perifericheskoi Nervnoi Sistemy.* Leningrad: 1967, 106.

Kogan, O. G. Rehabilitation of patients with traumas in spine and spinal cord injuries. Moscow: Medgiz, 1975.

Kolychev, V. P. Reflexes from the skeletal muscles on the vascular and the respiratory systems in the spinal cord injuries. *Fiziol. Zhurn. SSSR,* **45,** 10, 1959, 1247–1352.

König, M. P. Uber die Wirkung von Dinitrilen auf die Nervenregeneration. *Helv. Physiol. et Pharmacol. Acta,* **11,** 1953, 328–345.

Konorski, J. Mechanisms of learning. *Exptl. Biol.,* **4,** 409–431.

Kontsiovskaya, R. S. Treatment of severe eye burns with pyrogenal. In *Pirogenal.* Moscow: Meditsina, 1965, 273–277.

Koppani, T. Regeneration in the CNS of fishes. In *Regeneration in the CNS.* Springfield, Ill.: Charles C. Thomas, 1955, 3–19.

Koshtoyants, Kh. S. Osnovy Sravnitel'noi Fiziologii (Principles of comparative physiology). Moscow: AN SSSR, 1957.

Kosmarskaya, E. N. Reaction of the cortical nerve cells to prolonged stimulations by peripheral receptors. *Byull. Eksperim. Biol. i Med.,* **6,** 53, 1962, 88–91.

Kostyuk, P. G. Electrical phenomena in individual motoneurons during reciprocal excitation and inhibition. *Dokl. AN SSSR,* **119,** 6, 1958a, 1255-1258.

Kostyuk, P. G. Electrical phenomena in individual interneurons during reciprocal excitation and inhibition. *Dokl. AN SSSR,* **120,** 1, 1958b, 219-222.

Kostyuk, P. G. Dvukhneironnaya Reflektornaya Duga (Bineuronal reflex arc). Moscow: Medgiz, 1959.

Kostyuk, P. G. Pre- and postsynaptic changes in the degeneration of central synapses. *Fiziol. Zhurn. SSSR,* **48,** 11, 1962, 1316-1324.

Kostyuk, P. G. & A. A. Savos'kina. Peculiarities of transmission by the degenerated central synaptic terminals. *Fiziol. Zhurn. USSR,* **5,** 6, 1959, 718-727.

Kozak, W., W. V. Macfarlane & R. Westerman. Long-lasting reversible changes in the reflex responses of chronic spinal cats to touch, heat and cold. *Nature,* **193,** 4811, 1962, 171-173.

Kozak, W. & R. A. Westerman. Plastic changes of spinal nonsynaptic responses from tenotomized muscles in cats. *Nature,* **189,** 1961, 753-755.

Kozak, W. & R. Westerman. The plasticity problem of spinal reflexes in cats. In *Tsentral'nye Perifericheskie Mekhanizmy Dvigatel'noi Deyatel'nosti Zhivotnykh i Cheloveka.* Moscow: Nauka, 1964, 48-49.

Kozak, W. & R. Westerman. Basic patterns of plastic change in the mammalian nervous system. *Symposium Soc. Exptl. Biol.,* **20,** 1966a, 509-543.

Kozak, W. & R. Westerman. The plasticity problem of spinal reflexes in cats. In *Nervnye Mekhanizmy Dvigatel'noi Deyatel'nosti.* Moscow: Nauka, 1966b, 64-74.

Krasovskii, V. V. Restoration of abdominal cutaneous reflexes in patients with anatomical transection of the spinal cord. In *Voprosy Eksperimental'nogo i Klinicheskogo Izucheniya Posledstvii Spinnogo Mozga.* Moscow: AN SSSR, 1956, 103-105.

Kreutzberg, G. W. Autoradiographic study on incorporation of ^{3}H-leucine in peripheral nerves during regeneration. *Experientia,* **23,** 1, 1967, 33-34.

Krid, R., D. Deni-Brown, D. Eccles, E. Lidell & Ch. Sherrington. Reflektornaya Deyatel'nost Spinnogo Mozga (Reflex activity of the spinal cord). Moscow–Leningrad: Biomedgiz, 1935.

Krokhina, E. M. Sensory innervation of small and large intestine in mammals. In *Stroenie i Reaktivnve Svoistva Afferentnykh Sistem Vnutrennikh Organov.* Moscow: Medgiz, 1960, 73.

Kruglyi, M. M. Method of physical therapy during the postoperative period in patients with spinal cord trauma. In *Voprosy Eksperimental'nogo Izucheniya Posledstvii Travm Spinnogo Mozga.* Saratov: 1956, 193-197.

Kruglyi, M. M. Physical treatment as a method for the development of compensatory mechanisms at a late stage in patients of traumatic disease of the spinal cord. *Voprosy Kurortologii, Fizioterapii i Lechebnoi Fizkul'tury,* **1,** 1958, 63-67.

Kruglyi, M. M. Restoration of motor function in patients with spinal cord trauma by physical therapy. In *Problema Kompensatornykh Prisposoblenii.* Moscow: AN SSSR, 1960, 13-20.

Kudokotsev, V. P. Loss and restoration of regenerating capacity of the extremities in vertebrates. In *Tezisy Dokladov Tret'ego Vsesoyuznogo Soveshchaniya Embriologov.* Moscow: 1960, 86.

Kudokotsev, V. P. Stimulation of the regeneration of external organs by additional innervation in vertebrates. In *Osnovnye Usloviya Regeneratsii Organov i Tkanei u Zhivotnykh.* Moscow: 1966, 137-141.

Kuhn, R. A. Functional capacity of the isolated human spinal cord. *Brain,* **73,** 1, 1950, 1-51.

Kuhn, R. A. & M. B. Macht. Some manifestations of reflex activity in spinal man with particular reference to the occurrence of extensor spasm. *Bull. John Hopkins Hospital,* **84,** 1948, 43-75.

Kulenkampff, H. Das Verhalten der Neuroglia in den Vorderhörhern des Rückenmarke der wessen Maus unter dem Reiz Physiologischer Tätigkei. *Z. Anat. und Entwicklungsgesch,* **116,** 1952, 304-312.

Kul'vanovskii, M. V. Interoceptive reflexes from urinary bladder to respiration and blood pressure after the transection of pelvic and hypogastric nerves. *Trudy In-ta Fiziologii AN BSSR,* **1,** 1958, 220–232.

Kunstman, K. I. Effect of unilateral sympathectomy on cutaneous and tendon reflexes in dogs. *Izv. Nauchn. In-ta im. Lesgafta,* **14,** 1928, 1–21; 59–80.

Kuruma, I. Changes in the concentration of serotonin and catecholamines of the brain in febrile rabbits. The effect of high ambient temperature on the concentration of the serotonin and noradrenaline in the rabbit's brain stem. *Folia Pharmacol. Japan.,* **62,** 2, 1966, 8–10.

Kuruma, I. & H. Takagi. Changes in the concentration of serotonin and catacholamines of the brain in febrile rabbits. The degree of fever induced by the administration of pyrexal and changes in the constants of these amines in the brain stem. *Folia Pharmacol. Japan,* **60,** 6, 1964, 563–568.

Kustov, V. V. Action of pentoxyl on the nervous system. *Farmakologiya i Toksikologiya,* **22,** 1959, 387–391.

Kuz'menko, G. N. Effect of different doses of adrenaline and thyroxine on the higher nervous activity. *Uch. Zap. Leningradskogo Ped. In-ta,* **9,** 4, 1938, 215–232.

Lajtha, A. Protein metabolism of the nervous system. *Internat. Rev. Neurobiol.,* **6,** 1964, 1–98.

Lance, J. W. Behavior of pyramidal axons following section. *Brain,* **77,** 2, 1954, 314–324.

Lavrent'ev, B. I. Innervation mechanism (synapses) and patho-morphology of the synapses. In *Trudy Pervoi Gistologicheskoi Konferentsii.* Moscow: 1934a, 238–248.

Lavrent'ev, B. I. Some problems in the theory of the formation of nerve tissue. *Arkh. Biol. Nauk.,* **48,** 1934b, 1–2; 194–213.

Lazarev, N. V. Lektsiya po Farmakologii Sistemy Krovi (Lectures on the pharmacology of hemopietic system). Moscow: Medgiz, 1960.

Lazarev, N. V. & G. N. Felistovich. Pentoksil i Ego Primenenie pri Aleikiyakh (Pentoxyl and its application in leukopenia). Leningrad, 1954.

Lebedev, V. P. The mechanism of hind limb hypertoncity following a temporary ischaemia of caudal parts of the spinal cord. *Fiziol. Zhurn. SSSR,* **45,** 1959a, 1142–1147.

Lebedev, V. P. Pharmacology of experimental spasticity. Doctoral dissertation, Leningrad: 1959b.

Lebedev, V. P. Bioelectric peculiarities of anterior roots of the spinal cord in post-ischaemic spasticity. *Fiziol. Zhurn. SSSR,* **49,** 3, 1963, 322–329.

Lee, F. C. The regeneration of nervous tissue. *Physiol. Revs.,* **9,** 1929, 575–623.

Leites, S. M. Development of the regenerative process. *Khirurgiya,* **11,** 1945, 20–26.

Lekhtman, Ya. B. Vegetativnaya Nervnayà Sistema i Ee Rol'v Dvigatel'noi Deyatelnosti Chelveka (Somatic Nervous System and its role in the motor activity of man). Leningrad: Meditsina, 1969.

Lemas, V. B. Scientific conference on the regulation of inflamatory and regenerative processes. *Patol. Fiziol. i Eksperim. Terapiya,* **4,** 3, 1960, 83–84.

Leontyuk, A. S. Connections of intercostal nerves. In *Tezisy Dokladov Nauchnoi Sessii, Posvyashohennoi 35-letiyu Instituta Fiziologii AN BSSR.* Minsk, 1956, 162.

Levi-Montalcini, R. Growth stimulating effects of mouse sarcoma on the sensory and sympathetic nervous system of the chick embryo. *Anat. Rec.,* **109,** 1951, 59.

Levi-Montalcini, R. Effects of mouse tumor transplantation on the nervous system. *Ann. N. Y. Acad. Sci.,* **55,** 1952, 330–344.

Levi-Montalcini, R. & V. P. Angeletti. Nerve growth factor. *Physiol. Rev.,* **48,** 3, 1968, 534–569.

Levi-Montalcini, R. & B. Booker. Excessive growth of the sympathetic ganglia evoked by a protein isolated from mouse salivary glands. *Proc. Nat. Acad. Sci.,* **46,** 3, 1960, 373–384.

Levi-Montalcini, R. & S. Cohen. *In vitro* and *in vivo* effects of a nerve growth stimulating agent isolated from snake venom. *Proc. Nat. Acad. Sci.,* **42,** 1956, 695–702.

Levi-Montalcini, R. & V. Hamburger. A diffusible agent of mouse sarcoma producing hyperplasia of sympathetic ganglia and hyperneuretization of viscera in the chick embryo. *J. Exptl. Zool.*, **123**, 2, 1953, 233–239.

Levi-Montalcini, R., S. Cohen & V. Hamburger. *In vitro* experiments on a nerve growth promoting agent in mouse sarcoma 37 and 180. *Anat. Rec.*, **118**, 1954, 450–451.

Levi-Montalcini, R., H. Meyer & V. Hamberger. *In vitro* experiments on the effects of mouse sarcoma 180 and 37 on the spinal and sympathetic ganglia of the chick embryo. *Cancer Res.*, **14**, 1954, 49–57.

Levinson, L. V. Functional and histochemical study of nerve cells. Doctoral dissertation, Moscow, 1961.

Levitskaya, E. S. Conduction and sensitivity of internal organs and blood vessels. *Materialy po Evolyutsionnoi Fiziologii*, **1**, 1956, 174–182.

Lewin, M. G., R. R. Hansebout & H. M. Pappius. Chemical characteristics of traumatic spinal cord edema in cats. Effect of steroids on potassium depletion. *J. Neurosurg.*, **40**, 1974, 65–75.

Lhermitte, J. Sur la regeneration des recines posterieures dans la section complete de la moelle dorsale. *Rev. Neurol.*, **35**, 1919, 129–135.

Liozner, L. D. Regeneration and embryonal development. In *Problemy Sovremennoi Embriologii.* Leningrad: 1956, 330–340.

Liozner, L. D. Regenerating capacity in mammals. *Usp. Sovrem. Biol.*, **43**, 2, 1957, 224–238.

Liozner, L. D. Morphological investigation of the regenerative processes in mammals. *Usp. Sovrem. Biol.*, **51**, 2, 1961, 220–230.

Liozner, L. D. Vosstanovlenie Utrachennykh Organov (Restoration of lost organs). Moscow: AN SSSR, 1962.

Littrell, J. L. Apparent functional restitution in piromen treated spinal cats. In *Regeneration in the CNS.* Springfield, Ill.: Charles C. Thomas, 1955, 219–228.

Littrell, J. L., D. Bunnell, W. F. Agnew, I. O. Smart & W. F. Windle. Effects of a bacterial pyrogen on hind limb function in spinal cats. *Anat. Rec.*, **115**, 1953, 430.

Liu, C. N. Malonitril and nucleoprotein production in nerve cells. *Anat. Rec.*, **109**, 2, 1951, 320.

Liu, C. N. Fate of cells of Clarke's nucleus following axon section in cat, with evidence of spinal collaterals from dorsal spino-cerebeller tract. *Anat. Rec.*, **115**, 1953, 342.

Liu, C. N. Time pattern in retrograde degeneration after trauma of CNS of mammals. In *Regeneration in the CNS.* Springfield, Ill.: Charles C. Thomas, 1955, 84–93.

Liu, C. N. & W. W. Chambers. Intraspinal sprouting elicited from intact spinal sensory neurons by adjacent posterior root section. *Amer. J. Physiol.*, **18**, 3, 1955, 640.

Liu, C. N. & W. W. Chambers. Intraspinal sprouting of dorsal root axons. Development of new collaterals and preterminals following partial denervation of the spinal cord in the cat. *Arch. Neurol. and Pschiatry.*, **79**, 1, 1958, 46–61.

Liu, C. N. & D. Scott. Regeneration in the dorsal spinocerebeller tract of the cat. *J. Compar. Neurol.*, **109**, 2, 1958, 153–167.

Livshits, A. V. Electrical stimulation of urinary bladder during traumatic lesion of the spinal cord and cauda equina. Doctoral dissertation, Moscow, 1969.

Livshits, L. Yu., E. E. Melamud, V. I. Plotnyagina, A. A. Shul'dyakov, V. A. Kireev & A. I. Kózel'. Some fundamental questions regarding the rehabilitation of patients following a trauma of the vertebral column and the spinal cord. In *Reabilitatsiya Bol'nykh s Posledstviyami Povrezhdeniya Pozvonochnika i Spinnogo Mozga.* Kiev: Zdorov'e, 1969, 10–12.

Lobanova, M. V. Leukocytosis in the trauma of the spinal cord and cauda equina. In *Voprosy Eksperimental'nogo i Klinicheskogo Izucheniya Posledstvii Travmy Spinnogo Mozga.* Moscow: AN SSSR, 1956, 118–123.

Lockhart, W. S. Evidence of structural and functional regeneration of the CNS in man. In *Regeneration in the CNS.* Springfield, Ill.: Charles C. Thomas, 1955, 259–264.

Loiko, R. M. The connections of cervical nerves with sympathetic trunk. In *Tezisy Dokladov Nauchnoi Sessii Posvyashchennoi 35-letiyu Instituta Fiziologii AN BSSR.* Minsk, 1956, 167.

Long, Ch. & E. B. Lawton. Functional significance of spinal cord lesion level. *Arch. Phys. Med. and Rehabilit.*, **36**, 4, 1955, 249–255.

Lorento de No, R. La regeneracion de la medula espinal in las larvas de batracio. *Trab. Lab. Invest. Biol.*, **19**, 1921, 147–181.

Lorme, T. L. de. A restoration of muscle power by heavy resistance. *Arch. Phys. Med. and Rehabilit.*, **27**, 1946, 607–630.

Lubenskii, E. G. The experience and the results of the use of the preparations regulating the formation of glial scar during an operative interference in the trauma of the spinal cord. In *Priogenal.* Moscow: Meditsina, 1965, 244–250.

Lubenskii, E. G. & S. E. Narodovol'tseva. Treatment of closed injuries of the vertebral column and the spinal cord. In *Materialy Ob'edinennoi Nauchnoi Konferentsii Neirokhirurgov.* Leningrad, 1964, 3–9.

Lubinska, L. The physical state of axoplasm in teased vertebrate nerve fibers. *Acta. Biol. Exptl.*, **17**, 1, 1956, 135.

Lubinska, L. Sedentary and migratory states of Schwann cells. *Exptl. Cell Res.*, **S.8**, 1961, 74–90.

Lubinska, L. Axoplasmic streaming in regenerating and in normal nerve fibers. In *Progress in Brain Research,* 13. Amsterdam: Elsevier, 1964, 1–71.

Lubinska, L. Outflow from cut ends on 'nerve fibers. *Exptl. Cell Res.*, **10**, 1, 1965, 40–47.

Lubinska, L., S. Niemierko, B. Oderfeld, L. Szwara & J. Zelena. Bi-directional movements of axoplasm in peripheral nerve fibers. *Acta Biol. Exptl.*, **23**, 4, 1963, 239–247.

Lubinska, L., S. Niemierko & J. Zelena. Ascending and descending movements of axoplasm along axons. In *The Effect of Use and Disuse on Neuromuscular Function.* Prague: 1963, 197–202.

Leuscher, E. & A. Muralt. Der neuroregenerative Wuchsstoff "NR." *Helv. Physiol. et Pharmacol.* Acta, **5**, 1947, 17–25.

Lundberg, A. & Voorhoeve. Effects from the pyramdial tract on spinal reflex arcs. *Acta Physiol. Scand.*, **56**, 1962, 3–41; 201–219.

Maiorchik, V. E. Physiological peculiarties of lesion of the spinal cord. In *Sed'maia Sessia Neirokhirurgicheskogo Soveta.* Moscow: AMN SSSR, 1947, 176–179.

Maiorov, T. I. Changes in gastric secretion in patients following a trauma to the spinal cord and cauda equina. In *Voprosy Eksperimental'nogo i Klinicheskogo Izucheniya Posledstvii Travmy Spinnogo Mozga.* Moscow: AN SSSR, 1956, 130–133.

Mair, W. G. & R. Druckman. The pathology of spinal cord lesions and their relation to the clinical features in protrusion of cervical intervertebral discs. *Brain,* **76**, 1953, 70–91.

Maksimova, E. V. & Z. Afelt. Activity of fusimotor neurons in chronically isolated segments of the spinal cord. In *Materialy Nauchnoi Konferentsii Fiziologov, Biokhimikov, Patofiziologov i Farmakologov,* **1**. Makhachkala: 1970, 31–34.

Maksimova, E. V. & S. M. Sverdlov. Effect of pyramidal impulses on the motor nuclei of the spinal cord. In *Nervnye Mekhanizmy Dvigatel'noi Deyatel'nosti.* Moscow: Nauka, 1966, 115–129.

Malakhovskaya, D. B. Development of the inborn plantar reflex in early childhood. *Materialy po Evolyutsionnoi Fiziologii,* **4**, 1960, 14–22.

Manni, E. Persistenza nel piccione spinale di asimmetrie degli arti da lesions cerebellare. *Boll. Soc. Ital. Biol.*, **24**, 6, 1948a, 785–786.

Manni, E. L'Azione tonica della corteccia cerebrale e del mesencefalo sui centri spinal e in dipendente del cervelleto. *Boll. Soc. Ital. Biol.*, **24**, 4, 1948b, 590–591.

Markovich, N., S. Voinesku & G. Markovich. Effect of cortisone on the experimental traumatic scar of the cerebral cortex. *Voprosy Neirokhirurgii,* **2**, 1958, 15–19.

Martin, C. J. Trypsin, the pharmacology of the drug. *Exptl. Med. and Surg.*, **13**, 1955, 156–160.

Martin, C. J. Anti-inflamatory effect of trypsin. *Ann. N. Y. Acad. Sci.*, **68**, 1, 1957, 70–86.

Martin, C. J., R. Brendel & J. M. Beiler. Mechanism of anti-inflamatory action of trypsin. *Amer. J. Pharmacol.*, **127**, 1955, 125–128.

Matthews, P. B. C. Muscle spindles and their motor control. *Physiol. Revs.*, **44**, 1964, 219-288.

Matthews, P. B. C. & A. Dorfman. Inhibition of Hyaluronidase. *Physiol. Revs.*, **35**, 2, 1955, 381-402.

Matinyan, L. A. Compensatory adaptability after the transection of the posterior half of the spinal cord during phylogenesis. In *Problema Kompensatornykh Prisposoblenii.* Moscow: AN SSR, 1960, 357-363.

Matinyan, L. A. Complete transection of the spinal cord and the effect of enzymes on the restoration of functions. In *Materialy Ob'edinennoi Konferentsii Neirokhirurgov.* Leningrad: 1964, 250-252.

Matinyan, L. A. Complete transection of the spinal cord and effect of enzyme on the restoration of functions. In *Travma Pozvonochnika i Spinnogo Mozga.* Leningrad: 1965, 148-155.

Matinyan, L. A. & A. S. Andreasyan. Action of some preparations on the restoration of altered functions of the CNS. In *Eksperimental'nye Issledovaniya i Klinicheskoe Primenenie Pirogenala.* Moscow: 1961, 97-111.

Matinyan, L. A. & A. S. Andreasian. Enzymotherapeutics of organ injuries of the spinal cord. Erevan: 1973.

Matinyan, L. A., A. S. Andreasyan & G. A. Epremyan. Complete transection of the spinal cord and morphological and physiological studies after the administration of pyrogenal lidase and other substances. In *Priogenal.* Moscow: Meditsina, 1965, 104-115.

Matinyan, L. A. & Zh. S. Sarkisyan. Acid mucopolysaccharides of an intact spinal cord and after its complete transection during the administration of enzymes. In *Materialy XV Nauchnoi Konferentsii Fiziologov, Biokhimikov, Farmakologov Yuga RSFSR.* Makhachkala: 1965, 196-197.

Mats, V. N. The morphology and physiology of neuroglia. *Itogi Nauki. Morfologiya Cheloveka i Zhivotnykh.* Moscow: Nauka, 1968, 43-68.

Mats, V. N. Correlation between the nerve and glial cells in an increased activity of the nervous system. Doctoral dissertation, Moscow: 1969.

Matyushkin, D. I. Reflex excitation (trailing) of the spinal nerve centers. *Fiziol. Zhurn. SSSR,* **39**, 6, 1953, 689-698.

McCaman, R. E. & E. Robins. Quantitative biochemical studies of Wallerian degeneration in the peripheral and central nervous system. I. Chemical constituents. *J. Neurochem.*, **5**, 1959a, 18-31.

McCaman, R. E. & E. Robins. Quantitative biochemical studies of Wallerian degeneration in the peripheral and central nervous system. II. Twelve enzymes. *J. Neurochem.*, **5**, 1959b, 32-42.

McCouch, C. P., G. M. Austin & C. Y. Liu. Sprouting of new terminals as a cause of spasticity. *Amer. J. Physiol.*, **183**, 1955, 642-650.

McCouch, C. P., G. M. Austin, C. N. Liu & C. Y. Liu. Sprouting as a cause of spasticity. *J. Neurophysiol.*, **21**, 3, 1958. 205-216.

McCullough, A. W. Studies on peripheral nerve regeneration. Peripheral nerve regeneration in white rats of various ages when treated with a pyrogenic bacterial polysaccharide complex in various dosage. *J. Compar. Neurol.*, **113**, 3, 1959, 471-490.

McGreight, J. Regeneration of the spinal cord in the tail of *Diemyctulus Viridescens. Anat. Rec.*, **27**, 1924, 38.

McIntyre, A. K. Synaptic function and learning. *XIX Internat. Physiol. Congress,* 1953, 107-114.

Meerson, F. Z. O Vzaimosvyazi Fiziologicheskoi Funktsii i Geneticheskogo Apparata Kletki (Correlation between the physiological functions and the genetic apparatus of cells). Moscow: *AMN SSSR,* 1963.

Meerson, F. Z. Plasticheskoe Obespechenie Funktsii Organizma (Maintenance of plastic functions of an organism). Moscow: Nauka, 1967.

Meerson, F. Z. & R. I. Kruglikov. The correlation between the genetic apparatus and the physiological function of a neuron in conditioning and memory. *Zhurn. Vyssh. Nervn. Deyat.*, **16**, 2, 1966, 274-291.

Meerson, F. Z., R. I. Kruglikov & I. A. Kolmeitseva. Role of nucleic acids synthesis in reinforcing the conditioned reflexes and memory. *Byull. Eksperim. Biol. i Med.*, **60,** 12, 1965, 3–7.

Miani, N. Proximo-distal movement along the axon of protein synthesized in the perikaryon of regenerating neurons. *Nature,* **185,** 4712, 1960, 541–542.

Migliavacca, A. Kritische Beobachtungen über die Heilungsmöglichketi dez Rückenmarkverletzungen bei der experimentallen Rachiotomie des Fötus. *Z. Geburtschilfe,* **101,** 1931, 184–288.

Milyantsevich, E. P. Morphological changes of the mucus membrane of the stomach and solar plexus during experimental transection of the spinal cord in dogs. In *Voprosy Eksperimental'nogo i Klinicheskogo Izucheniya Posledstvii travmy Spinnogo Mozga.* Moscow: *AN SSSR,* 1956, 134–141.

Minchenko, A. G. Effect of pyrogenal, indole and chloralose on the metabolism of biogenic amines. Doctoral dissertation, Kiev: 1968.

Minkina, N. A. Histological changes in some organs of rats after the administration of pentoxyl. *Farmakologiva i Toksikologiya,* **21,** 6, 1958, 69–74.

Mitchell, S. Q. Numerical changes in circulating leucocytes in normal and chronically adrenalectomized cats after administration of Pyromen. *Amer. J. Physiol.*, **171,** 1952, 750–751.

Mitchell, S. Q. & E. G. Stuart. Role of adrenal gland in mechanism of leucocyte changes upon administration of Pyromen. *Amer. J. Physiol.*, **167,** 1951, 810.

Mokreeva, M. G. Physical therapy in diseases and following CNS trauma. Doctoral dissertation, Kiev: 1950.

Morozov, B. D. Problems of the regeneration of animal organs. *Usp. Sovrem. Biol.*, **4,** 1, 1935, 88–101.

Moruzzi, G. Somatic functions of the nervous system. *Annual. Rev. Physiol.*, **13,** 1951, 281–296.

Moshkov, V. N. Physical therapy as a method of restorative treatment in traumatic damage to the spinal cord. Doctoral dissertation, Moscow: 1944.

Moshkov, V. N. Obshchie Osnovy Lechebnoi Fizkul'tury (General principles of physical therapy). Moscow: Medgiz, 1963.

Moshkov, V. N., Kh. M. Freidin & M. Ya. Ratova. The application of physical therapy with mud bath as a method of restorative treatment in spinal injuries. *Gospit. Delo.*, **12,** 1944, 21–23.

Moyer, E. K. & D. L. Kimmel. The repair of severed motor and sensory spinal nerve roots by arterial sleeve method of anastomosis. *J. Compar. Neurol.*, **88,** 1, 1948, 285.

Moyer, E. K., D. L. Kimmel & L. W. Winborne. Regeneration of sensory spinal nerve roots in young and female rats. *J. Compar. Neurol.*, **98,** 2, 1953, 283.

Munro, A. F. & R. Robinson. Normal levels of plasma adrenaline and noradrenaline compared with those in subjects with complete transverse lesions of the spinal cord. *J. Physiol.*, **141,** 1958, 4.

Munro, A. F. & R. Robinson. The catecholamine content of the peripheral plasma in human subjects with complete transverse lesions of the spinal cord. *J. Physiol.*, **154,** 2, 1960, 244–253.

Muratov, S. N. The nerve regulation of tissue permeability. *Arkh. Patologii,* **22,** 5, 1960, 18–22.

Murrey, J. & Goldberger, M. E. Restitution of function and collateral sprouting in the cat spinal cord: the partially hemisected animal. *J. Comp. Neurol.*, **158,** 1974, 19–36.

Musalov, G. G. Effect of pyronin on the regeneration of intraspinal axons in dogs. In *Materialy XV Nauchnoi Konferentsii Fiziologov, Biokhimikov i Farmakologov Yuga RSFSR.* Makhachkala: 1965, 221–222.

Naidel', A. V. & E. I. Pal'tsev. Rearrangement of human spinal segmental apparatus in a conditioned reaction in time response. *Zhurn. Vyssh. Nervn. Deyat.*, **15,** 5, 1965, 940–942.

Naidin, V. L., A. A. Shlykov, N. I. Zakharchenko, L. G. Komolova, L. V. Kudryavtsev, V. I. Perov & N. S. Stolyarzh. Additional methods for compensating the motor functions in patients with traumatic lesions of the spinal cord in post-operative period. In *Reabilitatsiva Bol'nykh s Posledstviyami Povrezhdenii Pozvonochnika i Spinnogo Mozga.* Kiev: Zdorov'e, 1969, 60–61.

Nakamura, Y. Working ability of the paraplegia. *Paraplegia,* **2,** 2, 1973, 182–193.

Nasonov, D. N. & V. Ya. Aleksandrov. Causes of the appearance of bioelectric potentials. *Usp. Sovrem. Biol.,* 17, 1, 1944, 1–12.

Nasonov, N. V. Significance of cartilage in shaping the organ in axolotl. *Dokl. AN SSSR,* **1,** 6, 1935, 413–417.

Nasonov, N. V. Peculiarities and causes of the appearance of additional organs in amphibians. *Dokl. AN SSSR,* **2,** 5, 1936a, 201–205.

Nasonov, N. V. Various factors in formation of an organ in axolotl during subcutaneous implantation of homologous cartilagenous tissues. *Dokl. AN SSSR,* **4,** 2, 1936b, 97–100.

Nasonov, N. V. Dobavochnye Obrazovaniya, Razvivayushchiesya pri Vlozhenii Khryashcha pod Kozhu Vzroslykh Khvostatykh Amfibii (Formation and development of additional organs by subcutaneous implantation of cartilaginous tissue in adult tailed amphibians). Moscow: AN SSSR, 1941.

Needham, A. E. Regeneration and Wound Healing. New York: John Wiley & Sons, 1952.

Needham, A. E. Regeneration and growth. In *Fundamental Aspects of Normal and Malignant Growth.* Amsterdam: Elsevier, 1960, 588–663.

Neifakh, S. A. & E. P. Zdrodovskaya. Organic phosphorous metabolism in liver during burns and in experimental pyrexia. In *Ezhegodnik IEM AMN SSSR.* Leningrad: 1956.

Nesmeyanova, T. N. Inhibition in the transected spinal cord. In *Tezisy VIII Vsesoyuznogo S'ezda Fiziologov, Biokhimikov i Farmakologov.* Moscow: AN SSSR, 1955a, 446–447.

Nesmeyanova, T. N. Inhibition in the caudal part of the transected spinal cord. *Dokl. AN SSSR,* **105,** 3, 1955b, 610–613.

Nesmeyanova, T. N. Effect of work on the motor reflex of spinal dog. In *Tezisy Dokladov II Soveshchaniya, Posvyashchennogo Kompensatornym Prisposobleniyam pri Organicheskikh Porazheniyakh Tsentral'noi Nervnoi Sistemy.* Erevan: 1956, 11–13.

Nesmeyanova, T. N. Inhibition of motor reflexes in spinal dogs in the conditions of chronic experimentation. *Fiziol. Zhurn. SSSR,* **43,** 4, 1957, 301–309.

Nesmeyanova, T. N. Role of cutaneous stimulation for activating motor reflexes in the spinal dog. *Byull. Eksperim. Biol. i Med.,* **10,** 1959, 19–23.

Nesmeyanova, T. N. Peculiarities of the activity of the transected spinal cord in mammals and the possibility of the regeneration of its conducting paths. In *Symposium Internationale ad Rehabitation in Neurologie.* Prague: 1966.

Nesmeyanova, T. N. Some peculiarities of the activity of distal segment of the spinal cord in dogs. In *Vosstanovlenie Funktsii pri Porazheniyakh Tsentral'noi Nervnoi Sistemy.* Moscow: 1967, 97–98.

Nesmeyanova, T. N. Restoration of regenerating capacity of the conducting fibers in the mammalian central nervous system. In *Materialy v Konferentsii po Regeneratsii i Kletochnomu Razmnozheniyu.* Moscow: 1968a, 292–295.

Nesmeyanova, T. N. Some peculiarities of the reflex activity of the spinal cord after its separation from the higher parts of the CNS. In *Elektrofiziologicheskoe Issledovanie Kompensatsii Funktsii pri Povrezhdenii Tsentral'noi Nervnoi Sistemy.* Moscow: Nauka, 1968b, 140–152.

Nesmeyanova, T. N. Inhibition of muscular activity of the posterior extremities in the spinal dogs. In *Elektrofiziologicheskoe Issledovanie Kompensatsii Funktsii Tsentral'noi Nervnoi Sistemy.* Moscow: Nauka, 1968c, 153–159.

Nesmeyanova, T. N. Mechanisms of the restoration of motor functions in patients with complete or partial transection of the spinal cord. In *Reabilitatsiya Bol'nykh s Posledstviyami Povrezhdenii Pozvonochnika Spinnogo Mozga.* Kiev: Zdorov'e, 1969, 10–11.

Nesmeyanova, T. N. *New Develop. Electromyogr. & Clin. Neurophysiol.,* 1973, 1–3.

Nesmeyanova, T. N. Electromyography, as a method of prediction of recovering processes with trauma of spinal cord. *Bull. Eper. Biol. i Med.,* **10,** 1975.

Nesmeyanova, T. N. & N. M. Shamarina. Functional changes in the reflex responses in the spinal cord. In *Soveshchaniya po Voprosam Patofiziologii i Terpaii Travm Povrezhdennogo Spinnogo Mozga.* Moscow: 1953a, 36-37.

Nesmeyanova, T. N. & N. M. Shamarina. Functional changes in the reflex responses in the spinal cord. *Dokl. AN SSSR,* **89,** 4, 1953b, 185-188.

Nesmeyanova, T. N. & N. M. Shamarina. Functional changes in the reflex response in the spinal cord. *Dokl. AN SSSR,* **96,** 3, 1954a, 673-676.

Nesmeyanova, T. N. & N. M. Shamarina. Characteristic of reflex activity in the transected spinal cord. *Dokl. AN SSSR,* **97,** 3, 1954b, 547-549.

Nesmeyanova, T. N. & N. M. Shamarina. Functional changes in reflex responses in the spinal cord. In *Voprosy Eksperimental'nogo i Klinicheskogo Izucheniva Posledstvii Travmy Spinnogo Mozga.* Moscow: 1956, 86-97.

Nesmeyanova, T. N. & A. N. Trankvillitati. Electromyographic investigation of activity of the muscle of trunk and lower extremities in the spinal patients. In *Vosstanovlenie Funktsii pri Porazheniyakh Tsentral'noi Nervnoi Sistemy.* Leningrad: 1967, 108-110.

Nesmeyanova, T. N. & A. N. Trankvillitati. Electromyographic investigation of inclusion of muscles of trunk and lower extremities in the motor activity in patients with complete or partial transection of the spinal cord. *Byull. Eksperim. Biol. i Med.,* **4,** 1970, 40-44.

Nesmeyanova, T. N. & A. D. Vorob'eva. The neuroglial reaction and the regeneration of transected central conductors. *Dokl. AN SSSR,* **173,** 4, 1967, 967-970.

Nesmeyanova, T. N., E. N. Arnautova, F. A. Brazovskaya & V. M. Nikityuk. Action of subfebrile doses of pyrogenal on the formation of the spinal scar. In *Pirogenal.* Moscow: Meditsina, 1965a, 92-103.

Nesmeyanova, T. N., E. N. Arnautova & F. A. Brazovskaya. Stimulation of the regeneration of intraspinal axons in adult higher mammals. In *Materialy XV Nauchnoi Konferentsii Fiziologov, Biokhimikov i Farmakologov Yuga RSFSR.* Makhachkala, 1965b, 228-229.

Nesmeyanova, T. N., F. A. Brazovskaya & E. N. Arnautova. Effect of trypsin on the formation of a spinal scar. In *Mekhanizmy Kompensatornykh Prisposoblenii.* Moscow: Nauka, 1964a, 137-145.

Nesmeyanova, T. N., F. A. Brazovskaya & E. N. Arnautova. Stimulation of the regeneration of conducting paths of transected spinal cord in dogs. In *Mekhanizmy Kompensatornykh Prisposoblenii.* Moscow: Nauka, 1964b, 124-136.

Nesmeyanova, T. N., F. A. Brazovskaya & E. N. Arnautova. Transplants as stimulator of regenerations. In *Mekhanizmy Kompensatornykh Prisposoblenii.* Moscow: Nauka, 1964c, 115-123.

Nesmeyanova, T. N., F. A. Brazovskaya & E. N. Iordanskaya. Regeneration of conducting paths in the transected spinal cord. In *Tezisy Dokladov Konferentsii po Probleme Kompensatornykh Prisposoblenii.* Moscow: AN SSSR, 1958, 71.

Nesmeyanova, T. N., F. A. Brazovskaya & E. N. Iordanskaya. A case of partial regeneration of nerve fibers in the transected spinal cord of a dog. *Fiziol. Zhurn. SSSR,* **46,** 2, 1960a, 202-209.

Nesmeyanova, T. N., F. A. Brazovskaya & E. N. Iordanskaya. Regeneration of conducting paths in the transected spinal cord of a dog. In *Problemy Kompensatornykh Prisposoblenii.* Moscow: AN SSSR, 1960b, 304.

Nesmeyanova, T. N., F. A. Brazovskaya & E. N. Iordanskaya. Formation of the spinal scar and regeneration of nerve fibers under the action of pyrogenal. In *Eksperimental'noe Izuchenie i Klinicheskoe Primenenie Pirogenala.* Moscow: 1961, 54-73.

Nesmeyanova, T. N., F. A. Brazovskaya & E. N. Iordanskaya. Significance of improved tropism in the regeneration of the spinal conducting paths. *Fiziol. Zhurn. SSSR,* **49,** 3, 1963, 314-321.

Nesmeyanova, T. N., E. Yu. Gutmann & I. Gaek. Degeneration in central and peripheral conducting fibers. In *Nervnye Mekhanizmy Dvigatel'noi Deyatel'nosti.* Moscow: Nauka, 1966, 19-26.

Nesmeyanova, T. N., E. N. Iordanskaya & F. A. Brazovskaya. Action of different doses of pyrogenal on the formation of spinal scar. *Byull. Eksperim. Biol. i Med.*, **56**, 1963, 115–119.

Nesmeyanova, T. N., I. I. Pyatetskii-Shapiro & M. L. Shik. A method of evaluating the functional status of the spinal cord. In *Materialy X S'ezda Vsesoyuznogo Fiziologicheskogo Obshchestva im. Pavlova*, **2.** Erevan: Nauka, 1964, 125.

Nesmeyanova, T. N., I. I. Pyatetskii-Shapiro & M. L. Shik. Activity of motor units in the intact, spinal and the deafferented dogs. *Biofizika*, **10**, 2, 1965, 317–322.

Nesset, N. M., L. C. Ginger, & J. Byrne. Personal communication. *J. Lab. and Clin. Med.*, **37**, 5, 1951, 771–775.

Nezlina, N. I. Alteration and restoration of motor functions in dogs after hemisection of the brain stem. Doctoral dissertation, Moscow: 1957.

Nezlina, N. I. & B. P. Kazakova. Compensation of altered functions after the lateral hemisection of the spinal cord in cats. In *Elektrofiziologicheskie Issledovaniya Kompensatsii pri Povrezhdeniyakh Tsentral'noi Nervnoi Sistemy*. Moscow: Nauka, 1968, 208–214.

Noback, C., L. Basset & J. B. Campbell. Regeneration of axons across gaps in the transected spinal cords of adult cats. *Anat. Rec.*, **130**, 2, 1958, 349.

Nozdrachev, A. D. Kortikosteroidy i Simpaticheskaya Nervnaya Sistema (Corticosteroids and the sympathetic nervous system). Leningrad: Nauka, 1969.

Oganisyan, S. S. & L. A. Matinyan. Some clinical findings after the treatment of a spinal lesion with enzyme. In *Materialy X S'ezda Vsesovuznogo Fiziologicheskogo Obshchestva im. Pavlova*, **2.** Erevan: Nauka, 1964, 142–145.

Oivin, I. A. & K. N. Monakova. Qualitative method of evaluating the action of antiinflammatory agents. *Farmakologiya i Toksikologiya*, **16**, 6, 1953, 50–54.

Orbeli, L. A. Sympathetic innervation of the skeletal muscle. *Izv. Nauchn. In-ta im. Lesgafta*, **6**, 1923, 187–197.

Orbeli, L. A. Sympathetic innervation of traversely striated muscles. In *Yubileinyi Sbornik 75-letiya Akad. M. P. Pavlova*. Leningrad–Moscow: AN SSSR, 1924, 403.

Orbeli, L. A. The adaptation in a reflex apparatus (sympathetic innervation of the skeletal muscles, spinal cord and peripheral receptors). *Vrachebnaya Gazeta*, 1927, 163–169.

Orbeli, L. A. Correlation between the somatic and the sympathetic nervous system. *Vrachebonaya Gazeta*, 1930, 189.

Orbeli, L. A. Sympathetic innervation of skeletal muscles, sensory organs and the CNS. *Fiziol. Zhurn. SSSR*, **15**, 1, 1932, 5–14.

Orbeli, L. A. Lektsii po Fiziologii Nervnoi Sistemy (Lectures on the physiology of the nervous system). Leningrad: Medgiz, 1938.

Orbeli, L. A. Evolutionary principles in the physiology of the CNS. *Usp. Sovrem. Biol.*, **15**, 1942, 3.

Orbeli, L. A. Voprosy Vysshei Nervnoi Deyatel'nosti (Problems of the higher nervous activity). Moscow: AN SSSR, 1949, 448–463.

Orekhovich, V. N. Localization of the areas of increased activity of cathepsin in regenerating amphibian organs. *Byull. Eksperim. Biol. i Med.*, **3**, 2, 1937, 194–196.

Orekhovich, V. N. Changes in the activity of cathepsin in the regenerating liver of a rat. *Byull. Eksperim. Biol. i Med.*, **6**, 2, 1938, 230–232.

Orlova, B. L. Afferent innervation of the vessels of the thigh. In *Voprosy Morfologii Perefericheskoi Nervnoi Sistemy*, **3.** Minsk: 1956, 145.

Ortiz-Galvan, A. The effect of hydrocortisone on the healing of wounds of the brain. An experimental study on the cat. *Arch. Neurol. and Psychiatry*, **74**, 4, 1955, 407–413.

Ortiz-Galvan, A. Action of local hydrocortisone on spinal cord wounds. *Arch. Neurol. and Psychiatry*, **76**, 1, 1956, 34–41.

Osterholm, J. L. The pathophysiological response to spinal cord injury. The current status of related research. *J. Neurosurg.*, **40**, 1974, 3–33.

Osterholm, J. L. & G. J. Mathews. Altered norepinephrine metabolism following experimental spinal cord injury. I. Relationship to hemorrhagic necrosis and post-wounding neurological deficits. *J. Neurosurg.*, **36**, 1972, 386–394.

Osterholm, J. L. & G. J. Mathews. Altered norepinephrine metabolism following experimental spinal cord injury. II. Protection against traumatic spinal cord hemorrhagic necrosis by norepinephrine synthesis blockade with alpha metyl tyrosine. *J. Neurosurg.*, **36**, 1972, 395–401.

Owen, A. G. W. & C. S. Sherrington. Observations on strychnine reversal. *J. Physiol.*, **43**, 1911, 232.

Pal'tsev, E. I. Interaction of the tendon reflex arcs of lower extremities in man influencing the locomotor synergism. *Biofizika*, **12**, 5, 1967, 915–924.

Parin, V. V. The trophic maintenance of cardiac activity. In *Deistvie Neirotropnykh Sredstv na Troficheskie Protseessy i Tkanevyi Obmen.* Leningrad: 1966, 68–69.

Paskind, H. A. Regeneration of posterior root fibers in the cat. *Arch. Neurol. and Psychiatry*, **36**, 1936, 1077–1083.

Patskikh, E. V. Application of pyrogenal in opthalmology. In *Eksperimental'nye Issledovaniya i Klinicheskoe Primenenie Pirogenala.* Moscow: 1961, 234–245.

Patskikh, E. V. Application of pyrogenal in opthalmological practice in ambulatory cases. In *Pirogenal.* Moscow: Meditsina, 1965, 265–267.

Pavlov, I. P. Physiology of the higher nervous activity. *Poln. Sobr. Soch.*, **3.** Moscow–Leningrad: AN SSSR, 1951a, 219–234.

Pavlov, I. P. A trip of a physiologist in the field of psychiatry. *Poln. Sobr. Soch.*, **3.** Moscow–Leningrad: AN SSSR, 1951b, 126–132.

Pavlov, I. P. The problem of sleep. *Poln. Sobr. Soch.*, **3.** Moscow–Leningrad: AN SSSR, 1951c, 409–427.

Pchelkina, L. A. Intraspinal connections of the posterior root. *Uch. Zap. Vtorogo MMI, AMN, SSSR*, **2**, 1951, 203.

Penfield, W. Oligodendroglia and its relation to classical neuroglia. *Brain*, **47**, 10, 1924, 430–452.

Perkins, L., A. Babbini & L. W. Freeman. Distalproximal nerve implants in spinal cord transection. *Neurology*, **14**, 10, 1964, 949–954.

Person, R. S. The electromyographic investigation of patients with mild hemiparesis. *Zhurn. Nevrapatologii i Psikhiatsii*, **60**, 12, 1960, 1619–1621.

Person, R. S. Elektromiografika v Issledovaniyakh Cheloveka (Electromyograph investigations of humans). Moscow: Nauka, 1969.

Pevzner, L. Z. Effect of circulatory hypoxia on the concentration of nucleic acids in the cortical cells estimated by quantitative cytochemical method. *Nauchn. Soobshch. In-ta Fiziologii im. I. P. Pavlova AN SSSR*, **2**, 1959, 198–201.

Pevzner, L. Z. Concentration of nucleic acids in the nerve cells under different functional conditions. *Ukr. Biokhim. Zhurn.*, **35**, 1963, 448–477.

Pia, V. Diversito istochemiche nei nuclei gliali midollo spinale di ratto. *Sperimentale*, **113**, 6, 1963, 317–322.

Piatt, J. Regeneration in the CNS of amphibia. In *Regeneration in the CNS.* Springfield, Ill.: Charles C. Thomas, 1955, 20–46.

Pinto, T. & R. Bromiley. A search for spinal conditioning and for evidence that it can become a reflex. *J. Exptl. Psychol.*, **40**, 1950, 121–130.

Planel'es, K. K. Concluding remarks. In *Eksperimental'nye Issledovaniya i Klinicheskoe Primenenie Pirogenale.* Moscow: 1961, 252–253.

Planel'es K. K. Concluding remarks. In *Pirogenal.* Moscow: Meditsina, 1965, 458–467.

Planel'es, K. K. & Z. A. Popenenkova. Serotonin i Ego Znachenie v Infektsionnoi Patologii (Serotonin and its Significance in the Pathology of Infection). Moscow: Meditsina, 1965.

Plechkova, E. K. Reaktsiya Nervnoi Sistemy Organizma na Khronicheskoe Povrezhdenie Perifericheskogo Nerva (Reaction of the nervous system to chronic damages of the peripheral nerve). Moscow: Meditsina, 1961.

Polak, M. Morphological and functional characteristics of the central and peripheral neuroglia (light microscopic observations). In *Progress in Brain Research*, **15.** Amsterdam: Elsevier, 1965, 12–34.

Polezhaev, L. V. Resorption, proliferation and changes in the respective tissues during the regeneration of extremities in axolotls. *Biol. Zhurn.*, **2**, 1933a, 4–5; 368–373.

Polezhaev, L. V. The revival of regenerative capacity in the tailless amphibians. *Biol. Zhurn.*, **2,** 1933b, 4-5; 357-367.

Polezhaev, L. V. Significance of vestiges of an organ in the regeneration of extremity in axolotl. *Arkh. Anat. Gistol. i Embriol.*, **13,** 1, 1934, 91-98; 1935, **14,** 384-403.

Polezhaev, L. V. Investigation into the mechanism of regeneration in the USSR. *Usp. Sovrem. Biol.*, **24,** 1947, 375-402.

Polezhaev, L. V. Replacement of the bone defects in the skull of mice. *Dokl. AN SSSR*, **77,** 1951, 525.

Polezhaev, L. V. Change of regeneration capacity in animals. *Izv. AN SSSR, Seriya Biol.*, **1,** 1956, 68-83.

Polezhaev, L. V. Restoration of nonregenerative skull bones in mammals. *Izv. AN SSSR. Seriya Biol.*, **5,** 1957, 556-571.

Polezhaev, L. V. Regeneration of dental tissue in dogs. *Dokl. AN SSSR*, **119,** 5, 1958a, 1039-1042.

Polezhaev, L. V. Restoration of regeneration capacity in mammals. Regeneration capacity in mammals and man. *Folia Biol. Pol.* **6,** 3, 1958b, 203-238.

Polezhaev, L. V. Restoration of regeneration capacity of the extremities in axolotl after X-ray irradiation. *Dokl. AN SSSR*, **127,** 3, 1959a, 713-716.

Polezhaev, L. V. Some difficulties in the study of regeneration. *Folia Biol. Pol.* **7,** 1959b, 215-237.

Polezhaev, L. V. Conditions determining the regeneration capacity of organs and tissues in animals. In *Usloviya Regeneratsii Organov i Tkanei u Zhivotnykh.* Moscow: 1966a, 185-192.

Polezhaev, L. V. Restoration of regenerating capacity suppressed by X-ray irradiation. *Izv. AN SSSR, Seriya, Biol.*, **1,** 1966b, 37-58.

Polezhaev, L. V. Utrata i Vosstanovlenie Regeneratsionnoi Sposobnosti Organov i Tkanei u Zhivotnykh (Loss and restoration of the regeneration capacity of organs and tissues in animals). Moscow: Nauka, 1968. [English trans., Harvard Univ. Press, 1972.]

Polezhaev, L. V. & E. P. Karnaukhova. Stimulation of the multiplication of nerve cells in the mammalian cerebral cortex. *Dokl. AN SSSR*, **150,** 1963, 430-433.

Polezhaev, L. V. & I. I. Morozov. A new method of prolonging the regeneration capacity of extremities in the tail-less amphibians. *Dokl. AN SSSR*, **30,** 1941, 670-672.

Polezhaev, L. V. & G. P. Ramenskaya. Regeneration of extremities in jerlyanka by hydrolytic cartilage products). *Dokl. AN SSSR*, **70,** 1950, 141-144.

Polezhaev, L. V. & K. Yu. Reznikov. Changes in cortical nerve tissue after its partial removal in kittens. *Arkh. Anat. Gistol. i Embriol.*, **51,** 12, 1966, 9-21.

Polezhaev, L. V., A. I. Matveeva & N. A. Zakharova. Regeneration of skull by transplanting bone pieces in mammals. *Byull. Eksperim. Biol. i Med.*, **42,** 4, 1957, 94-98.

Polezhaev, L. V., N. A. Teplits & I. I. Ernakova. Restoration of regeneration capacity of the extremities suppressed by X-ray irradiation in axolotls with proteins, nucleic acids and lyophilized tissues. *Dokl. AN SSSR*, **138,** 2, 1961, 477-480.

Polezhaev, L. V., N. A. Teplits & S. Ya. Tuchkova. Significance of nucleic acids from proteins in the restoration of the regeneration capacity of extremities in axolotls, suppressed by X-ray irradiation. *Dokl. AN SSSR*, **144,** 4, 1962, 930-933.

Polezhaev, L. V., A. V. Akhabadze, N. A. Muzlaeva & M. N. Yavich. Stimulyatsiya Regeneratsii Myshtsy Serdtsa (Stimulation of regeneration of cardiac muscles). Moscow: Nauka, 1965.

Polezhaev, L. V., A. V. Akhabadze, N. A. Zakharova & V. L. Mant'eva. The myocardial regeneration in mammals. *Dokl. AN SSSR*, **119,** 5, 1958, 1039-1042.

Polezhaev, L. V., A. V. Akhabadze, N. A. Zakharova & V. L. Mant'eva. Stimulation of regeneration of cardiac muscles in mammals. *Dokl. AN SSSR, Seriya Biol.*, **1,** 1959, 16-33.

Pollock, L. J. & L. Davis. The reflex activities of a decerebrated animal. *J. Compar. Neurol.*, **50,** 1930, 377-411.

Pollock, L. J. & L. Davis. Studies in decerebration. VI. *Amer. J. Physiol.*, **98,** 1934, 47-49.

Pompeiano, O. & J. E. Swett. EEG and behavioral manifestations of sleep induced by cutaneous nerve stimulation in normal cats. *Arch. Ital. Biol.*, **100,** 3, 1962a, 311–342.

Pompeiano, O. & J. E. Swett. Identification of cutaneous and muscle afferent fibers producing EEG synchronization or arousal in normal cats. *Arch. Ital. Biol.*, **100,** 3, 1962b, 343–374.

Pool, J. L. Electrospinogram (ESG). Spinal cord action potentials recorded from a paraplegic patient. *J. Neurosurg.*, **3,** 3, 1946, 192–198.

Pope, A. Implication of histochemical studies for metabolism of the neuroglia. In *The Biology of the Neuroglia.* Springfield, Ill.: Charles C. Thomas, 1958, 211.

Pribytkova, G. N. Effect of different doses of adrenaline on the higher nervous activity. *Byull. Eksperim. Biol. i Med.*, **2,** 2, 1936, 117–119.

Prikhod'ko, A. K. Funktsionel'noe Lechenie Povrezhdenii i Zabolevanii Dvigatel'nogo Apparata (Treatment of damages and diseases of the motor apparatus). Kiev: 1940.

Pronko, N. H. & W. N. Kellogg. The phenomenon of the muscle twitch in flexion conditioning. *J. Exptl. Psychol.*, **31,** 1942a, 232–238.

Pronko, N. H. & W. N. Kellogg. Reflex mechanisms and the case of conditioning. *Amer. J. Psychol.*, **55,** 1942b, 371–384.

Prosser, C. L. & W. S. Hunter. The extinction of startle responses and spinal reflexes in the white rat. *Amer. J. Physiol.*, **117,** 1936, 609–618.

Pryakhina, A. I. Functional status of the patients following the treatment of trauma of the spinal cord and cauda equina. In *Voprosy Eksperimental'nogo i Klinicheskogo Izucheniya Posledstvii Travmy Spinnogo Mozga.* Moscow: AN SSSR, 1956, 139–141.

Raker, Ch. W. Use of enzymes in veterinary medicine. *Ann. N. Y. Acad. Sci.*, **69,** 1, 1957, 144–150.

Ranson, S. & P. Billigsley. An experimental analysis of the sympathetic trunk and great splanchnic nerve in the cat. *J. Compar. Neurol.*, **29,** 1918, 3.

Rasskazov, E. V. Rehabilitation of patients with closed injury of the vertebral column and lesion of the spinal cord with the help of lidase and pyrogenal. In *Vosstanovlenie Funktsii pri Porazheniyakh Tsentral'noi i Perifericheskoi Nervnoi Sistemy.* Leningrad: 1967, 129.

Razdol'skii, I. Ya. The clinical history of bullet injuries and the lesions of the vertebral column and the spinal cord. In *Opyt Sovetskoi Meditsiny v Velikoi Otechestvannoi Voine,* **11.** Moscow: Medgiz, 1952, 72–123.

Rensch, B. & L. Franzisket. Lang andauernde bedingte Reflexe bei Rückenmarksfroschen. *Z. Vergl. Physiol.*, **36,** 1954, 318–326.

Reznikov, K. Yu. A quantitative method of evaluating the multiplication of nerve cells in the rat cerebral cortex. *Dokl. AN SSSR,* **164,** 1, 1965, 187–190.

Reznikov, K. Yu. Cytophotometric investigation of DNA concentration in the nuclei of rat cortical cells both in the normal state and after intracerebral RNA administration. *Dokl. AN SSSR,* **176,** 2, 1967, 449–451.

Riddoch, C. The reflex function of the completely divided spinal cord in man, compared with those associated with less severe lesions. *Brain,* **40,** 1937, 264–272.

Roaf, R. International classification of spinal injuries. *Paraplegia,* **10,** 1972, 78.

Robertis, E. de. Submicroscopic morphology of the synapse. *Internat. Rev. Cytol.*, **8,** 1959, 61–96.

Robertis, E. de. Histopathology of Synapses and Neurosecretion. London: Pergamon Press, 1964.

Robinson, R. & A. F. Munro. Adrenocortical activity in subjects with complete transverse lesions of the spinal cord. *Nature,* **182,** 1958, 805.

Rosner, S. The action of piromen on certain neuropathologic states. *J. Nervous and Mental Disease,* **120,** 1–2, 1954, 22–26.

Rossi, O. & G. Castaldi. La rigerazione del tessuto nervoso neivertebrati superiori. *Riv. Patol. Nerve Ment.*, **46,** 1935, 1–369.

Roux, J. Note Sur l'origine et la terminaison des arosses fibers a myeline du grand sympatique. *Compt. Rend. Soc. Biol.*, **1,** 1900, 52.

Rumyantsev, G. E. Tkanevaya Terapiya (Tissue therapy). Rostov-on-Don: Rosizdat, 1951.

Rusetskii, I. M. Kolennyi refleks (The knee jerk). Tatgosizdat, 1935.

Rushworth, G. The pathophysiology of spasticity. *Proc. Roy. Soc. Med.*, **57**, 8, 1964, 715-720.

Rusk, H. A. Rehabilitation Medicine, **33**. St. Louis: 1958.

Ryvkina, D. E. & A. R. Striganova. Local and general changes of proteolysis during the regeneration of an organ. *Izv. AN SSSR, Seriya Biol.*, **5**, 1939a, 789-799.

Ryvkina, D. E. & A. R. Striganova. Tissue metabolism in burn injuries. *Izv. AN SSSR, Seriya Biol.*, **3**, 1939b, 445-456.

Saf'yants, V. I. Contralateral inhibitory and exaltatory influence on flexor reflex centers. Doctoral dissertation, Leningrad: 1964a.

Saf'yants, V. I. Reflex response and the contralateral influence on the different components of a flexor center. *Fiziol. Zhurn. SSSR*, **50**, 1, 1964b, 73-80.

Samarin, N. Zur Frage uber Regeneration des Ruckenmarknervengewebes nach aseptischen Verletaungen. *Virchows Arch. Pathol. Anat. und Physiol.*, **260**, 2, 1926, 369-397.

Samarin, N. N. Healing of aseptic spinal injuries in rabbits. *Vestn. Khirur. i Pogranich. Obl.*, **48/49**, 1929, 129-138.

Schimert, J. Das Verhalten der Hinterwurzelleteralen in Ruckenmark. *Z. Anat. und Entwichlungsgesch.*, **109**, 1939, 665-687.

Schmitt, F. O. The structure and properties of nerve membranes. In *Metabolism of the Nervous System.* London: Pergamon Press, 1957, 44.

Schotte, O. Systeme nerveauz et regeneration chez le triton. *Rev. Suisse Zool.*, **33**, 1926, 1-211.

Scott, D. Condition over regenerated CNS neurons. In *Regeneration in the CNS.* Springfild, Ill.: Charles C. Thomas, 1955, 181-194.

Scott, D. & C. D. Clemente. Conduction of nerve impulses in regenerated fibers of the spinal cord of the cat. *Amer. J. Physiol.*, **167**, 1951, 825-832.

Scott, D. & C. D. Clemente. Conduction of nerve impulses in regenerated fibers of the spinal cord of the cat. *Arch. Neurol. and Psychiatry*, **67**, 1952a, 830.

Scott, D. & C. D. Clemente. Mechanism of spinal cord fibers in the cat. *Federat. Proc.*, **11**, 1952b, 143-144.

Scott, D. & C. D. Clemente. Regeneration of spinal cord fibers in the cat. *J. Compar. Neurol.*, **102**, 3, 1955, 633-670.

Scott, D. & C. N. Liu. Effect of nerve growth factor on regeneration of spinal neurons in the cat. *Exptl. Neurol.*, **8**, 4, 1963, 279-289.

Scott, D. & C. N. Liu. Factors promoting regeneration of spinal neurons. positive influence of nerve growth factor. In *Progress in Brain Research*, **13**. Amsterdam: Elsevier, 1964, 127-150.

Scott, D., E. Gutmann, & P. Horsky. Regeneration in spinal neurons: proteosynthesis following nerve growth factor administration. *Science*, **152**, 3723, 1966, 787-788.

Schotle, O. Systeme nerveaux et regeneration chez le trilen. *Rev. Suisse Zool.*, **133**, 1, 1926, 1-211.

Sechenov, I. M. (1868). Electrical and chemical stimulation of sensory spinal nerves of frogs. In *Fiziologiya Nervnoi Sistemy*, **3**. Moscow: AN SSSR, 1952a, 117-122.

Sechenov, I. M. (1864). A new addition in the mechanisms inhibiting the movements. In *Fiziologiya Nervnoi Sistemy*, **3**. Moscow: AN SSSR, 1952b, 61-66.

Selawry, O. & C. Kraus. Reaction of dogs to hypothermia and fever. *J. Appl. Physiol.*, **13**, 2, 1958, 231-236.

Selezneva, L. G. Experience of treating scars following burn injuries with pyrogenal. In *Pirogenal.* Moscow: Meditsina, 1965, 209-212.

Selezneva, L. G. & L. A. Drize. Use of pyrogenal for treating corneal opacities. In *Pirogenal.* Moscow: Meditsina, 1965, 268-272.

Selye, H. *Stress.* Montreal: Acta Press, 1950.

Sergeev, Yu. V. Permeability of skin capillaries with hyaluronidase during ether anesthesia. In *Materialy po Patogenezu Vospaleniva i Patologiya Sosudistoi Pronitsaemosti*, **13**, 1, 1954, 77-82.

Shamarina, N. M. Possibility of reinforcement in the lower section of the CNS in experimentally produced changes in innervation. *Fiziol. Zhurn. SSSR*, **46**, 4, 1960a, 418-428.

Shamarina, N. M. Possibility of reorganization of the nervous relations in antagonist muscles in decorticated rabbits. *Fiziol. Zhurn. SSSR,* **46,** 10, 1960b, 1236-1242.

Shamarina, N. M. & T. N. Nesmeyanova. Reconstruction of reflex reactions of the spinal cord under experimental conditions. *Fiziol. Zhurn. SSSR,* **39,** 5, 1953, 601-609.

Sharpless, S. K. Reorganization of function in the nervous system–use and disuse. *Ann. Rev. Physiol.,* **26,** 1964, 357-388.

Shchitkov, K. G. Changes in the spinal motor cells in the unilateral amputation of an extremity. *Arkh. Patologii,* **21,** 1, 1959, 29-33.

Sherrington, S. S. Decerebrated rigidity and reflex coordination of movements. *J. Physiol.,* **22,** 1898, 319-332.

Sherrington, C. S. The Integrative Action of the Nervous System. London, 1906a.

Sherrington, C. S. Observation of scratch reflex in the spinal dog. *J. Physiol.,* **34,** 1906b, 1-12.

Sherrington, C. S. On plastic tonus and proprioceptive reflexes. *J. Exptl. Physiol.,* **2,** 1909, 109-156.

Sherrington, C. S. Flexion reflex of the limb, crossed extension reflex and reflex stepping and standing. *J. Physiol.,* **40,** 1910, 28.

Sherrington, C. S. Reflex inhibition as a factor in the coordination of movements and postures. *Quart. J. Physiol.,* **6,** 1913, 251-310.

Shreder, V. N. Biochemistry of leukocytes in an injury. *Usp. Sovrem. Biol.,* **3,** 1949, 461-474.

Shurin, S. P. Role of heparin in cellular metabolic and enzymatic processes. *Voprosy Fiziologii i Patologii Geparina.* Novosibirsk: Nauka, 1965, 13-38.

Shurrager, P. S. Conditioning in the Spinal Dog. Urbana, Ill.: 1939a.

Shurrager, P. S. Further observation on "conditioning" and "extinction" in the spinal dog. *Psychol. Bull.,* **36,** 1939b, 660-665.

Shurrager, P. S. A comment on "an attempt to condition the chronic spinal dog." *J. Exptl. Psychol.,* **37,** 1947, 261-263.

Shurrager, P. S. Walking in spinal kittens and puppies. In *Regeneration in the CNS.* Springfield, Ill.: Charles C. Thomas, 1955, 208-218.

Shurrager, P. S. & E. A. Culler. Phenomenon allied to conditioning in the spinal dog. *Amer. J. Physiol.,* **123,** 1, 1938, 186-187.

Shurrager, P. S. & E. A. Culler. Conditioning in the spinal dog. *J. Exptl. Psychol.,* **26,** 2, 1940, 133-159.

Shurrager, P. S. & E. A. Culler. Conditioned extinction of a reflex in the spinal dog. *J. Exptl. Psychol.,* **28,** 4, 1941, 287-303.

Shurrager, P. S. & R. A. Dykman. Walking spinal cernivores. *J. Compar. and Phsyiol. Psychol.,* **44,** 1951, 252-262.

Shurrager, P. S. & H. C. Shurrager. Converting a spinal CR into a reflex. *J. Exptl. Psychol.,* **29,** 3, 1941, 217-224.

Shurrager, P. S. & H. C. Shurrager. The rate of learning measured at a single synapse. *J. Exptl. Psychol.,* **36,** 4, 1946, 347-354.

Shurrager, P. S. & H. C. Shurrager. Comment on a search for spinal conditioning and for evidence that it can become a reflex. *J. Exptl. Psychol.,* **40,** 1, 1950, 135-137.

Shuster, S. & J. Flynn. Pituitary response to pyrogen in Cushing's syndrome. *Lancet.,* **1,** 7189, 1961, 1256-1266.

Siedek, H., A. Mostbeck, & El. Schnetz. Uber die Ausscheidung von 17-Ketosteroiden und 17-Hydroxycorticoiden bei kunstlichen Fieber. *Wiener Klin. Wochenschr.,* **71,** 45, 1959, 860-865.

Singer, M. The influence of the nerve in regeneration of the amphibian extremity. *Quart. Rev. Biol.,* **27,** 1952, 169-200.

Singer, M. The influence of nerves on regeneration. In *Regeneration in Vertebrates.* Chicago, Ill.: C. S. Thornton Univ. Press, 1955a, 59-80.

Singer, M. Nervous mechanisms in the regeneration of body parts in vertebrates. In *Developing Cell Systems and Their Control.* New York: Ronald Press, 1955b, 115.

Singer, M. Nervous control of the regrowth of body parts in vertebrates. In *The Effect of Use and Disuse on Neuromuscular Functions.* Prague: Czech. Acad. Sci., 1963, 83-93.

Singer, M. A theory of the trophic nervous control of amphibian limb regeneration, including a reevaluation of quantitative nerve requirements. In *Regeneration in Animals and Related Problems.* Amsterdam: North-Holland, 1965, 20–30.

Sjostrand, J. Studies on glial cells in the hypoglossal nucleus of the rabbit and morphological changes in glial cells during nerve regeneration. *Acta Physiol. Scand.*, 67, S. 270, 1966, 1–7.

Skorobogatova, L. I. Disintegration of tissue proteins in animal extremities with varying regeneration capacity in different periods after amputation. *Dokl. AN SSSR,* **81,** 5, 1951a, 957–960.

Skorobogatova, L. I. Proteolysis in the extremities in some vertebrates with varying regeneration capacity in different periods after amputation. *Dokl. AN SSSR,* **79,** 6, 1951b, 1053–1056.

Skotnikov, V. P. Neurodystrophy after spinal and para-articular fixation in patients with trauma to the spinal cord. In *Voprosy Eksperimental'nogo i Klinicheskogo Izucheniya Posledstvii Travmy Spinnogo Mozga.* Moscow: AN SSSR, 1956, 157–164.

Skuratova, S. A. Development of a stable center of excitation in the spinal cord of warm-blooded animals. In *Tazisy Dokladov na Konferentsii Molodykh Uchenykh Instituta Normal'noi Patologicheskoi Fiziologii AMN SSSR.* Moscow: 1956, 37.

Snesarev, P. E. Obshchaya Gistopatologiya Mozgovoi Travmy (General histopathology of brain injury). Moscow, 1946.

Snesarev, P. E. Teoreticheskie Osnovy Patologicheskoi Anatomii Psikhicheskikh Boleznei (Theoretical basis of the pathological anatomy of mental diseases). Moscow: Medgiz, 1950.

Sokolov, E. N., G. G. Arakelov & L. B. Levinson. Neurological mechanisms of "adaptation." In *Sovremennye Problemy Elektrofiziologii Tsentral'noi Nervnoi Sistemy.* Moscow: Nauka, 1967, 262–272.

Sorokin, A. N. Pyrogenic properties of some bacterial and endogenous pyrogens. In *Tezisy Dokladov Simpoziuma po Rezul'tatam Eksperimental'nogo Izucheniya i Klinicheskogo Primeniya Pirogenala.* Moscow: 1964, 3–4.

Sorokin, A. N. Pirogeny (Pyrogens). Leningrad: Meditsina, 1965.

Sozon-Yaroshevich, A. Yu. Treatment of open injuries of the spinal cord. *Sov. Khirurgiya,* **6,** 1934, 3–4.

Spenser, W. A., R. F. Thompson & D. R. Neilson. Alterations in responsiveness of ascending and reflex pathways activated by iterated cutaneous afferent volleys. *J. Neurophysiol.*, **29,** 2, 1966a, 240–252.

Spenser, W. A., R. F. Thompson & D. R. Neilson. Decremental of ventral root electrotonus and intracellularly recorded PSP, produced by iterated cutaneous afferent volleys. *J. Neurophysiol.*, **29,** 2, 1966b, 253–274.

Sperry, R. V. Mechanism of maturation of the nervous system. In *Eksperimental'naya Psikhologiya.* Moscow: IL, 1960, 319–374.

Stefantsov, B. D. Vliyanie Simpaticheskoi Nervnoi Sistemy na Funktsional'noe Sostoyanie Povrezhdennoi Tsentral'noi Nervnoi Sistemy (Influence of the sympathetic nervous system on the functional status of the damaged CNS). Moscow: AN SSSR, 1961.

Stefantsov, B. D. Somatic nervous system and the problem of restoration of altered functions. In *Voprosy Fiziologii Vegetativnoi Nervnoi Sistemy i Mozzhechka.* Erevan: AN Arm. SSR, 1964, 513–523.

Steinberg, F. U. The management of patients with spinal cord injury by a hospital based home care programme. *Paraplegia,* **12,** 2, 1975, 245.

Stepanyan-Tarakanova, A. M. Travmaticheskaya Bolezn' Spinnogo Mozga (Traumatic disease of the spinal cord). Moscow: Medgiz, 1959.

Strel'tsov, V. V. Direct motor effect of a spinal nerve on the skeletal muscle. *Russk. Fiziol. Zhurn.*, **9,** 1926, 333–336.

Stuart, E. G. Alterations in connective tissue mast cells induced by bacterial pyrogens. *Amer. J. Physiol.*, **163,** 1950, 753–754.

Stuart, E. G. Accelerating effect of pyromen in contrast to inhibitory effect of cortisone on the arthus phenomenon in rabbits. *Federat. Proc.*, **10,** 1951a, 133.

Stuart, E. G. Connective tissue mast cell responses to bacterial pyroges, ovalbumin and cortisone. *Anat. Rec.,* **109,** 1951b, 351.

Stuart, E. G. Possible mechanisms of action of the bacterial polysaccharide complex pirogen. *Amer. J. Physiol.,* **171,** 1952, 771.

Stuart, E. G. Tissue reactions and possible mechanisms of pyromen and desoxycorticosterone acetate in CNS regeneration. In *Regeneration in the CNS.* Springfield, Ill.: Charles C. Thomas, 1955, 162–169.

Studitskii, A. N. Fundamentals of the biological theory of regeneration. In *Voprosy Vosstanovleniya Organov i Tkanei Pozvonochnykh Zhivotnykh,* **11,** 1954, 7–40.

Studitskii, A. N. New theoretical and experimental basis of the biological theory of regeneration. In *Usloviya Regeneratsii Organov i Tkanei u Zhivotnykh.* Moscow: 1966, 281–287.

Studitskii, A. N. & A. R. Striganova. Vosstanovitel'nye Protsessy v Skeletnoi Muskulature (Restorative processes in skeletal muscles). Moscow: AN SSSR, 1951.

Studitskii, A. N., R. P. Zhenevskaya & O. A. Rumyantseva. Principle of the techniques of restoration of muscles following the transplantation of minced muscle tissue. *Ceskosloveska Morfologia,* **4,** 4, 1956, 331–340.

Stuteville, O. H., R. L. Lanfranchi, & S. Wallach. Trypsin in the treatment of swellings of the head and neck. *Amer. J. Surg.,* **96,** 6, 1958, 287.

Sugar, O. & R. W. Gerard. Spinal cord regeneration in the rat. *J. Neurophysiol.,* **3,** 1940, 1–19.

Sumi, T. Repetitive excitation of motoneurons by afferent shock stimulus to muscle nerve in the previously spinalized cats. *Japan. J. Physiol.,* **9,** 4, 1959, 498–505.

Sundbland, L., N. Egelius, & E. Jensson. Action of hydrocortisone on the hyaluronic acid of joint fluids in rheumatic arthritis. *Acta. Med. Scand.,* **154,** S.312, 1956, 424.

Sunderland, S. Rate of regeneration in human peripheral nerves. *Arch. Neurol. and Psychiatry,* **58,** 3, 1947, 251–295.

Suponitskaya, M. A. Restoration of functions of traumatic spinal cord depending on the degree of permeability of the subdural space. In *Voprosy Eksperimental'nogo i Klinicheskogo Ucheniya Posledstvii Travmy Spinnogo Mozga.* Moscow: AN SSR, 1956, 190–192.

Szentagothai, J. Short propriospinal neurons and intrinsic connections of the spinal gray matter. *Acta Morphol. Hung.,* **1,** 1, 1951, 81–94.

Szentagothai, J. Anatomical aspect of inhibitor pathways and synapses. In *Nervous Inhibition.* Oxford: Pergamon Press, 1961, 32–45.

Szentagothai, J. & K. Rajkovits. Die Rückwerkung der spezifischen funtion auf die Struktur der Nervenelemente. *Acta Morphol. Hung.,* **5,** 1955, 3–4; 253–274.

Tabenhous, M. Mechanism of corticosteroid actions in disease processes. *Ann. N. Y. Acad. Sci.,* **26,** 1953, 623–814.

Takeba, K., C. Setaishi, & M. Hirama. Effects of bacterial pyrogen on the pituitary adrenal axis at various times during 24 hours. *J. Clin. Endocrinol. and Metabol.,* **26,** 4, 1966, 437–442.

Tarlov, I. M. Rigidity in man due to spinal interneuron loss. *Arch. Neurol.,* **16,** 5, 1967, 536–543.

Taylor, A. G. Autonomic dysreflexia in spinal cord injury. *Nurs. Clin. North Am.,* **9,** 1974, 717–725.

Tayushev, K. G. Morphological changes in spinal cords and sympathetic ganglions and in nerves supplying the pancreas and suprarenal glands in experimental transection of the spinal cord. In *Travma Pozyorochnika i Spinnogo Mozga,* **3.** Leningrad: 1965, 158–164.

Tello, J. F. La influencia del neurotropismo en la regeneracion de los centros nerviosos. *Trab. Lab. Invest. Biol.,* **9,** 4, 1911, 123–159.

Tello, J. F. Gegenwärtige Anschaungen über den Neurotropismus. *Vortr. Ehtwickl. Mechan. Org.,* **33,** 1923, 1–73.

Teplits, N. A. Change in the concentration of nucleic acids in limb tissues after X-ray irradiation and during normal regeneration in axolotl. *Dokl. AN SSSR,* **159,** 2, 1964a, 442–445.

Teplits, N. A. Changes in the concentrations of nucleic acids during X-ray irradiation, suppression and restoration of regenerating capacity in the limbs of axolotl. *Dokl. AN SSSR,* **156,** 1964b, 1207–1209.

Thompson, R. E. & W. A. Spencer. Habituation: A model phenomenon for the study of neuronal substrates of behavior. *Psychol. Rev.,* **73,** 1, 1966, 16–43.

Thulin, C. A. Bioelectrical characteristics of regenerated fibers in the feline spinal cord. *Exptl. Neurol.,* **2,** 1960, 533-546.

Tkach, E. V. & S. N. Kassovskaya. Electromyographic and biochemical studies and the results of treatment of spasticity in patients with lesions of the spinal cord. In. *Vosstanovlenie Funktsii pri Porazheniyakh Tsentral'noi i Perifericheskoi Nervnoi Sistemy.* Leningrad, 1967, 110.

Tkach, E. V. & O. G. Kogan. Functional status of nerve-muscle apparatus in traumas of the spinal cord. In *Travma Pozvonochnika i Spinnogo Mozga,* **3.** Leningrad: 1965, 121–129.

Tonkikh, A. V. Effect of the sympathetic nervous system on spinal reflexes of frogs. *Russk. Fiziol. Zhurn.,* **8,** 1925, 5–6; 31–42.

Tonkikh, A. V. Participation of the sympathetic nervous system in Sechenov type inhibition. *Russk. Fiziol. Zhurn.,* **10,** 1927, 85–94.

Tonkikh, A. V. New data in the Sechenov type inhibition. *Russk. Fiziol. Zhurn.,* **12,** 1930, 11–20.

Tonkikh, A. V. Mechanisms of adaptation and trophic effect of the sympathetic nervous system. In *Evolyutsiya Funktsii.* Moscow–Leningrad: Nauka, 1964, 135–141.

Tower, S. Function and structure in the chronically isolated lumbosacral spinal cord of the dog. *J. Compar. Neurol.,* **67,** 1, 1937, 109.

Trankvillitati, A. N. Importance of functional therapy and massage in the development of compensatory adaptability after compression fracture of the spinal cord. In *Problema Kompensatornykh Prisposoblenii.* Moscow: AN SSSR, 1960, 21–24.

Trankvillitati, A. N. Compensatory method of restoration of motor signs in patients following compression of the spinal cord. In *Pirogenal.* Moscow: Miditsina, 1965a, 234–244.

Trankvillitati, A. N. Physical therapy in compression fractures of vertebral column with the spinal cord lesion. In *Materialy Konferentsii Kafedry Lechebnogo Kontrolya i Lechebnoi Fizicheskoi Kul'tury.* Moscow: 1965b, 22–23.

Trankvillitati, A. N. Physical therapy and massage in combination with pyrogenal for the treatment of compression fracture with the spinal cord lesion. In *Sportivnaya Meditsina i Lechebnaya Fizkul'tura.* Moscow: 1966, 61–64.

Trankvillitati, A. N. Restoration of voluntary movements of the lower extremities in patients with transection of the spinal cord. In *Vosstanovlenie Funktsii pri Porazheniyakh Tsentral'noi i Perifericheskoi Nervnoi Sistemy.* Leningrad: 1967, 107.

Trankvillitati, A. N. Method and organization of physical therapy for treating patients with lesions of the spinal cord at the thoraco-lumbar region. In *Reabilitatsiya Bol'nykh s Posledstviyami Povrezhdenii Pozvonochnika i Spinnogo Mozga.* Kiev: Zdorov'e, 1969, 115.

Trankvillitati, A. N. & T. N. Nesmeyanova. Treatment of patients with compression fracture of the vertebral column. In *Eksperimental'noe Izuchenie i Klinicheskoe Primenenie Pirogenala.* Moscow: 1961, 143–152.

Traugott, N. N., L. Ya. Balashov & D. A. Kaufman. Mechanism of action of animazin on the higher nervous activity of man. *Zhurn. Vyssh. Nervn. Deyat.,* **11,** 5, 1961, 814–822.

Trevor, H. Factors promoting regeneration of spinal neurons: positive influence of nerve growth factor. In *Progress in Brain Research,* **13,** Amsterdam: Elsevier, 1964, 148.

Tschirjew, S. Sur les terminaisons nerveuses dans les muscles stries. *Compt. Rend. Akad.,* **87,** 1878, 604.

Tuge, H. A. & S. Hanzowa. Physiological and morphological regeneration of the sectioned spinal cord in adult teleosts. *J. Compar. Neurol.,* **67,** 1937, 343–365.

Turbes, C. C. & L. W. Freeman. The use of peripheral nerve in spinal cord anastomosis for surgical treatment of experimental spinal transection in the dog. *Neurology,* **8,** 10, 1958, 857–861.

Turbes, C. C. & L. W. Freeman. Morphological findings in studies of regeneration of synapses in the mammalian spinal cord. *Neurology,* **11,** 11, 1961, 970–976.

Turren, L. L. Effect of experimental temporary vascular occlusion on the spinal cord. *Arch. Neurol. and Psychiat.,* **35,** 1936, 748.

Tushnov, M. P. Problema Spermatoksinov i Lizatov (Problem of sperm toxins and lysates). Moscow: Sel'khozgiz, 1938.

Uarova-Yakobson, S. I. Physical therapy in spastic paralysis. In *Trudy.* Moscow: GIF, 1940, 103–126.

Uflyand, Yu. M. Fiziologiya Dvigatel'nogo Apparata Cheloveka (Physiology of motor apparatus in man). Leningrad: Meditsina, 1965.

Ugryumov, V. M. Functional changes in several internal organs during trauma of the spinal cord. In *Voprosy Eksperimental'nogo i Klinicheskogo Izucheniya Posledstvii Travmy Spinnogo Mozga.* Moscow: AN SSSR, 1956a, 124–129.

Ugryumov, V. M. Remnants of trauma of the spinal cord in man and some problems relating to their surgical treatment. In *Voprosy Eksperimental'nogo i Klinicheskogo Izucheniya Posledstvii Travmy Spinnogo Mozga.* Moscow: AN SSSR, 1956b, 21–35.

Ugryumov, V. M. Treatment and restoration of function in trauma of the spinal cord. In *Problema Kompensatornykh Prisposoblenii.* Moscow: AN SSSR, 1960, 7–12.

Ugryumov, V. M. Povrezhdeniya Pozvonochnika i Spinnogo Mozga i ikh Khirurgicheskoe Lechenie (Injuries and surgical treatment of the spinal column and cord). Moscow–Leningrad: Medgiz, 1961.

Ugryumov, V. M. & E. I. Babichenko. Closed injuries of the spine and spinal cord. Leningrad: Medgiz, 1973.

Ugryumov, V. M., M. M. Kruglyi & E. N. Vinarskaya. Lechebnaya Gimnastika pri Povrezhdeniyakh Pozvonochnika i Spinnogo Mozga (Physical therapy in the injuries of the vertebral column and the spinal cord). I. Moscow: Meditsina, 1964, 4–22.

Ugryumov, V. M., E. G. Lubenskii & S. E. Narodovol'tseva. Restoration of functions in closed injuries of the vertebral column and the spinal cord. In *Vosstanoblenie Funktsii pri Porazheniyakh Tsentral'noi i Perifericheskoi Nervnoi Sistemy.* Leningrad: 1967, 104.

Ugryumova, R. I. Bladder reflex as an objective sign of the revival of functional disorders of the spinal cord and cauda equina. In *Voprosy Eksperimental'nogo i Klinicheskogo Izucheniya Posledstvii Travmy Spinnogo Mozga.* Moscow: AN SSSR, 1956, 106–110.

Ukhtomskii, A. A. Parabioz i Dominanta (Parabiosis and dominant). *Sobr. Soch.,* **1.** Leningrad: LGU, 1950, 232–289.

Urbani, E. Proteolytic enzymes in regeneration. In *Regeneration in Animals.* Amsterdam: North-Holland, 1965, 39–55.

Urgandzhyan, T. G. Role of cerebral cortex in compensatory adaptation after transection of anterior half of the spinal cord in dogs. Doctoral dissertation, Moscow: 1953.

Urgandzhyan, T. G. Role of the sympathetic nervous system in the process of compensation of functions. *Fiziol. Zhurn. SSSR,* **48,** 9, 1962, 1064–1070.

Urgandzhyan, T. G. Progressing features of compensatory adaptability in combined hemisection of the ventral and dorsal halves of the spinal cord. Doctoral dissertation, Erevan: 1967.

Urgandzhyan, T. G. & Z. N. Bakhchieva. Sympathoadrenal system and compensatory adaptability. In *Voprosy Fiziologii Vegetativnoi Nervnoi Sistemy i Mozzhechka.* Erevan: AN SSR, 1964, 535–549.

Van Crevel, H. The rate of secondary degeneration in the CNS. Doctoral disseration, Leiden: 1958, 1–90.

Van Harreveld, A. On the mechanism of the "spontaneous" reinnervation in paretic muscles. *Amer. J. Physiol.,* **150,** 1947, 670–676.

Van Harreveld, A. Spinal asphyxiation and spasticity. In *Basic Research in Paraplegia.* Springfield, Ill.: Charles C. Thomas, 1962, 127.

Van Harreveld, A. Effect of spinal cord asphyxiation. In *Progress in Brain Research,* **12.** Amsterdam: Elsevier, 1964, 280–303.

Van Harreveld, A. & J. Schade. Nerve cell destruction by asphyxiation of the spinal cord. *J. Neuropathol.,* **21,** 1962, 410–423.

Van Harreveld, A. & D. Spinelli. Reflex activity in spinal cats with postasphyxial rigidity. *Arch. Internat. Physiol. et Biochim.*, **73**, 2, 1965, 209–230.

Vasilenko, D. A. & P. G. Kostyuk. The neuronal organization of the pyramidal motor system. In *Nervnye Mekhanizmy Dvigatel'noi Deyatel'nosti.* Moscow: Nauka, 1966, 105–115.

Vasil'ev, P. V. & P. P. Saksonov. The pharmacology of pyrogenic bacterial polysaccharides. *Byull. Eksperim. Biol. i Med.*, **44**, 8, 1957, 77–80.

Vera, C. L. & J. V. Luco. Synaptic transmission in spinal cord during Wallerian degeneration of dorsal root fibers. *J. Neurophysiol.*, **21**, 4, 1958, 334–344.

Veremeenko, K. N. Proteoliticheskie Fermenti Podzheludochnoi Zhelezy i ikh Primenenie v Klinike (Pancreatic proteolytic enzymes and their application in clinical practice). Kiev: Zdorov'e, 1967.

Vereshchagin, S. M. Study of the processes of excitation and inhibition of motor activities in the invertebrates. Doctoral dissertation, Leningrad: 1967.

Veselkin, P. N. Biological significance of the febrile reaction. *Arkh. Patologii,* **19,** 1, 1957, 13–20.

Veselkin, P. N. Energy metabolism in febrile conditions. In *Fosforilirovanie i Funktsiya.* Leningrad: 1960, 327–332.

Veselkin, P. N. Mechanism of the therapeutic action of pyrogenal. In *Pirogenal.* Moscow: Meditsina, 1965, 7–16.

Vishnevskii, A. A., A. V. Livshits & B. I. Khodorov. Electrical stimulation of the urinary bladder. *Eksperim. Khirurgiya i Anesteziol.*, 1, 1965, 5–9.

Vishnevskii, A. A., A. V. Livshits & B. I. Khodorov. Electrical stimulation of the urinary bladder in traumatic transection of the spinal cord in man. *Eksperim. Khirurgiya i Anesteziol.*, **1**, 1967, 46–50.

Vlanskaya, N. D. Kidney functions in patients following trauma of the vertebral column and the spinal cord. In *Voprosy Eksperimental'nogo i Klinicheskogo Izucheniya Posledstvii Travmy Spinnogo Mozga.* Moscow: AN SSSR, 1956, 146–147.

Vogt, M. Distribution of adrenaline and noradrenaline in the CNS and its modification by drugs. In *Metabolism of the Nervous System.* London: Pergamon Press, 1957, 553–565.

Voino-Yasenetskii, V. V. Tissue incompatibility in corneal transplantation. Doctoral dissertation, Leningrad: 1961.

Volokhov, A. A. Zakonomernosti Ontogeneza Nervnoi Deyatel'nosti v Svete Evolyutsionnogo Ucheniya (Laws governing the ontogenesis of nervous activity in the light of evolution). Moscow–Leningrad: AN SSSR, 1951.

Vorob'ev, V. P. Atlas Anatomii Cheloveka (Atlas of human anatomy), **2.** Moscow–Leningrad: 1938.

Vorontsova, M. A. Regeneratsiya Organov u Zhivotnykh (Regeneration of organs in animals). Moscow: Nauka, 1949.

Vorontsova, M. A. Vosstanovlenie Utrachennykh Organov u Zhivotnykh i Cheloveka (Restoration of lost organs in animals and man). Moscow: Nauka, 1953.

Vorontsova, M. A. & L. D. Liozner. Fiziologicheskaya Regeneratsiya (Physiological regeneration). Moscow: Nauka, 1955.

Vvedenskii, N. E. (1912). The status of nerve centers during prolonged stimulation of the sensory nerve. *Sobr. Soch. LTU,* **41,** 1938, 2.

Vysheslavtseva, K. A. Treatment of the diseases of peripheral nervous system and cerebral arachnoiditis with pyrogenal. In *Pirogenal.* Moscow: Meditsina, 1965, 337–340.

Wedell, G. & C. Zander. The fragility of nonmyelinated nerve fibers. *J. Anat.*, **85,** 1951, 242–250.

Weiler, K. Untersuchung des Knieschnenreflexes beim Menschen. *Z. ges. Neurol. und Psychiat.*, **1,** 1910, 118–132.

Weiss, M. & J. Beck. Sport as part of therapy and rehabilitation of paraplegia. *Paraplegia,* **2,** 1973, 166–172.

Weiss, P. Abhängigkeit der Regeneration enhwicnebter Amphibienestremitäten von Nervensystem (Der Begriff des "Gestultungstonus"). *Roux' Arch Entwickl. Mechan. Org.*, S. P. 104, 1925.

Weiss, P. *In vitro* experiments on the factors determining the course of the outgrowing nerve fiber. *J. Exptl. Zool.*, **68**, 1934, 393–448.

Weiss, P. An introduction to genetic neurology. In *Genetic Neurology*. Chicago: Univ. Chicago Press, 1950.

Weiss, P. Nervous system (Neurogenesis). In *Analysis of Development*. Philadelphia: 1955a, 346–401.

Weiss, P. Parameters of nerve regeneration. In *Regeneration in the CNS*. Springfield, Ill.: Charles C. Thomas, 1955b, 131–134.

Weiss, P. and H. Hiscoe. Experiments on the mechanism of nerve growth. *Exptl. Zool.*, **107**, 1948, 1315.

Weiss, P. & A. Hoag, Competitive reinnervation of rat muscles by their own and foreign nerves. *J. Neurophysiol.*, **9**, 5, 1946, 413–418.

Weiss, P. & A. C. Taylor. Further experimental evidence against "Neurotropism" in nerve regeneration. *J. Exptl. Zool.*, **95**, 1944, 233–237.

Weiss, P., O. Taylor & P. Pillai. The nerve fiber as a system in continuous flow: microcinematographic and electronmicroscopic demonstration. *Science*, **136**, 1962, 330–331.

Westerman, R. Regeneration of olfactory paths in carp. *Experientia*, **20**, 519, 1964, 1–5.

Wexler, B. C. Effects of a bacterial polysaccharide (Piromen) on the pituitary-adrenal axis. Modification of ACTH release by morphine and salicylate. *Metabolism*, **12**, 1, 1963, 49–56.

Wexler, B., A. Dolgin & E. W. Tryczinsky. Effects of a bacterial polysaccharide (pyromen) on the pituitary-adrenal axis: adrenal ascorbic acid, cholesterol and histologic alterations. *Endocrinology*, **61**, 3, 1957, 300–308.

Wexler, B. C., J. Faehnrich, M. E. Weiss & O. D. Grace. The use of bacterial polysaccharide (Piromen) as a pituitary-adrenal stimulator in dogs. *Amer. J. Veterin. Res.*, **18**, 68, 1957, 642–647.

Wichman, B. E. The mast cell count during the process of wound healing. *Acta Pathol. et Microbiol. Scand.*, S.108, 1955, 1–35.

Windle, W. F. Endocrine and connective tissue cellular responses to administration of bacterial pyrogen. *Abstracts and Communications XVIII International physiological Congress.* Copenhagen: 1950, 518.

Windle, W. F. Activities of certain bacterial polysaccharides. *Ann. N. Y. Acad. Sci.*, **14**, 3, 1952, 159–161.

Windle, W. F. Comments on regeneration in the human CNS. In *Regeneration in the CNS.* Springfield, Ill.: Charles C. Thomas, 1955, 265–271.

Windle, W. F. Regeneration of axons in the vertebrate CNS. *Physiol. Revs.*, **36**, 4, 1956, 427–440.

Windle, W. F. Some observations on the regeneration of CNS in man. In *Regeneratsiya Tsentral'noi Nervnoi Sistemy*, Moscow: IL, 1959, 206–211.

Windle, W. F. & W. W. Chambers. Regeneration in the spinal cord of the cat and dog. *J. Compar. Neurol.*, **93**, 1950, 241–257.

Windle, W. F. & W. W. Chambers. Regeneration in the spinal cord of cat and dog. *Arch. Neurol. and Psychiatry*, **65**, 1951, 261–262.

Windle, W. F. & H. H. Wilcox. Extramedullary hemopoiesis in rabbit and cat induced by bacterial pyrogens. *Amer. J. Physiol.*, **163**, 1950, 762–769.

Windle, W. F., C. D. Clemente & W. W. Chambers. Inhibition of formation of glial barrier as a means of permitting a peripheral nerve to grow in the brain. *J. Compar. Neurol.*, **96**, 1952, 359–369.

Windle, W. F., C. D. Clemente, D. Scott & W. W. Chambers. Structural and functional regeneration in the CNS. *Arch. Neurol.*, **67**, 1952, 553–559.

Windle, W. F., L. Littrell, J. Smart & J. Joralemon. Regeneration in the cord of spinal monkeys. *Neurology*, **6**, 6, 1956, 420–428.

Windle, W. F., H. H. Wilcox, R. Rhines & C. D. Clemente. Changes in endocrine organs induced by bacterial pyrogens. *Federat. Proc.*, **9**, 1950, 137–146.

Windle, W. F., W. W. Chambers, W. A. Ricker, L. G. Cinger & H. Koenig. Reaction of tissues to administration of a pyrogenic preparation from a pseudomonas species.

Amer. J. Med. Sci., **219**, 1950, 422–426.

Wischnevsky, A. A. & A. W. Livshits. Electrostimulation of the bladder. Moscow: Medgiz, 1973.

Woll, P. Two systems of transmission of cutaneous sensations. In *Teorii Scyazi v Sensornykh Sistemakh.* Leningrad: Mir, 1964, 116–184.

Woods, H. W., H. Landy & M. I. Shear. Effects of endotoxic polysaccharides on tumor glycolysis. *Federat. Proc.*, **18**, 1959, 355–363.

Woods, H. W., H. Landy, J. L. Whitby & D. Burk. Symposium on bacterial endotoxins. *Bacteriol. Revs.*, **25**, 4, 1961, 447–456.

Yakimovich, R. I. Interoceptive conditioned reflexes from urinary bladder in rabbits before and after transection of the spinal cord. *Trudy Inist. Fiziologii AN BSSR,* **2**, 1958, 188–194.

Yakovleva, L. A. Regeneration and repair of the spinal cord after trauma. Doctoral dissertation, Leningrad: 1951.

Yakovleva, L. A. Replacement of the spinal damage with homotransplant prepared from degenerated sciatic nerve. *Dokl. AN SSSR,* **98**, 5, 1954, 1041–1044.

Yakovleva, L. A. Regeneration of nerve fibers in the spinal cord of albino rats. In *Problemy Morfologii Nervnoi Sistemy.* Leningrad: Medgiz, 1956, 37–42.

Young, J. Z. Structure, degeneration and repair of nerve fibers. *Nature,* **156**, 1945, 132.

Young, J. Z. Growth and plasticity in the nervous system. *Proc. Roy. Soc.*, **139**, 1951, 18–37.

Young, J. Z. Morphological and histochemical studies of partially and totally deafferented spinal cord segments. *Exptl. Neurol.*, **14**, 1966, 238–248.

Young, J. Z., W. Holmes & F. K. Sanders. Nerve regeneration. Importance of the peripheral stump and the value of nerve grafts. *Lancet,* 2, 1940, 128–130.

Yuan Li-Young. Histochemical analysis of the changes in nucleic acids during the regeneration of oral mucous membrane epithelium after damage. In *Tezisy Dokladov Nauchnoi Konferentsii po Probleme Determinatsii i Plastichnosti Tkanei,* 1959, 117.

Yusevich, Yu. S. Elektromiografiya v Klinike Nervnykh Boleznei (Electromyography in clinical cases with nerve diseases). Moscow: Medgiz, 1958.

Yusevich, J. S. Clinical electromyography and some questions relating to the neurophysiology of movements. *Electromyography,* **10**, 2, 1970, 123–144.

Zdrodovskaya, E. A. Phosphorus metabolism in rabbit liver during hyperthermia induced by dinitrophenol and in experimental pyrexia. In *Fiziologicheskie Mekhanizmy Likhoradochnoi Reaktsii.* Leningrad: 1957, 310.

Zelena, J. & L. Lubinska. Early changes of acetylcholinesterase activity near the lesion in crushed nerves. *Physiol. Bohemosl.*, **11**, 4, 1962, 261–268.

Zelikina, T. I. Regeneration of the nerve tissue in higher and lower vertebrates. *Trudy In-ta. Morfol. Zhivotn.*, **11**, 1954, 356–397.

Zelinskii, N. D. Chemical nature of the factor causing the growth of accessory limbs in axolotl in the works of N. V. Nasonov. *Zhurn. Obshch. Biol.*, 7, 3, 1946, 161–170.

Zelinskii, N. D. & D. M. Fedotov. The works of academician N. V. Nasonov on the problem of organization. In *Dobavochnye Obrazovaniya, Razvivayushchiesya pri Vlozhenii Khryashcha pod Kozhu Vzroslykh Khvostatykh Amfibii.* Moscow: AN SSSR, 1941, 3.

Zemlyanskaya, A. A. Study of traumatic lesions of the spinal cord. *Trudy Saratovskogo Med. In-ta,* 3, 1940, 1–2.

Zhabotinskii, Yu. M. Normal'naya i Patologicheskaya Morfologiya Neirona (Normal and pathological morphology of the neuron). Moscow: Meditsina, 1965.

Zimkin, N. V. Regulation of the function of the spinal cord by the cerebral cortex. *Fiziol. Zhurn. SSSR,* **33**, 1947, 147–152.

INDEX

O

P

R

S

T

U

W